Diabetes
For Canadians

FOR

DUMMIES®

A Wiley Brand

3RD EDITION

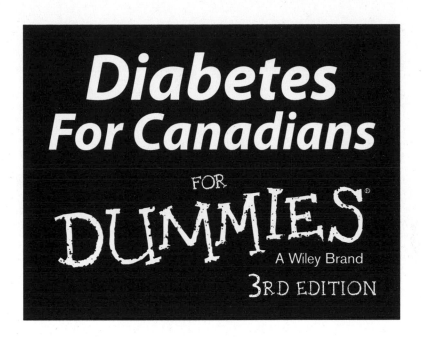

Diabetes For Canadians

FOR

DUMMIES®

A Wiley Brand

3RD EDITION

**by Ian Blumer, MD, FRCPC
and Alan L. Rubin, MD**

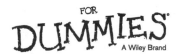

Diabetes For Canadians For Dummies®, 3rd Edition

Published by
John Wiley & Sons Canada, Ltd.
6045 Freemont Blvd.

Mississauga, ON L5R 4J3
www.wiley.com

For general information on John Wiley & Sons Canada, Ltd., including all books published by Wiley Publishing Inc., please call our distribution centre at 1-800-567-4797. For reseller information, including discounts and premium sales, please call our sales department at 416-646-7992. For press review copies, author interviews, or other publicity information, please contact our publicity department, Tel. 416-646-4582, Fax 416-236-4448.

Wiley also publishes its books in a variety of electronic formats. Some content that appears in print may not be available in electronic books.

Library and Archives Canada Cataloguing in Publication Data

Blumer, Ian
    Diabetes for Canadians for dummies / Ian Blumer, Alan L.
Rubin. – 3rd ed.
Includes index.
Issued also in electronic formats.
ISBN 978-1-118-39956-9
    1. Diabetes–Popular works. I. Rubin, Alan L II. Title.
RA645.D5B48 2013   616.4'62   C2013-901610-4

ISBN 978-1-118-39956-9 (pbk); 978-1-118-41416-3 (ebk);
978-1-118-41415-6 (ebk); 978-1-118-41417-0 (ebk)

Printed in the United States

About the Authors

Ian Blumer, MD, FRCPC, is a diabetes specialist in the Greater Toronto Area of Ontario. He has a teaching appointment with the University of Toronto and is a medical advisor and board member of the Charles H. Best Diabetes Centre in Whitby, Ontario.

Dr. Blumer is a member of the executive of the Clinical and Scientific Section of the Canadian Diabetes Association (CDA), and is a recipient of the CDA Special Dedication Award. He is also chair of the Endocrine Society Diabetes and Pregnancy Clinical Practice Guidelines. Dr. Blumer has the great honour and pleasure of being a faculty member of Taking Control of Your Diabetes (www.tcoyd.org); an American organization whose mission is to empower people living with diabetes and to educate diabetes health care providers.

An enthusiastic and highly regarded lecturer, Dr. Blumer has spoken about diabetes to numerous professional and lay audiences around the world.

Dr. Blumer is the author of *What Your Doctor* Really *Thinks: Diagnosing the Doctor-Patient Relationship* (Dundurn), and is the co-author of three other For Dummies titles: *Diabetes Cookbook For Canadians For Dummies* (co-written by Cynthia Payne RD, CDE), *Understanding Prescription Drugs For Canadians For Dummies* (co-written by Dr. Heather McDonald-Blumer), and *Celiac Disease For Dummies* (co-written with Dr. Sheila Crowe). Under the pen name of Sidney Gale, Dr. Blumer has recently published his first novel, *Unto the Breach*, a young adult story of adventure and overcoming adversity.

Dr. Blumer's website (www.ourdiabetes.com) offers practical patient-oriented advice on how to manage one's diabetes.

Ian welcomes your comments about this book diabetes@ianblumer.com

Alan L. Rubin, MD, is one of the United States' foremost experts on diabetes. He is a professional member of the American Diabetes Association and the Endocrine Society and has been in private practice specializing in diabetes and thyroid disease for more than 35 years. Dr. Rubin was assistant clinical professor of medicine at the University of California Medical Center in San Francisco for 20 years. He has spoken about diabetes to professional medical audiences and non-medical audiences around the world. He has been a consultant to many pharmaceutical companies and companies that make diabetes products.

Dr. Rubin was one of the first specialists in his field to recognize the significance of patient self-testing of blood glucose, the major advance in diabetes care since the advent of insulin. As a result, he has been on numerous radio and television programs, talking about the cause, the prevention, and the treatment of diabetes and its complications.

Since publishing *Diabetes For Dummies,* Dr. Rubin has had six other bestselling For Dummies books: *Diabetes Cookbook For Dummies, Thyroid For Dummies, High Blood Pressure For Dummies, Type 1 Diabetes For Dummies, Prediabetes For Dummies,* and *Vitamin D For Dummies.* His seven books cover the medical problems of 150 million Americans.

Dedication

Ian: This 3rd edition of *Diabetes For Canadians For Dummies* is dedicated to Marlene Grass, RN, CDE, the founder of the Charles H. Best Diabetes Centre, and to the Best Centre staff. A pioneer in type 1 diabetes education, Marlene saw the path long before the rest of the world knew which way to turn.

Alan: *Diabetes For Dummies* is dedicated to my wife, Enid. She has been the perfect helpmate, always there with a smile and encouragement. There is no question that she promotes all my books better than anyone else. She even listens to my recommendations.

Diabetes For Dummies is also dedicated to the thousands of people with diabetes who have written to thank me for helping them to understand what they are dealing with and for telling me where I need to provide more information and emphasis to make this an even better book.

Author Acknowledgements

Ian: I would like to express my thanks and gratitude to those folks at Wiley that have helped me steer this book along its journey: Anam Ahmed (editor), Heather Ball (copy editor), and Pamela Vokey (production editor).

I would also like to thank my colleagues who provided such helpful tips and suggestions for this 3rd edition of *Diabetes For Canadians For Dummies*: Diana Balicsak, Irma Carson, Alice Cheng, Bin Chin, Denice Feig, Jonathon Fowles, Marlene Grass, Sandy Hubbard, Jill Milliken, Bill Polonsky, Michael Riddell and, especially, Maureen Clement, a physician of immense knowledge, a leader in diabetes care in Canada, and a kind and thoughtful friend who I have somehow once again managed to corral into reviewing my manuscript.

And, as always, I would like to once again thank my wonderful wife, Heather, for her constant support through this book's journey and all the others we have undertaken during three wonderful decades of marriage.

Alan: For *Diabetes For Dummies*, acquisitions editor Michael Lewis deserves major thanks. I have had the pleasure of working with him for several years. He is supportive, encouraging, and fun, and I look forward to a long association with him. I am also blessed with another great project editor, Chrissy Guthrie, and copy editor, Caitie Copple, who not only made sure that everything was readable and understandable but also offered excellent suggestions to improve the information. My thanks also to Dr. Lori Brame for reviewing the book for scientific accuracy.

Ronnie and Michael Goldfield should definitely be considered the godparents of *Diabetes For Dummies*.

Publisher's Acknowledgments

We're proud of this book; please send us your comments through our online registration form located at http://dummies.custhelp.com. For other comments, please contact our Customer Care Department within the U.S. at 877-762-2974, outside the U.S. at 317-572-3993, or fax 317-572-4002.

Some of the people who helped bring this book to market include the following:

Acquisitions and Editorial

Associate Acquisitions Editor: Anam Ahmed

Production Editor: Pamela Vokey

Copy Editor: Heather Ball

Editorial Assistant: Kathy Deady

Cartoons: Rich Tennant (www.the5thwave.com)

Cover photo: © Godfried Edelman / iStockphoto

Composition Services

Senior Project Coordinator: Kristie Rees

Layout and Graphics: Jennifer Creasey, Joyce Haughey

Proofreaders: John Greenough, Wordsmith Editorial

Indexer: Christine Karpeles

John Wiley & Sons Canada, Ltd.

    Deborah Barton, Vice President and Director of Operations

    Jennifer Smith, Vice-President and Publisher, Professional Development

    Alison Maclean, Managing Editor

Publishing and Editorial for Consumer Dummies

    Kathleen Nebenhaus, Vice President and Executive Publisher

    David Palmer, Associate Publisher

    Kristin Ferguson-Wagstaffe, Product Development Director

Publishing for Technology Dummies

    Andy Cummings, Vice President and Publisher

Composition Services

    Debbie Stailey, Director of Composition Services

Contents at a Glance

Table of Contents

Part II: How Diabetes Can Affect Your Body................ 59

Introduction

Recently, a friend of Ian's developed diabetes and, being a resourceful person, had borrowed the second edition of this book from the library and read it cover to cover. "So, Ian," he said when they met for dinner shortly thereafter, "I've read your book. It was very helpful, but I'm just wondering if there is anything new in the world of diabetes since you wrote that edition."

Ian picked up the dog-eared copy that his friend had brought and thumbed through it. "Well," Ian said as he looked at the book, "we've got new information on nutrition and exercise. And a whole bunch of new types of medications. And a whole slew of new blood glucose meters. And the whole field of continuous glucose monitoring is burgeoning. And . . ."

"Whoa," Ian's friend interrupted. "I had no idea so much could change so quickly. You should write a new edition."

Ian smiled as he turned on his computer and showed him the draft chapters of this, the third edition of *Diabetes For Canadians For Dummies*. "You're right, a new edition *was* necessary. And here it is."

Each edition of *Diabetes For Canadians For Dummies* has been based on the most recent version of the Canadian Diabetes Association Clinical Practice Guidelines. This third edition is based on the 2013 version of these guidelines. And, as is true of any For Dummies book, this one is imbued with tips and advice that Ian (and Alan) have found particularly helpful for people living with diabetes to successfully manage this condition.

Being diagnosed with diabetes is, of course, not the most welcome of news. But it is also an opportunity to look at your lifestyle and make those changes that may have been due anyhow. It's never too late to start leading a healthier life!

About This Book

We've designed *Diabetes For Canadians For Dummies* so you don't have to read it cover to cover, but if you know nothing about diabetes, doing so may be a good approach. (Indeed, many readers of our earlier editions have told us this is exactly what they did!) We want this book to provide you with the most important information you need to know about your diabetes: what leads to it, how it affects you, and, most importantly, how to effectively deal with diabetes so that you can achieve and maintain good health.

Canada has a long and proud history of being at the forefront of diabetes research and therapy. *Diabetes For Canadians For Dummies* looks at the special issues that Canadians with diabetes have to face (like Ian's patient who returned to his car one February morning after his son's hockey practice, only to find his insulin frozen solid!). Also, as noted above, this book is based on the Canadian Diabetes Association Clinical Practice Guidelines, guidelines which are respected and used around the world.

In this book you will find frequent references to websites that offer excellent information. If you don't have Internet access at home, you can get online at your neighbourhood library. As Internet addresses change frequently, if you find that a recommended link isn't working, try going to the home page of the site and checking the site map to find the new page.

Conventions Used in This Book

Diabetes, as you know, is associated with sugar problems. But sugars come in many types, so doctors avoid using the words *sugar* and *glucose* interchangeably. In this book, we use the word *glucose* rather than *sugar* (unless we're talking about things such as table sugar or sweets you have in your diet). As well, because adding mmol/L (which is short for millimoles per litre) after every blood glucose value gets redundant, we sometimes omit the units. So for example, if we say that a fasting blood glucose of 7.0 (or higher) is indicative of diabetes, you can safely assume we mean 7.0 *mmol/L*. Similarly when we talk about a test called the A1C (which you'll learn all about in this book) and mention a value of, say 8.5, we mean 8.5 *percent*.

What You Don't Have to Read

We hope you'll enjoy reading everything in this book; however, throughout the book, you'll find shaded areas, which are called sidebars, containing material that's interesting but not essential. Feel free to skip them if the material they cover is of no particular interest to you. You'll still understand everything else.

In addition, we've noted some paragraphs that have a more technical nature with the Technical Stuff icon (see "Icons Used in This Book," later in this Introduction for more on icons). Although these paragraphs deepen your knowledge of diabetes, you can still understand the text without reading them.

Foolish Assumptions

This book assumes that you know nothing about diabetes. We provide fundamental information so that you will become familiar with the most important measures available to keep you healthy with your diabetes. However, if you already know a lot about diabetes, you'll find more in-depth explanations. You can pick and choose how much you want to know about a subject. The key points are clearly marked.

How This Book Is Organized

This book is divided into six parts to help you find out all you can about the topic of diabetes.

Part 1: Dealing with the Diagnosis of Diabetes

To slay the dragon, you have to be able to identify it. This part sorts out the different types of diabetes and looks at how you get diabetes and how you can help protect your family from developing it. In this part, you also find out how to deal with the emotional and psychological consequences of the diagnosis.

Part II: How Diabetes Can Affect Your Body

Diabetes may be associated with sugar, but to say that it's the *same* as sugar is like saying that a car is the same as a spark plug. Diabetes is far more than that and can affect every part of you. If you understand diabetes, you understand how your body works both when it's healthy and when it's not.

In this part, you find out what you need to know about both the acute and long-term problems that diabetes can cause. You also find out about sexual problems related to diabetes and about how diabetes can affect pregnancy.

Part III: Rule Your Diabetes: Don't Let It Rule You

In this part, you discover all the tools available to treat diabetes. You find out about the health care team that is there to assist you and about the ways you can make effective use of good nutrition and exercise to keep yourself healthy. You also discover the medications that may assist you with controlling your blood glucose.

Part IV: Particular Patients and Special Circumstances

Diabetes affects people differently depending on their age group. In this part, you hear about those differences and how to manage them. You also find out about diabetes in Aboriginal peoples.

We look at employment and insurance difficulties that people with diabetes can face and how to address them. This part also discusses diabetes and driving and offers suggestions to help you maintain a driver's licence and to obtain a commercial licence.

And so that you are always prepared, we discuss precautions you can take so that you can look after your diabetes if disaster strikes.

Part V: The Part of Tens

This part presents a concise summary of the most crucial stuff you need to know. Find out not only Ten Ways to Stay Healthy and Prevent Complications, but also Ten Frequently Asked Questions — and their answers, of course.

Part VI: Appendixes

This is where you find information on the Food Group System used in diabetes meal planning. We also look at some terrific diabetes-oriented websites and, last, we present a glossary. (We define words as we go along, but in case you forget what a term means, you can quickly flip to the back of the book.)

Icons Used in This Book

The icons tell you what you must know, what you should know, and what you might find interesting but can live without.

This icon indicates a story about one of our patients. (The names and other identifiers have been changed to maintain confidentiality.)

When you see this icon you know the information that follows is particularly important.

This icon gives you technical information or terminology that may be helpful, but not necessary, to your understanding of the topic.

When you see this icon, it means the information is *critical* and is not to be missed.

This icon points out when you should contact your health care team (for example, if your blood glucose control needs improving or if you need a particular test done). Your health care team includes your family doctor, your diabetes specialist, your diabetes nurse educator, your dietitian, your eye doctor (optometrist or ophthalmologist), your pharmacist, and, when necessary, other specialists (such as a podiatrist, dentist, cardiologist, kidney specialist, neurologist, emergency room physician, and so forth). We let you know which member of your team you should contact. (Incidentally, the most important member of your health care team is *you.*)

This icon is used when we share a practical, timesaving piece of advice, sometimes providing some additional detail on an important point.

Part I
Dealing with the Diagnosis of Diabetes

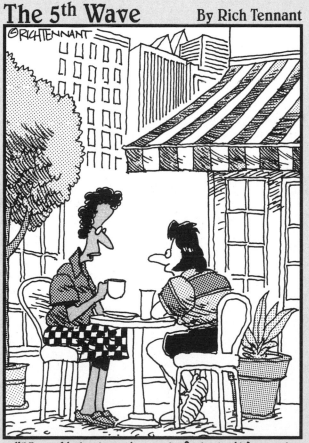

The 5th Wave   By Rich Tennant

"No, diabetes is not fatal, it's not contagious, and it doesn't mean you'll always get half my desserts."

In this part . . .

Υou have found out that you or a loved one has diabetes. What do you do now? This part looks at what organ malfunction leads to diabetes and how diabetes can make you feel.

Chapter 1

Membership in a Club You Didn't Ask to Join

As a person with diabetes, you already know that diabetes isn't "just a sugar problem." In fact, the moment you were told you had diabetes, many different thoughts may have run through your mind. You have feelings, and you have your own personal story. You're not the same person as your next-door neighbour or your sister or your friend, and your diabetes and the way you respond to its challenges are unique to you.

And unless you live alone on a desert island, your diabetes doesn't affect just you. Your family, friends, and co-workers are influenced by your diabetes and by their desire to help you.

In this chapter we consider how you might feel after you first find out you have diabetes, and we also look at some coping strategies to help you deal with this unwelcome news.

Figuring Out What Diabetes Is

Because we spend so much time discussing diabetes in this book, we want to start by defining the condition. *Diabetes* is a *metabolic disorder* (a problem with the body's internal chemistry) characterized by the presence of high blood glucose because the pancreas is unable to make enough insulin hormone or because the insulin the pancreas makes is not working properly, or both. (We take a closer look at glucose in Chapter 2.)

That may be the technically correct definition of diabetes, but to leave it at that would be akin to defining Paris as "a city with a metal tower located in France." France does indeed have a metal tower — and diabetes does indeed have high blood glucose — but to limit your perspective to such simple definitions would be to miss out on so, so much. Diabetes isn't just a sugar problem; it's a whole body problem. But fortunately this is a problem with many available ways to tackle it head on.

Diabetes is actually the short form for diabetes *mellitus.* The Romans noticed that the urine of certain people was *mellitus,* the Latin word for "sweet." The Greeks noticed that when people with sweet urine drank, fluids came out in the urine almost as fast as they went in the mouth, like a siphon. They called this by the Greek word for "siphon" — *diabetes.* Hence "diabetes mellitus." Nonetheless, we think the essence of diabetes is much better captured by the 17th-century definition of diabetes: "the pissing evil." Talk about calling it the way you see it!

You may have done some searching in books or on the Internet and come across another form of diabetes called *diabetes insipidus.* This term refers to an entirely different condition than diabetes mellitus. The only thing they have in common is a tendency to pass lots of urine. And now that we've clarified that, you won't see diabetes insipidus mentioned again in this book.

You're Not Alone

It seems unimaginable, but the number of people worldwide living with diabetes has risen from an estimated 30 million in 1985 to a mind boggling 366 million in 2011 and, by 2030, it is predicted 552 million people will be living with diabetes. In Canada, currently over 2.5 million people are living with diabetes. Clearly, as the title of this section says, you are most definitely not alone.

Hardly a day goes by when a person with diabetes isn't in the news. Even better, so far as we're concerned, is that their diabetes is not part of the news. Clearly the media and society in general have come to recognize that living with diabetes is, in and of itself, not the newsworthy part of most stories. We couldn't have found a better example of this than the 2009 appointment of Sonia Sotomayor to the US Supreme Court. Nearly all the news stories spoke of her intelligence and education and hard work and abilities. Her having diabetes was hardly mentioned. And those stories that did mention it did so in passing. Diabetes didn't — and doesn't — define her life.

It is not hard to find other examples of people living with diabetes who have achieved the loftiest of goals. Sebastien Sasseville (www.sebinspires.com) did so quite literally when he successfully climbed Mount Everest. And Gary Hall Junior is one of the most successful athletes in Olympic history with a bucketful of medals to his credit. Ian remembers meeting John Chick when John was playing with the CFL's Saskatchewan Roughriders (he now plays in the NFL). (Ian never felt so small in his life than he did that day, standing beside the towering athlete!) John is a past winner of the CFL Most Outstanding Defensive Player award. All these amazing individuals have diabetes.

Away from the sports arena, Ernest Hemingway, Thomas Edison, Jack Benny, Elizabeth Taylor, Drew Carey, and — Ian's all-time favourite piece of diabetes lore — Elvis Presley have all lived with diabetes.

You may not have spoken to Stephen Steele, but he has quite possibly spoken to you. Stephen is a commercial pilot with a major Canadian airline. And if you've ever had the bad luck to be on some sinking vessel off the Atlantic coast, the hero who plucked you from the ocean may have been none other than Major Chuck Grenkow, a Medal of Bravery-winning former Canadian Forces pilot and aircraft commander, who performed search and rescue operations with the Canadian military. Oh, by the way, they both have diabetes.

Diabetes is a common disease, so it's bound to occur in some very uncommon people. But you don't have to be famous to be considered exceptional. Indeed, every day of the week in our practices we see special people, people who have diabetes yet look after families, work in automotive plants or office buildings, write exams, go to movies, and do their best to live life to the fullest — people, perhaps, just like you.

The point is, diabetes shouldn't define your life. You're the same person the day after you found out you had diabetes as you were the day before. But you've been given an additional challenge to contend with. Diabetes shouldn't stop you from doing what you want to do with your life. Certainly, it does complicate things in some ways. But if you follow the principles of good diabetes care that we discuss in this book, you may actually be healthier than people without diabetes who smoke, overeat, under-exercise, or engage in other unhealthy activities.

Handling the News

If you are like most people, you were likely quite shocked when you were first told you had diabetes. Nobody wants to have diabetes and your first thought may well have been, "How can this be?" But, alas, it did come to be and you have had to deal with it ever since. You may have had your share of emotional ups and downs in coming to terms with your diabetes. For each person with this condition the journey toward acceptance is unique.

Hopefully, you not only came to accept your diabetes diagnosis, but also shared the news with your family and other people close to you. Having diabetes isn't something to be ashamed of, and it isn't something that you should have to hide from anyone. Your diabetes isn't your fault. You didn't want to have diabetes. You didn't try to get diabetes. And no one can catch it from you.

The Impact of Your Diabetes on Your Relationships

Everyone is involved in relationships with others. These might be family relationships, relationships with friends or workmates or, with some other people. And although living with diabetes needn't be front and centre in your interactions with people, it needn't be a secret either. In this section we look at how having diabetes may affect your relationships.

Looking at the impact of your diabetes on your relationships with your family

If one person in a family has diabetes, then, in a sense, everyone in the family has diabetes. Or at least has to live with it and deal with it.

If you've recently been diagnosed with diabetes, your family likely has had as many questions as you. What is diabetes? How can it affect you? How is it treated? Will you be okay? Some of the answers are simple. Some are complicated. (To help answer their questions we'd suggest you let your family members borrow this book from you and read it, too.) The fact your family is asking these questions isn't, of course, to play J. Edgar Hoover on you. Rather, it is simply a reflection of their concern and caring.

Ultimately, your diabetes is, well, *your* diabetes, and you need to take ownership of it. It is — and always will be — your decision about how you eat, if and how you exercise, if you test your blood glucose levels, attend doctors' appointments, and so forth. But all of this will be easier if you see your family as partners in your journey with diabetes. This may not, however, always be easy or straightforward.

Here are some ways you can help maintain positive, mentoring family relationships:

- **Don't keep your feelings about your diabetes to yourself.** Let your family members know if your diabetes is getting you down. Let them know if you are feeling positive about how things are going.

- **Feel free to test your blood glucose and, if you're giving insulin, inject this in front of family members.** You're the one *doing it*; it's a far lesser deal for someone else to *watch* when you're doing it. (And even at that, it will soon become routine enough to your family that they won't even notice.)

- **Remember that your blood glucose results are *yours*.** You only need to share the numbers if you want to. (We discuss this further later in this chapter.)

- **Make grocery shopping a collective experience and share your knowledge about healthy food with your family members.** Indeed, you can help ensure the whole family is eating healthfully because, as we discover in Chapter 10, a "diabetic diet" is, basically, a healthy eating diet.

- **Make exercising a family experience.** As we look at in Chapter 11, diabetes loves exercise and should be a regular part of your existence. But it should also be a part of *everyone's* existence, whether or not they have diabetes.

- **If you feel you'd like a supportive "extra set of ears" when you see a member of your health care team, bring a sufficiently mature family member with you to your appointment.** This is especially helpful for appointments with your diabetes educator or dietitian. (We discuss the members and roles of the diabetes health care team in Chapter 8.)

- **Remember that your family cares about you and wants to help you.** This is especially important when helping you in an emergency situation. Teach your family members what to do if ever you should need their help to treat a bad episode of low blood glucose. We discuss this in detail in Chapter 5.

Looking at the impact of your diabetes on your relationships with your friends

Your friends are your friends for a reason. Maybe you share the same interests in music or sports or hobbies, or perhaps you share opposite sides of the same picket fence. Whatever the case, your diabetes needn't interfere with your relationships with your friends. If anything, it can strengthen friendships and even foster developing new relationships. Indeed, we know many people living with diabetes who developed friendships *because of* their diabetes. For example, they met new friends at meetings of the CDA (Canadian Diabetes Association) or JDRF (Juvenile Diabetes Research Foundation) or at local diabetes support groups.

Here are a couple of ways that diabetes may affect your friendships:

✓ **As with family (see the preceding section), your friends care about you.** Therefore, if you want to share your thoughts or feelings about your diabetes with your friends, do so. And if you need to test your blood glucose or you need to give yourself an injection of insulin, don't feel obliged to do this in private. (You're welcome to, of course, but we hope you won't feel you *have* to.)

✓ **Keep right on doing the same activities with your friends that you've always done.** You may have to modify to some degree the way in which you do the activities, but your friends won't mind. For example, if you like to bike, because of your diabetes you may need to sometimes stop to check your blood glucose or to take some extra fluid to keep hydrated. Your friends will likely enjoy the excuse to rest; Ian sure does when he bikes with his friends who have diabetes!

We never recommend drinking alcohol to excess. But it is a fact of life — especially among teenagers and young adults — that overindulging with friends may happen. If you and your friends like to drink together and you've had more than your share, make sure your friends know the difference between being drunk and having low blood glucose. If ever your friends are unsure if you're drunk or having low blood glucose — especially if you are getting sleepy or confused and are unable to check your blood glucose — then your friends should call 9-1-1. We discuss the treatment of low blood glucose in Chapter 5.

Looking at the impact of your diabetes on your relationships with your workmates

Although we encourage you to share the fact of your diabetes (and its impact on you) with your family and friends, it's not quite as straightforward with your workmates.

Of course, some of your workmates may also be your friends; people you play hockey with, have over for a barbeque, and so forth. For these particular workplace relationships our advice is the same as in the preceding section about friends. Most of your workmates, however, are probably not your friends. They're more likely to be people that you work with, but do not socialize with much, if at all. Regarding these relationships and your diabetes, we suggest the following:

- ✔ **Be as open or as closed about your diabetes as you wish.** If you want to share the fact of your diabetes, feel free to do so. If you want to keep it private, do that. It is no one else's business unless you want it to be. (Exceptions do apply, however. For example, if you have a job in which you can be endangered or can endanger others if you have a diabetes emergency, you may be obliged to let your workplace know you have diabetes.)

- ✔ **If you are on medication — particularly insulin — that can cause your blood glucose level to go low, and especially if you have previously experienced bad episodes of hypoglycemia that required someone to assist you, try to find at least one workmate you can confide in and who can help you out if you run into a bad low.** Show this person where you keep your diabetes emergency supplies (such as dextrose tablets or juice). Also keep a glucagon kit at work (we discuss glucagon kits in Chapter 5) and teach your trusted workmate when and how to use it.

Juggling Your Diabetes and Your "Real Life"

Most people these days feel like they are constantly run off their feet. They juggle work (in or out of the home) and family life. They run here, run there, and try to squeeze in time for friends, sports, hobbies, volunteering, and so on. This never-ending rush of activity, often accompanied by stress, leaves very little time or energy for anything else. Oh, but wait, you have diabetes. How in the world are you going to fit managing your diabetes into your life? We look at that in this section.

Juggling your diabetes and your family life

Many of Ian's patients — especially the mothers of young children — tell us that they are so busy looking after their family that they have no time or energy to look after themselves. Time and again we see young women who manage their diabetes beautifully leading up to and during pregnancy, only to see it go off the rails when the realities of having a newborn (then infant then toddler. . .) are added to the mix. Whether you are the mother of a youngster or the father of a teenager or live in some other sort of family relationship, you likely find that sometimes family commitments get in the way of paying close attention to your diabetes. That makes perfect sense. However, your diabetes isn't going away and you have to deal with it. Here are some tips you may find helpful for juggling your diabetes and your family life:

- ✔ **Involve your family in your diabetes.** Take your kids grocery shopping (okay, sure, it will double the time it takes . . . maybe don't do this every time), have your child help you write down your blood glucose readings, and so on.

- ✔ **Exercise with your family.** Make it a collective experience. Or go out for a walk after you've dropped your kids off at hockey or soccer practice.

- ✔ **Make time for yourself.** Looking after your own health isn't selfish. Quite the opposite: Keeping yourself healthy is one of the *very best* things you can do for your whole family.

Juggling your diabetes and your work life

Depending on your occupation and where you work, time constraints or other challenges can make looking after your diabetes difficult while on the job. Table 1-1 illustrates some examples of these challenges and possible options available to help. (In Chapter 16 we look in detail at diabetes, employment issues, and your rights.)

Table 1-1	Dealing with Challenges at Work
If Your Work . . .	*We Recommend You . . .*
Provides no or insufficient breaks for eating, blood glucose testing, or injecting insulin	Speak to your employer. It is your legal right to be given sufficient time to perform these health-related tasks.
Makes it impossible to do fingerstick blood glucose tests because your hands are always dirty or greasy	Talk to your pharmacist about alternative-site blood glucose meters that allow you to test your blood glucose from, for example, your forearm. (We discuss this topic in more detail in Chapter 9.)
Does not have a discrete place for you to give your insulin and you're not comfortable injecting yourself in front of others	Speak to your diabetes specialist or diabetes educator about discrete ways to give your insulin.
Is in a hot environment and you do not have access to a fridge to store your insulin	Bring an insulated container to work in which to keep your insulin. (We discuss insulin storage in Chapter 13.)

Putting Your Energies into Your Diabetes

Living with diabetes is a time-consuming, energy-demanding, unceasing commitment. Diabetes doesn't take holidays, breaks, or any time off. Indeed, living with diabetes can sometimes feel like a full-time job. So if ever anyone has the audacity to tell you that your diabetes is no big deal, ask them if they want to try having diabetes for a while! Anyhow, the fact remains that you do have diabetes, it's not going away, and you have to invest time and energy to keep yourself healthy. This isn't easy, but it is essential.

How much energy goes into managing your diabetes? Well, you need to invest energy into choosing the right foods and preparing them in the right way. You need to check your blood glucose and take your medicines. You need to attend appointments with doctors and nurses and dietitians and other health care professionals. You need to visit the pharmacy regularly and you need to do lab tests and go for eye exams and check your feet. And you need to put physical energy into expending energy; that is, exercising. And you need to do all this in addition to doing everything else that goes on in your life. To effectively juggle and manage all these many things is, for most people, simply going to be impossible at times and something will, for a time, slip through the cracks. This is perfectly understandable, but for many people leads to feelings of guilt. We discuss this next.

Feeling guilty with your diabetes

Given what we say in the preceding sections, sometimes you'll find that you simply can't muster all the energy you need, and something has to give. If you've been living with diabetes for a while, you probably can recall different times when you let your diabetes slide. Perhaps you didn't eat as healthfully as you knew you should, or you tested your blood less often, or you stopped exercising. If so, we hope you didn't feel guilty about it. Or at least kept your guilt to a minimum. It is perfectly normal to have stages where your energy feels sapped and looking after your diabetes seems like more effort than you can muster. The key is to recognize that although this is both understandable and normal, you need to get back on track — preferably sooner than later. Your diabetes demands it and you deserve it. And as for feelings of guilt, don't beat yourself up over what you think you should've done better in the past; instead think about how you're going to better manage your diabetes in the future. Just like driving a car, you should be spending a lot more time looking forward than in your rear-view mirror.

We provide coping tips later in this chapter.

Feeling frustrated with your diabetes

The fact that you have diabetes doesn't change day-to-day, but lots of other things do. We're talking changes in the workplace, stresses at home, short-term illnesses, travel, and so forth. And that, in turn, will impact on your diabetes and in particular on your blood glucose control. It can be frustrating, indeed, when factors often beyond your control adversely impact your diabetes. Longer-term changes can also impact on your diabetes and lead to feelings of frustration. For example, perhaps you have developed arthritis and cannot exercise as much. Or, as typically happens if you have type 2 diabetes, the medications that were working just fine at first start to work less well.

Faced with all these changes that affect your glucose control, you may feel like you're trying to hit a moving target. Actually, it's not *like* trying to hit a moving target. It *is* trying to hit a moving target! Everything can seem to be going well, your blood glucose levels in check, your diet on track, your daily walks a well-honed ritual, then, *Wham!* A few holiday dinners or a sprained ankle or a bout of bronchitis or trouble at the office, and all of a sudden your blood glucose levels are up. Or pills that were working well start to be ineffective, and your blood glucose levels are on the rise. Or the insulin dose you give seems to work beautifully one day, and poorly the next. Feeling frustrated? Who wouldn't! Although your diabetes isn't going away, coping strategies can help you deal with the frustrations that diabetes presents. We look at this topic in the very next section. (As for bringing your glucose levels back in check, we discuss this in Chapters 10 to 13.)

Coping with diabetes

Whether you've had diabetes for ten days or ten years (or much longer), sometimes you will feel frustrated, discouraged, or simply fed up with dealing with it. This is perfectly understandable. Diabetes is a full-time job that you didn't apply for and would rather not have been hired for, thank you very much.

If your diabetes is getting you down, you can do a whole host of things to help lift yourself out of the doldrums. Here are some options:

- **Don't deny your feelings.** They are not unjustified and in any event, your feelings are your feelings.

- **Don't bottle up your emotions.** Share your feelings with those that are close to you, especially your family.

- **Seek support.** Participate in a support group (whether virtual or in-the-flesh).

✔ **Don't be too hard on yourself if your blood glucose levels are not as good or as consistent as they should be**. Perfect blood glucose control is not possible given that we have *imperfect* therapy. (Speaking of which, one of Ian's dictums is that the word "perfect" and the word "diabetes" should never be used in the same sentence.)

✔ **Think positively.** Focus on your successes (be they eating a healthy meal, going out for a walk, and so on) and pat yourself on the back more often.

✔ **Exercise regularly.** If you're feeling stressed and tired and burnt out with your diabetes, the idea of exercising may be the furthest thing from your mind. But exercise can hugely improve one's energy level and well-being.

✔ **Speak to your doctor about how you're feeling.** Discuss temporarily lightening some of your diabetes workload. For example, ask if for a period of time you can safely test your blood glucose less often. Or, if you're on four times daily insulin, ask if you can safely, temporarily, switch to a different insulin that is given twice per day.

✔ **Know that help is available.** Your doctor, depending on your specific situation, may recommend antidepressant medication or other forms of psychological support.

Feeling at wits' end with diabetes is common enough that an entire book is devoted to the subject. *Diabetes Burnout* by Dr. William Polonsky is an excellent resource to help you cope.

Diabetes etiquette

If you have diabetes, you've probably run into situations where people have offered you well-intentioned, but unsolicited and unhelpful advice. (We love the term for these people — especially those who question your food choices when you're in the cafeteria lineup or at a restaurant: the diabetes police!) The Behavioral Diabetes Institute (BDI; www.behavioraldiabetes institute.org) has developed etiquette cards for people with diabetes to give out to others (who don't have diabetes). With the BDI's kind permission, here's what the card says:

1. DON'T offer unsolicited advice about my eating or other aspects of diabetes. You may mean well, but giving advice about someone's personal habits, especially when it is not requested, isn't very nice. Besides, many of the popularly held beliefs about diabetes ("you should just stop eating sugar") are out of date or just plain wrong.

2. DO realize and appreciate that diabetes is hard work. Diabetes management is a full-time job that I didn't apply for, didn't want and can't quit. It Involves thinking about what, when, and

(continued)

(continued)

how much I eat, while also factoring in exercise, medication, stress, blood sugar monitoring, and so much more — each and every day.

3. DON'T tell me horror stories about your grandmother or other people with diabetes you have heard about. Diabetes is scary enough, and stories like these are not reassuring! Besides, we now know that with good management, odds are good you can live a long, healthy and happy life with diabetes.

4. DO offer to join me in making healthy lifestyle changes. Not having to be alone with efforts to change, like starting an exercise program, is one of the most powerful ways that you can be helpful. After all, healthy lifestyle changes can benefit everyone!

5. DON'T look so horrified when I check my blood sugars or give myself an injection. It is not a lot of fun for me either. Checking blood sugars and taking medications are things I must do to manage diabetes well. If I have to hide while I do so, it makes it much harder for me.

6. DO ask how you might be helpful. If you want to be supportive, there may be lots of little things I would probably appreciate your help with. However, what I really need may be very different than what you think I need, so please ask first.

7. DON'T offer thoughtless reassurances. When you first learn about my diabetes, you may want to reassure me by saying things like, "Hey, it could be worse; you could have cancer!" This won't make me feel better. And the implicit message seems to be that diabetes is no big deal. However, diabetes (like cancer) IS a big deal.

8. DO be supportive of my efforts for self-care. Help me set up an environment for success by supporting healthy food choices. Please honor my decision to decline a particular food, even when you really want me to try it. You are most helpful when you are not being a source of unnecessary temptation.

9. DON'T peek at or comment on my blood glucose numbers without asking me first. These numbers are private unless I choose to share them. It is normal to have numbers that are sometimes too low or too high. Your unsolicited comments about these numbers can add to the disappointment, frustration and anger I already feel.

10. DO offer your love and encouragement. As I work hard to manage diabetes successfully, sometimes just knowing that you care can be very helpful and motivating.

Chapter 2

You and Your Blood Glucose

The ancient Greeks and Romans knew about diabetes. Fortunately, the way they tested for the condition — by tasting the urine — has gone by the wayside. (So has the other old way of testing for diabetes — urinating near an anthill and seeing if the ants came scurrying for takeout.)

For most people, diabetes is diagnosed when they have their blood glucose level measured either as part of a routine checkup with their family doctor, or for some other coincidental reason (such as when tests are taken for an insurance application or in preparation for surgery). Others have their diabetes discovered when they seek medical attention after they've started to feel unwell due to symptoms of high blood glucose (which we discuss later in this chapter).

In this chapter you discover how diabetes is diagnosed, how you may feel if your blood glucose is too high, and what you can do to bring things under control.

What Is Glucose?

The sweetness of the urine with which the ancients had first-hand experience comes from *glucose,* the body's predominant form of sugar. Glucose is the fuel that your body uses to provide instant energy so that muscles can move and important chemical reactions can take place. Glucose is a *carbohydrate*, one group of the three sources of energy in the body. The others are protein and fat, which we discuss in greater detail in Chapter 10.

Many different kinds of sugar exist, but the important one regarding diabetes is glucose. Unlike in high school chemistry class, here we let you off easy and, apart from our discussion about nutrition therapy, we don't talk about all the other sugars that are around. But just in case you're wondering, some examples of other sugars are *fructose* (the sugar found in fruits and vegetables) and *sucrose* (or table sugar, which is actually a combination of glucose and fructose).

Diagnosing Diabetes

Diagnosing diabetes should be simple. You likely know by now that you have diabetes when your glucose level is too high. But what, exactly, is too high? One way to think of "too high" is to think of the level of blood glucose that can cause damage to your body. The Canadian Diabetes Association considers people to have diabetes if they meet *any* one of these four criteria (these are summarized in Table 2-1):

✔ A **random** blood glucose level equal to or greater than 11.1 millimoles per litre (mmol/L). *Random* is defined as any time of day or night, without regard to how long it's been since the last time you ingested anything containing calories.

✔ A **fasting** blood glucose level equal to or greater than 7.0 mmol/L. *Fasting* is defined as eight or more hours without calorie intake.

✔ A blood glucose level equal to or greater than 11.1 mmol/L, when tested two hours after ingesting 75 grams of glucose as part of what is called a **glucose tolerance test.**

✔ An **A1C** level equal to or greater than 6.5 percent. The A1C is measured on a blood test and allows for an estimate of one's average blood glucose level for the preceding three months. The A1C should *not* be used as a diagnostic test for diabetes if you are a child, an adolescent, are pregnant, if type 1 diabetes is suspected, or if you have a condition which can affect its accuracy. We discuss the A1C test in detail (including a discussion of these other conditions) in Chapter 9.

Table 2-1	Diagnostic Criteria for Diabetes
Test	*Level Diagnosing Diabetes*
Random blood glucose	11.1 mmol/L or higher
Fasting blood glucose	7.0 mmol/L or higher
Two-hour blood glucose level on a glucose tolerance test	11.1 mmol/L or higher
A1C	6.5% or higher

Testing positive for one of the previously mentioned criteria on a single occasion is not enough to make a diagnosis of diabetes (although important exceptions exist, which we discuss next). Any one of the tests must be also be positive on another day to establish the diagnosis. More than one patient has come to us with a diagnosis of diabetes after having been tested only once, and then when we retested their blood glucose it turned out to be normal. They didn't have diabetes after all.

The diagnosis of diabetes should be based on a blood sample taken *from a vein* and *analyzed at a laboratory.* If you borrow your friend's blood glucose meter, prick your finger to get a blood glucose sample, and find your blood glucose level to be high, see your doctor to have a blood sample drawn from a vein at a laboratory. Don't diagnose yourself based on a glucose meter result.

Waiting for another day to have a second test performed after having an initial high blood glucose discovered is *not* required — and indeed, can be dangerous in two circumstances:

- ✔ If your initial blood glucose level is 11.1 mmol/L or higher *and* you have symptoms of high blood glucose (frequent urination, increased thirst, loss of weight)

- ✔ If your doctor thinks you may have type 1 diabetes (especially if you are a child)

In either of these circumstances, the diagnosis of diabetes is made without a second test, and you need to start treatment *immediately.*

If you have visited U.S. websites, you may have noticed that in the United States they use different units — called milligrams per decilitre (abbreviated mg/dL). To convert mg/dL to mmol/L you divide mg/dL by 18. For example, 200 mg/dL divided by 18 equals 11.1 mmol/L.

How High Blood Glucose Makes You Feel

Knowing a bit about how your body normally handles blood glucose will help you understand the symptoms of high blood glucose. In this section we look at both these issues.

Understanding how your body handles blood glucose

The pancreas makes a hormone called *insulin*. (We talk more about the pancreas in Chapter 3.) A *hormone* is a chemical substance made in one part of the body that travels (usually through the bloodstream) to another part of the body where it performs its work. Insulin finely controls the level of glucose in your blood. Insulin acts like a key to open the lining of a cell so that glucose can enter the cell. If glucose can't enter the cell, it can't provide energy to the body.

Insulin is an amazing substance. Not only does it allow glucose to enter cells, but it also enables fat and muscle to form and allows the liver to store glucose (in a form called *glycogen*) for use when you may not be eating properly.

Without insulin, the body's tissues start to break down. Perhaps you have seen a heart-rending photo of an ill-looking child with diabetes from before insulin was discovered, and the thrilling photo of that same child, now the picture of health, after starting insulin therapy. (We talk more about the discovery of insulin — and Canada's important contribution — in Chapter 3.)

The pancreas normally functions like a precision tool. It releases just the right amount of insulin to keep your body's blood glucose in a remarkably tight range seldom exceeding 7.5 mmol/L or so. If the pancreas isn't able to produce the proper amount of insulin, or if the insulin it makes isn't working effectively, then your blood glucose level will start to rise. If it goes up just a bit, you won't have any symptoms. But if it reaches as high as 10.0 mmol/L or so, glucose begins to filter through the kidneys and spill into the urine. At that stage you may begin to experience symptoms (see the next section for more).

It's a shame that people don't get symptoms until the glucose level is almost 50 percent higher than the normal level, because by the time symptoms arise, damage may already have occurred to the body. We would be much better off if even slightly high glucose levels made our skin glow bright green, identifying the problem right away.

Examining symptoms caused by high blood glucose

The following list contains the most common symptoms of high blood glucose. You may find that some of these remind you of what you were feeling when you first found out you had diabetes:

- ✔ **Frequent urination and thirst:** High blood glucose makes more urine form, and the more urine you make, the more fluid you lose from your body. The large quantity of urine makes you feel the need to urinate more frequently during the day and to get up at night to empty your bladder, which keeps filling up. As the amount of fluid in your body declines, you feel thirsty and drink much more frequently. Many people with newly diagnosed diabetes believe that they are urinating more often because they are drinking more, but it is actually the other way around.

- ✔ **Blurred vision:** When the blood glucose level changes substantially, it causes the amount of fluid in the lens of the eye to change also. This alters the way that light passes through your eye, making it bend more than usual and making things look blurry. Have you ever noticed how a knife in a glass of water looks bent? The same sort of thing is going on in your eye.

  In the same way that your eyesight can become blurry as your blood glucose rises, it can become blurry as your blood glucose falls. Many people with diabetes become understandably alarmed when their vision gets worse after they first start diabetes therapy, but in fact this is typically a good sign that their blood glucose is improving. If this happens to you, be reassured that your eyesight will return to its usual state within a few weeks. Don't waste your hard-earned money buying new, expensive prescription glasses if you've very recently been diagnosed with diabetes. Instead, if you need to, purchase inexpensive over-the-counter glasses at your neighbourhood drugstore, and you'll likely find that within a month you can give them away.

- ✔ **Hunger:** Inability to get energy in the form of glucose into the muscle cells that need it leads to a feeling of hunger despite all the glucose that is present in the blood stream.

- **Fatigue:** Because glucose can't enter most cells in the absence of insulin or with ineffective insulin (see Chapter 3 for more), if you have uncontrolled diabetes glucose can't be used as a fuel to move muscles and help other tissues function properly. And just like when you try to pedal a bike with deflated tires, you get tired awfully quickly.

- **Weight loss:** Because you can't nourish your cells without sufficient or effective insulin (see the preceding bullets), weight loss is common among people with newly diagnosed diabetes (especially if you have type 1 diabetes, as we discuss in Chapter 4). You lose muscle tissue and you lose fat tissue. And as these tissues are lost, the body wastes away (again, this is especially true of type 1 diabetes). Your blood glucose level is high, but the glucose just can't work. It's as if your car has a full gas tank but the fuel line is blocked. The gauge reads "full" but the car stalls anyhow.

- **Persistent vaginal infections:** When blood glucose rises, it rises in all the fluids in your body. For women, this means higher glucose levels in their vaginal secretions. Yeast organisms thrive in a high-glucose environment and as a result women with elevated glucose levels are prone to vaginal yeast infections. Symptoms include vaginal itching or burning, an abnormal discharge from the vagina, and sometimes an odour.

Although people with high blood glucose commonly experience the symptoms in this list, many people with undiagnosed diabetes don't have these symptoms. It's no wonder, therefore, that the diagnosis of diabetes can be especially surprising to them.

ANECDOTE

Doctor, my eyes!

Sam O'Reilly was a 60-year-old man who had just been diagnosed with diabetes. This was discovered shortly after he developed bothersome thirst and frequent urination and had gone to the hospital to get checked out. His blood glucose level was found to be 25 mmol/L. He was immediately started on pills to reduce his glucose level, and an appointment was arranged to see Ian two weeks thereafter.

About five days before his appointment, Mr. O'Reilly called Ian's office in a near panic. He was sure he was going blind. Days after starting his new pills, his thirst and urine problems had improved, but now he could no longer read his daily newspaper or even see the television; everything had become one big blur. Ian had him come to the office right away, not because he was worried about Mr. O'Reilly but to reassure him. The only additional prescription Mr. O'Reilly needed turned out to be "tincture of time," and this worked perfectly. Indeed, within a week or so, Mr. O'Reilly's eyesight was back to normal.

Controlling Your Blood Glucose

Anyone with diabetes can have excellent blood glucose control. It may not always be easy to achieve, but it can be achieved and indeed *must* be achieved if you are going to keep healthy.

These are three key strategies used to control blood glucose:

- ✔ Healthy eating (more aptly called *nutrition therapy*; see Chapter 10)
- ✔ Exercise (see Chapter 11)
- ✔ Medication (see Chapters 12 and 13)

What You Can Do If You Lose Control of Your Blood Glucose

You will find that when you improve your blood glucose control, you will feel better. You won't be running to the bathroom around the clock, your energy level will improve, and you'll have a better sense of well-being. At times, however, your blood glucose control may worsen and some of your symptoms may start to return. You may find that your blood glucose levels go up if you're under greater stress, if you've come down with an infection, if you've gotten off track with your nutrition plan, or if you're unable to go out for your daily walk because of yet another February snowstorm.

When your glucose control worsens, remember two things:

- ✔ If you're feeling reasonably well, even if your blood glucose levels climb up into the high teens (or even somewhat higher), you're not in immediate danger. (The exception is if you have type 1 diabetes and are developing ketones. See Chapter 5 for a discussion of ketoacidosis.) A few days of blood glucose readings of 20 mmol/L will not damage your organs.

- ✔ Look at the higher glucose levels as a message that something is wrong and take corrective action. This may be as simple as adjusting your diet or restarting your exercise plan. Perhaps you've forgotten to refill a prescription for your diabetes medicines, in which case a trip to the pharmacy is in order. Or if you're unsure what has triggered the problem and what to do about it, then call your doctor or diabetes educator.

If your blood glucose readings have risen to the high teens or higher *and you're feeling unwell* (or if you have type 1 diabetes and you have developed ketones — see Chapter 5), then you need to seek *immediate* medical assistance. If you're very ill, proceed to the nearest emergency department. If you're not feeling all that bad, you may first contact your physician or diabetes educator. (As we discuss in Chapter 8, some diabetes educators are trained and empowered to assist you with these situations.)

Chapter 3

Discovering the Cause of Your Diabetes

. . . .

In This Chapter

▶ Understanding how your organs maintain glucose control

▶ Discovering how organ malfunction has led to your diabetes

. . . .

You may not think that having a personal relationship with one of your body's organs is possible or even desirable. Then again, maybe you just haven't had a chance to meet some of them up close and personal. In which case, this chapter is for you.

Ask most people what organ is involved with diabetes and a typical response would be "the pancreas." Indeed, the pancreas *is* a key player in diabetes, but it isn't the only one.

In this chapter, we take a look at the role each of the key participants plays in diabetes. (Incidentally, given the important role of genetics — as we discuss in Chapter 4 — two key participants are your parents. Which of course adds to the importance of picking your parents carefully, though that remains a bit impractical, even with modern technology.)

How Your Organs Make Music

You may not think of your organs as being music makers (singing and other, ruder noises notwithstanding), but when controlling your blood glucose, your body is engaged in a wonderfully intricate symphony with each organ playing its part.

Glucose regulation starts the moment you begin to eat. When you ingest certain types of food, they get broken down inside your gut into glucose, which is then absorbed across the lining of the small intestine into your blood. When inside your blood, the glucose travels around your body looking for a nice place to go. Some of the glucose gets used by your brain and some gets taken up and stored in your liver and muscles (in a form called glycogen). Your muscles use some of the glucose straight away as they do their work. And fat cells store some of it as, well, fat.

As sophisticated as glucose metabolism is, with every passing year new research — including important Canadian contributions — comes out shedding additional light (and complexity!) on our understanding of this finely honed mechanism. In particular the important role of intestinal hormones is now recognized.

So, with baton at the ready, let us now look in more detail at the players in this orchestra.

Presenting your pancreas

Unless you have diabetes, you probably don't ever think about that funny-looking organ tucked behind your stomach. Well, even if you do have diabetes, your dinnertime conversation likely doesn't centre on this tadpole-shaped (yuck!), 25.5-centimetre (10-inch) long, 80-gram (3-oz) organ. Figure 3-1 shows its location in your body.

The pancreas has two main functions. One is to produce enzymes, which are then released into your small intestine to assist with the breakdown of food. That is called the pancreas's *exocrine* function. The cells responsible for this take up 95 percent of the pancreas. People with diabetes seldom have a problem with this pancreas function.

Your pancreas's second task is called its *endocrine* function, and that has everything to do with your diabetes. Within the pancreas are clusters of hormone-producing cells called *islet cells*. The most important of these islet cells when it comes to diabetes is the beta cell. It is the *beta cell* that produces and releases into the blood stream a hormone called insulin. A normal pancreas has about 1.5 million islet cells. (If extracted and lumped together, these cells could fit inside a thimble. ***Note:*** Please do not try this at home!)

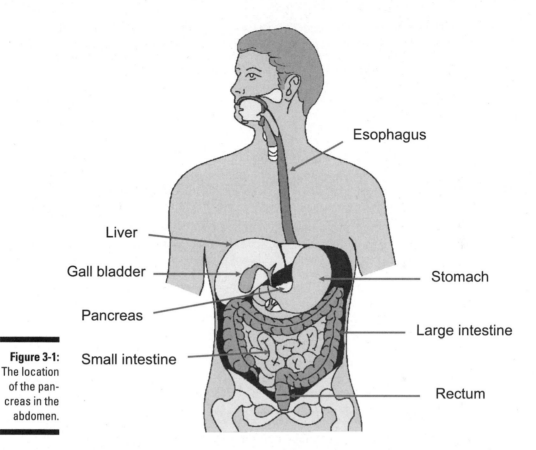

Esophagus

Liver

Gall bladder

Stomach

Pancreas

Large intestine

Figure 3-1:
The location
of the pan-
creas in the
abdomen.

Small intestine

Rectum

The pancreas also produces other hormones. One of these is glucagon. *Glucagon* can be thought of as an anti-insulin hormone because it acts in ways that oppose what insulin does. *Amylin,* another pancreatic hormone, works as a partner with insulin in keeping blood glucose under control. We discuss these hormones in more detail later in this section. Other pancreatic hormones (somatostatin and others) are either not involved with diabetes or are less important for blood glucose control and we don't discuss these further.

Looking at your liver

Perhaps we're biased, but we feel bad for the liver. Apart from when people cook liver (and most people don't even like it), the only time it seems to get attention is when someone is suffering from liver diseases like hepatitis or cirrhosis.

Your liver has many, many tasks to fulfill, including helping to rid your body of certain toxins and producing crucial proteins, such as clotting factors that prevent you from bleeding. The liver's role in glucose metabolism is to serve as a highly sophisticated storage depot for glucose, removing it from or delivering it to the blood in precise amounts, depending on your body's needs at any given time.

Going on about your gut

The intestine is the place where the carbohydrates you ingest get broken down and glucose gets absorbed into your body. That used to be pretty well all we knew about the gut and glucose metabolism. Over the past few years, however, pioneering research (much of it by Dr. Daniel Drucker in Toronto) has shed light on the powerful endocrine functions of the gut and what goes awry when one has diabetes (as we discuss later in this chapter). When a person eats, K and L cells in the intestine release hormones called *incretins* (specifically, GLP-1 and GIP). These incretin hormones stimulate the pancreas to make insulin (which will allow for glucose to leave the blood and enter the body's cells) and to make less glucagon (which will prevent the liver from releasing extra glucose into the blood). Incretin hormones also reduce appetite and slow down how quickly food is absorbed into your body from your intestine.

Mentioning your muscles

When you walked over to your favourite chair before plunking yourself down to read this book, you were using your muscles and, without even thinking about it, your muscles were actively using glucose to do their work. Some of this glucose comes from stores within muscle and some comes from actively extracting glucose from your blood. When we think of muscles, we tend to think of power or strength. We should also think of fuel, because glucose is a key energy source that your muscles need to work properly.

Chewing the fat

You may know that if you're overweight, you're more prone to getting type 2 diabetes. But not all fat tissue is the same. Fat inside the abdomen is called *visceral fat*, and fat in the abdominal wall and legs and arms is called *non-visceral fat*. (How creative is that?) Depending on how much of each of these types of fat you have, your risk for getting diabetes will vary. We discuss this further in the next section.

The fat cells' role in glucose metabolism is to store extra glucose (as fat). For this reason, even if you were to entirely avoid ingesting fats, you could still gain excess weight if you were eating excess calories (such as ingesting too many carbohydrates). Imagine eating two dozen apples and drinking a litre of maple syrup a day. You wouldn't see an ounce of fat — not right away, that is. The fat would appear soon enough, though, but about a foot and a half lower than your lips!

Being brainy

The role of the brain in controlling glucose metabolism (apart from regulating appetite) is still largely unknown, but recent research has provided evidence that nerve connections link the central nervous system (that is, the brain and spinal cord) to the islet cells in the pancreas and help control their function. No doubt much more on this story will emerge in the coming years.

Playing a beautiful melody

In order for the body to function properly, it needs to maintain a normal blood glucose level both when you've eaten and when you've not recently eaten. We look at these two scenarios here.

Maintaining a normal blood glucose level after you've eaten

When things are going right, as soon as your blood glucose level rises after eating, your pancreas

- **Releases insulin into the bloodstream.** The insulin attaches to the lining of certain cells (such as muscle cells) and, as if a key has opened a door, the cells then allow the glucose to enter.

- **Releases amylin into the bloodstream.** Scientists haven't fully sorted out how amylin helps control blood glucose, but a main action appears to be slowing down how quickly food is absorbed into your body from the intestine.

- **Reduces how much glucagon it releases into the bloodstream.** The less glucagon in your bloodstream, the less glucose your liver will release. Your glucose goes up after eating, so having a lower amount of glucagon in your body as you eat is helpful because you don't need your liver to make additional glucose at that time.

At the same time that your pancreas is doing all those clever things, your intestines are releasing incretin hormones. These hormones, as we discuss in the preceding section, help control blood glucose through a variety of mechanisms, including stimulating your pancreas to make insulin.

As soon as your glucose level falls back to normal, the pancreas shuts off production of insulin (good thing, too; otherwise we would always have low blood glucose — a condition called *hypoglycemia*) and your glucose level immediately stabilizes.

Maintaining a normal blood glucose level when you've not recently eaten

The body requires a certain level of glucose in the blood at all times so if you haven't eaten recently (and, therefore, you've not ingested nutrients to fuel your body), your body has to look elsewhere for energy. In this situation your pancreas will increase its release of glucagon which, in turn, will stimulate your liver to both make more glucose (out of protein) and to release some of its stored glucose into the bloodstream. Your organs then use the glucose as fuel. (At the same time, your pancreas will reduce how much insulin it is making since if you're not eating and your glucose level is not elevated your body will not need much insulin.)

Your body even has a backup plan. Say you've been feeling unwell for a few days and haven't been eating properly. You may not have been eating enough to keep up with your body's demands for glucose, and your liver's stores of glucose (in the form of glycogen) and its ability to produce glucose may already have been exhausted. So where will your body turn for its source of fuel? Well, your clever body will, like a hybrid car, look for alternative fuels and start to break down fat tissue, which releases fatty acids into the blood. These fatty acids serve as an alternative source of energy to keep you and your organs going.

What Happens When Your Organs Hit the Wrong Notes?

The intricate system we describe in the previous section is the way things are supposed to work. And if they did, you wouldn't have diabetes. But you do have diabetes, so something has gone wrong. That's not your fault. You didn't want things to go wrong and you sure as heck didn't intentionally make things go wrong. So don't feel guilty.

If you have type 1 diabetes then the main problem is that you are unable to make any insulin (or make, at best, such tiny amounts that it is insignificant).

If you have type 2 diabetes (far and away the most common form, as we discuss further in Chapter 4), then you typically have two different problems with insulin: You don't make enough insulin, and the insulin you do make does not work sufficiently well. Also, your incretin hormones don't work as well as they should. We look at these issues in this section.

Insulin resistance

Almost all people with type 2 diabetes have *insulin resistance*, which means that certain tissues (such as fat and muscle) in your body resist the action of insulin. As a result, when you eat, even though your pancreas makes insulin, it doesn't work sufficiently well. Using the earlier analogy (see "Playing a beautiful melody" in the preceding section), your insulin can't unlock the key on the cell lining, so the glucose has a hard time entering your cells.

The degree to which you have insulin resistance is significantly related not just to how much fat tissue you have, but also to where it's located. Visceral fat (the fat within the abdomen) is the type of fat most likely to cause insulin resistance, followed by fat within the abdominal wall and fat elsewhere on your body. Insulin resistance (and type 2 diabetes) is, therefore, more common in people with an apple-shaped physique rather than a pear-shaped physique.

(Although we do not know for certain why someone has insulin resistance, rapidly emerging evidence shows that fat cells are responsible by causing inflammation in the body; indeed, some theories suggest that diabetes, heart disease, and many other health problems share this common denominator.)

If you have a healthy pancreas, it can overcome a problem with insulin resistance simply by making more insulin. But if you have diabetes, your pancreas is unable to produce sufficient insulin. We look at this next.

Insulin deficiency

Although the initial problem if you have type 2 diabetes is insulin resistance, with time your pancreas's ability to produce insulin wanes so you now have two problems: insulin resistance and insulin deficiency. This one-two punch leaves you unable (without treatment) to move sufficient glucose from your blood into your cells. Instead, the glucose hangs around in your bloodstream and eventually it gets so high that it spills out into the urine, making both you and your urine the sweet things that you are.

Unfortunately, there is no proven way to prevent insulin deficiency from worsening; as a result, almost all people with type 2 diabetes require more and more medication (including insulin therapy) as time goes by. ***Remember:*** This is not your fault!

If you have type 1 diabetes (which we discuss further in Chapter 4), your main problem is that your pancreas is unable to make insulin. As you eat, your blood glucose level goes up, and, try as it might, your pancreas is unable to respond. For this reason, all people with type 1 diabetes require insulin therapy. If you have type 1 diabetes and you're also overweight, you may also have insulin resistance; this is sometimes informally referred to as *double diabetes*.

Defective incretin action

As we discuss in the previous section, normally when one eats, the intestines quickly respond by releasing incretin hormones into the blood. These incretins assist with glucose regulation in several ways including stimulating insulin secretion and reducing glucagon secretion. If you have type 2 diabetes, however, your body's incretin function is impaired. As a result, despite your blood glucose level rising as the food you eat is absorbed into your body, your incretin system lets you down and fails to sufficiently stimulate your pancreas to release more insulin and less glucagon.

The problems that we have just discussed are often relative. In other words, if you have type 2 diabetes, your organs can partially respond to the insulin you have. And if you have only recently acquired type 1 diabetes, your body may still have *some* ability to produce insulin, but far less than you need.

Regardless of which type of diabetes you have, if you're not able to use glucose properly for fuel, your body starts to use other tissues for this purpose. You break down fat and, eventually, you break down muscle. The excess glucose that accumulates in your blood spills into the urine. And that is why, if you have uncontrolled *hyperglycemia* (high blood glucose), you may have noticed that you're losing weight and muscle bulk. But, of course, that either already is — or soon will be — behind you, because from this point on you're going to make sure that you control your blood glucose levels and stay healthy.

The discovery of insulin

Until not too long ago, type 2 diabetes was uncommon. To have diabetes was to have type 1 diabetes. And to have type 1 diabetes before the discovery of insulin was to have a terminal illness. Imagine, therefore, the euphoria that greeted the discovery of insulin. It must surely have been equal to what the discovery of a universal cure for cancer would be nowadays. And it happened right here in Canada.

In 1889, a scientist discovered that if a dog's pancreas was removed, the dog immediately developed diabetes. This was the first strong clue that the pancreas and diabetes were intimately related. But how they were related remained a mystery.

In 1920, Dr. Frederick Banting, a Canadian surgeon from Alliston, Ontario, was working as a very junior lecturer at the University of Western Ontario in London. While preparing for a class, he read an article on diabetes and the pancreas, and that sparked an interest — soon to be an obsession — in finding out what secretion the pancreas might be making that prevents diabetes.

Dr. Banting, all of 29 years of age at the time, approached Dr. John Macleod, a professor at the University of Toronto, and asked permission to use a laboratory. Dr. Macleod agreed and assigned Charles H. Best, a science student, to assist. How was Best chosen for a role that was soon to make him world-famous? Through a rigorous selection process, you might think. Well, it wasn't quite like that. In fact, Best was picked by virtue of winning a coin toss!

Dr. Banting and Mr. Best (he wasn't a doctor yet) began their work in May 1921, and in December they were joined by J. B. Collip, a biochemist from the University of Alberta. After some initial setbacks (what would science be without setbacks?), they eventually purified a pancreatic extract that they felt could be given to people with diabetes.

On January 11, 1922, their extract was administered to Leonard Thompson, a 14-year-old boy in the Toronto General Hospital. The treatment was a dismal failure. Thankfully, the young scientists and Leonard were not deterred and, after some further work in the laboratory, they tried again on January 23. We do not know if they shouted "Eureka!" but they must have wanted to when they saw Leonard's glucose level fall and his well-being suddenly improve. The boy had been rescued from death. Insulin was born.

That is the end of one story and the beginning of another, for the subsequent personal rivalries between Banting and Best on the one side and Collip and Macleod on the other is the stuff of legend. The Nobel Prize in physiology or medicine was awarded to Banting and Macleod in 1923. Banting shared his portion with Best, and Macleod did likewise with Collip. Michael Bliss, a Canadian historian, has written an absolutely wonderful book, *The Discovery of Insulin,* which chronicles the story and is as entertaining and fascinating to read as any detective novel.

Chapter 4

Looking at the Different Types of Diabetes

. . . .

In This Chapter

▶ Identifying the symptoms and causes of type 1 diabetes

▶ Identifying the symptoms and causes of type 2 diabetes

▶ Looking at LADA

▶ Comparing type 1 and type 2 diabetes

▶ Reviewing gestational diabetes

▶ Understanding the Metabolic Syndrome

▶ Finding out the importance of prediabetes

▶ Exploring other types of diabetes

. . . .

You might think that diabetes is diabetes is diabetes. And, true enough, in many ways the various forms of diabetes have much in common. Most importantly, everyone with diabetes is combating a tendency to have high blood glucose levels. And everyone with diabetes has to strive to keep these blood glucose levels in check through a combination of lifestyle efforts and, when necessary, medications. Having said that, certain things are unique to the different forms of diabetes and require special attention.

Jim, a 50-year-old assembly-line worker at a car plant, had always been healthy. Indeed, he never saw doctors. He was a hard-working man who enjoyed playing ball in the summer and hockey in the winter. Over the past few months he had noticed that he was going to the bathroom night and day. And he was constantly thirsty. Thinking that he needed better nutrition, he had started to drink glass after glass of orange juice. But that didn't make him feel better. One day he got on the scale and realized that, although he was still overweight, during the past six months he had lost 7 kilograms (15 pounds) without even trying. Jim was hesitant to see a doctor, but his wife finally convinced him that he had to get checked out. He went to see his family physician, a blood test was done, and a day later Jim got a call at work that he had to come in to see the doctor right away. His blood glucose level was 25 mmol/L. Jim's doctor told him the result and what it meant. Jim had type 2 diabetes.

Mary was a 5-year-old girl. She was a beautiful, healthy, and happy child, but had suddenly become irritable and in just a matter of days had started to look increasingly unwell. She was quickly losing weight and had started to wet her bed. Mary's parents became alarmed and took her to the local emergency department, where doctors found that she had a blood glucose level of 15 mmol/L and that her urine contained a substance called ketones. Mary was diagnosed as having type 1 diabetes.

Fatima was pregnant with her third child. She had had no problems during the first two pregnancies, and with this one she also felt fine. As a matter of routine procedure, when Fatima reached her 24th week of pregnancy, her doctor sent her for a glucose tolerance test in which she drank a sugar-rich liquid and her blood glucose level was checked a couple of hours later. Her result was 11.2 mmol/L. Fatima's doctor diagnosed her as having gestational diabetes.

What do Jim, Mary, and Fatima have in common? That's easy to answer and takes but one word: diabetes. But if we were to write about how they differ, that would take a whole chapter. This chapter! Here we look at the different forms of diabetes, what they have in common, and how they differ.

Type 1 Diabetes and You

Type 1 diabetes is caused by destruction of the insulin-producing (beta) cells in the pancreas. This results in insulin deficiency which, without treatment, leads to a dangerous buildup of acid in the body called *ketoacidosis* (which we discuss in Chapter 5). Children, teenagers, and young adults are the most likely to develop type 1 diabetes, but it can occur at virtually any age. If you have type 1 diabetes, you need to inject insulin into your body if you are to stay healthy (or even alive!).

Type 1 diabetes used to be called *juvenile-onset diabetes* or *insulin dependent diabetes*. The problem with these old terms is that many people don't fit the descriptive titles. For example, many children who get diabetes actually have type 2 diabetes. And many adults who get diabetes actually have type 1 diabetes. Unfortunately, you're still likely to come across the outdated names because many people — including, sigh, some health care providers — haven't caught up with the current terminology.

Identifying the symptoms of type 1 diabetes

Symptoms of undiagnosed or insufficiently treated type 1 diabetes are directly related to high blood glucose caused by lack of insulin. Symptoms of type 1 diabetes tend to come on quite quickly, usually over a matter of days or weeks. These symptoms include

- **Blurred vision:** When the glucose levels in your body undergo a big change, the fluid content of the lens of your eyes also changes. That, in turn, alters the way that light bends as it passes through your eyes and leads to blurring. Maybe you have noticed the way that a knife in a glass of water looks bent. It's much the same phenomenon. Your blurred vision will correct soon after you start insulin.

- **Fatigue:** When type 1 diabetes first strikes, you suddenly start to lose body fluids, muscle mass, and fat tissue, and you quickly become malnourished and are on the verge of being (or actually are) dehydrated. In the face of this onslaught, it's no wonder you feel fatigued. If you have type 1 diabetes, you probably recall how quickly your energy improved when you started insulin therapy.

- **Frequent urination:** As we explain in Chapter 3, passing lots of urine is a typical symptom of high blood glucose. You experience frequent urination because when your blood glucose level rises to above 10 mmol/L or so (people without diabetes seldom have values above 7.5 mmol/L or so), glucose passes through the kidneys and spills into the urine, drawing extra fluids along the way.

- **Increased thirst:** Because you're losing excess fluids in the urine, you're at risk of getting dehydrated. Your clever body tries to prevent this by making you feel thirstier, which, of course, encourages you to drink more.

- **Weight loss and increased hunger:** If you have uncontrolled type 1 diabetes, you're passing urine that's rich in glucose and, thus, rich in calories. This wasted nutrition is going down the drain, in a manner of speaking. The body then starts to break down muscle and fat tissue. As your body wastes away, you become hungry as your brain encourages you to eat to make up for these losses.

- **Fruity breath:** When your body can't use glucose as a fuel, it looks for alternative sources of energy, one of which is fat tissue. As fat tissue breaks down, it releases acids called *ketones* and these typically make the breath smell fruity, very much like a candy mint. If lots of ketones are present, this can be a sign of a dangerous condition called ketoacidosis, which we discuss further in Chapter 5.

Investigating the causes of type 1 diabetes

If you or someone you love has type 1 diabetes, after you get over the shock of hearing the news, the next thing you'll probably ask is "How could this have happened?" And that's an excellent question. In fact, that is the same question scientists and physicians have been asking for many, many years, and it still goes unanswered.

Type 1 diabetes isn't contagious, and you can rest assured that you didn't get it from someone with diabetes sneezing on you or coughing on you. And you didn't get type 1 diabetes from eating the wrong foods, not exercising enough, or being under stress. In fact, you did nothing wrong at all. Type 1 diabetes is not something that you brought on; it is something that happened *to* you.

Type 1 diabetes is almost always an *autoimmune* disease, meaning that your body has been unkind enough to react against itself. (We say *almost* always because occasionally the insulin-producing beta cells are destroyed by unknown mechanisms.) Many different types of autoimmune disease exist, including certain types of thyroid disease and arthritis conditions such as lupus and rheumatoid arthritis.

Everyone makes antibodies to fight off infections, but in the case of type 1 diabetes, your body creates antibodies that have decided that your own insulin-producing islet cells of your pancreas are the enemy and have attacked these cells. This can be demonstrated by checking for certain antibodies in the blood stream, including islet cell antibodies, insulin antibodies, and glutamic acid decarboxylase (GAD) antibodies. Routinely testing for these antibodies is not necessary; the diagnosis of type 1 diabetes is usually evident without these tests. (Also, these tests are often only available in research laboratories and their costs are usually not covered by provincial health insurance plans.)

Why your immune system would turn against your pancreas is unknown, but a number of theories exist:

> ✔ **A virus infection triggering an abnormal immune system response:** At various times in our lives we develop viral infections and our bodies fight these off by producing antibodies. It could be that one of these viruses shared something in its appearance with an islet cell and the body's antibodies couldn't separate out the good guys (your islet cells) from the bad guys (the virus) and attacked both.

✔ **Early exposure to cow's milk:** Non-breastfed babies have a higher risk of developing type 1 diabetes. It could be that a protein in cow's milk causes the same sort of response as a virus and, just as we discuss in the preceding paragraph, leads to an antibody attack on your own pancreas. Bear in mind, however, that an association is not the same as cause and effect. (For example, if you have blonde hair and blue eyes, your blonde hair did not cause your blue eyes, they simply occurred together). In other words, the fact that non-breastfed babies have a higher risk of type 1 diabetes may have nothing to do with their not having been breastfed.

✔ **A virus damaging the pancreas by directly attacking it:** Indeed, some small outbreaks of type 1 diabetes have supported this idea.

✔ **Exposure to oxygen free radicals:** As a result of normal chemical reactions in our bodies, we produce molecules called *oxygen free radicals*. Oxygen free radicals can be produced in excess numbers by exposure to air pollution and smoking. Oxygen free radicals could possibly accumulate in the pancreas and cause damage.

✔ **Exposure to certain chemicals:** Certain chemicals are known to cause type 1 diabetes. One such example is a rat poison called Vacor, which, if ingested, can damage the pancreas.

Other theories exist as well (including the recently proposed, provocative idea that insufficient vitamin D due to lack of sun exposure in northern climates leads to type 1 diabetes), but the simple truth is that the cause of your type 1 diabetes is unknown. One thing, however, that *is* known is that certain underlying genetic characteristics may make you more susceptible to getting type 1 diabetes. Individually they would not cause you to develop diabetes, but when taken together with some other trigger, they might.

The best possible illustration of how getting type 1 diabetes must be a combination of a genetic susceptibility *and* an environmental trigger is found in one extraordinarily simple fact. If you have type 1 diabetes and you have an identical twin (who would, therefore, have the same genes as you do), the likelihood of your identical twin getting type 1 diabetes is somewhere between 25 to 50 percent. If the cause was purely genetic, the odds would be 100 percent. Something else clearly must be at play here. But what? At this time, the answer is simply a mystery.

The great British prime minister Benjamin Disraeli may have been right when he said there are "lies, damn lies, and statistics," but regarding the inheritance of type 1 diabetes, certain statistics do seem to be true. In particular, if you have a parent or a (non-identical) sibling with type 1 diabetes, you have approximately a 5 percent risk of developing type 1 diabetes. This risk rises to about 30 percent if both your parents have type 1 diabetes.

Latent autoimmune diabetes of adults

Latent autoimmune diabetes of adults (abbreviated as LADA) refers to a slowly onsetting form of type 1 diabetes in adults. The most important thing to know about LADA is that because it slowly develops and because people with it generally feel fairly well initially, doctors often mistake it for type 2 diabetes and treat it (unsuccessfully) with oral medications when, in fact, insulin is required.

One key difference between LADA and type 2 diabetes is that most people with LADA (like most people with type 1 diabetes) are lean at the time of diagnosis, whereas most people with type 2 diabetes are overweight at the time of diagnosis.

Marcel was a 65-year-old man diagnosed with type 2 diabetes by his family physician when, during a routine physical, his fasting blood glucose was found to be 9.2 mmol/L and A1C 7.9 percent. He felt fine, exercised regularly, and was not overweight. He was treated with metformin initially, but his blood glucose control worsened and, soon thereafter, gliclazide and sitagliptin (Januvia) were added. Nonetheless his blood glucose levels kept climbing and he then developed increased thirst, frequent urination, and weight loss. Four months after the diagnosis of diabetes had been made, Marcel was referred to Ian who immediately diagnosed him as having the LADA form of type 1 diabetes, prescribed insulin, discontinued his oral diabetes medications and in a matter of a few weeks Marcel's blood glucose levels were down to normal and he was feeling immensely better.

Marcel's case in the preceding anecdote is typical of the situation where a person with LADA is mislabelled as having type 2 diabetes and appropriate therapy (with insulin) gets delayed. Did he have a "bad" family doctor? Not in the least. In fact, he had a conscientious, caring family doctor who had quite rightly been vigorously trying to help his patient get his blood glucose control in check. The problem was that his family physician, like many physicians, was unfamiliar with LADA and hadn't considered that type 1 diabetes could develop in someone in their middle (or later) years.

If you have been diagnosed with type 2 diabetes yet you are not overweight and your blood glucose control is inadequate with your non-insulin blood glucose-lowering therapy then ask your doctor if you might have LADA. Show this page to your doctor if he or she is unfamiliar with the term LADA. Your doctor may thank you for the insight.

Preventing type 1 diabetes

Although medical science currently has no proven way of preventing type 1 diabetes, very exciting research studies are underway looking at this very thing. Researchers are evaluating two types of preventative strategies:

- **Primary prevention:** This type of prevention aims to prevent diabetes before it starts. Possible candidates for primary prevention are people who are at particularly high risk of developing type 1 diabetes. They have a close family member (or members) with the condition, have certain antibodies in the blood (we discuss these in the previous section), and/or have genes that put them at increased risk.

  An example of primary prevention is not giving infants cow's milk in case it contains certain proteins that may trigger diabetes. (The TRIGR study is evaluating this possibility: www.trigr.org.)

- **Secondary prevention:** This type of prevention aims to administer treatment to a person with diabetes as soon as possible after the disease is diagnosed, with a view to getting it to go away immediately. (And if it stayed away — without requiring further treatment — this would be a cure.) An example of secondary prevention is taking a medicine that targets the immune system to try to get it to stop making antibodies that destroy the insulin-producing beta cells of the pancreas. (Although people with type 1 diabetes lack insulin, early on in the course of the disease they often still retain the ability to make *some* insulin. The goal of secondary prevention would be to maintain and enhance this ability.) As we say, this is experimental; at present neither a proven means of preventing type 1diabetes nor a cure for type 1 diabetes exists.

Researchers routinely pool their resources to improve their odds of success. TrialNet (www.diabetestrialnet.org) is an organization that has a specific mandate to "perform intervention studies to preserve insulin-producing cells in individuals at risk for type 1 diabetes and in those with new onset type 1 diabetes." If you are interested in seeing if you or a family member may be a candidate to participate in a research study on type 1 diabetes, visit the TrialNet website for more information and to find the contact information for Canadian research centres (click the "Locations" tab).

Type 2 Diabetes and You

Type 2 diabetes is caused by a combination of insulin resistance and insufficient insulin. (We discuss this in detail in Chapter 3.) Type 2 diabetes is much, much more common than type 1 diabetes (ten times more common, in fact). Whereas type 1 diabetes tends to develop in children and young adults, type 2 diabetes typically affects middle-aged or older people. Your likelihood of developing type 2 diabetes increases as you get older. Also, being overweight and sedentary put you at particularly high risk of developing type 2 diabetes.

Although adults are most likely to be affected by type 2 diabetes, increasing numbers of children are also developing the condition. This appears to be directly related to affected children not being sufficiently physically active and being overweight. If you have type 2 diabetes and want to help protect your young children or grandchildren from also getting type 2 diabetes, consider giving them a membership to the YMCA or local community recreation centre rather than a video game for their next birthday. Even better, get a membership for yourself, too, and go together!

Type 2 diabetes used to be called *adult-onset diabetes* or *non-insulin dependent diabetes.* But because children can develop type 2 diabetes, the former term didn't make sense, and because many people with type 2 diabetes require insulin therapy, the latter term didn't make sense either. For these reasons, these older terms have been abandoned. Nonetheless, not everyone has caught on, so you may still come across the older terms.

If you have type 2 diabetes and require insulin, you *still have type 2 diabetes,* not type 1 diabetes.

In Chapter 3 we talk about the cause of type 2 diabetes and how, with this condition, the pancreas is able to make insulin but the body's tissues aren't able to use it properly. This is called *insulin resistance,* and we look at it in more detail later in this chapter.

If you have type 2 diabetes, you don't have a less severe or less important form of diabetes than type 1 diabetes. You don't have a "touch of diabetes"; you have the real thing, and you require intensive therapy and equally intensive monitoring to keep yourself healthy. Don't let anyone try to convince you that if you're being treated with nutrition (diet) and exercise therapy alone, your diabetes is less serious than if you were on insulin. On the other hand, don't let anyone try to convince you that if you're on insulin, your condition must be worse than someone with diabetes who doesn't require insulin. All forms of diabetes are serious. And all people with diabetes are at risk of complications. But — and this is a big *but* — equally important, working with their health care team, all people with diabetes have the means to reduce that risk.

Type 2 diabetes is written as, well, type 2 diabetes, not type II diabetes. The little in-joke among diabetes specialists is that this nomenclature was chosen so that doctors wouldn't think it was to be called type *eleven* diabetes!

Identifying the symptoms of type 2 diabetes

Unlike type 1 diabetes, the symptoms of type 2 diabetes tend to come on gradually; often so gradually that people who later discover they have the condition have discounted the symptoms, blaming them on something else. Perhaps before you were diagnosed as having type 2 diabetes, you attributed your weight loss to a new diet. Or maybe you remember blaming your thirst on a particularly hot summer. Indeed, the symptoms of type 2 diabetes can come on so gradually and so imperceptibly that by the time it is discovered, your blood glucose may be extraordinarily high. Moreover, it may have been high for so long that damage has already occurred to your body.

Many people with newly diagnosed type 2 diabetes already have some degree of damage to their bodies. That's why the Canadian Diabetes Association recommends people at risk for type 2 diabetes be screened for it routinely; the goal is to try to make the diagnosis as early as possible so people can get treatment before damage to the body occurs. We discuss screening for type 2 diabetes later in this chapter.

Type 2 diabetes gets a foot in the door

Nicholas had always been a very healthy man. Indeed, the last time he had seen a doctor was when he had his appendix taken out 10 years ago, when he was 40 years of age. The only reason he was now in the family doctor's office was at his wife's insistence. Starting a year ago, he had noticed some mild numbness in his right big toe. A month or two later, the same thing developed in his left big toe.

Nicholas wasn't a complainer and he figured it was just because of some new, overly tight-fitting shoes he had yet to break in. Nonetheless, as the months passed, things got worse and worse and now the numbness involved all his toes and had started to feel increasingly painful.

When his doctor examined Nicholas's feet, they looked healthy enough, but when the doctor pressed on the toes with a thin nylon rod, Nicholas hardly noticed. A few tests later and the doctor had made her diagnosis. Nicholas had nerve damage in his feet due to diabetes. It was a shock for Nicholas. He had no recollection of having been overly thirsty or passing excessive quantities of urine. Indeed, he had felt perfectly fine otherwise. Not in a million years had he imagined that diabetes could show itself in such an unusual way.

Many of the symptoms of (uncontrolled) type 2 diabetes are common to type 1 diabetes, including the following:

- Blurred vision
- Fatigue
- Frequent urination
- Increase in thirst
- Weight loss (more common with newly onsetting type 1 diabetes than with newly discovered type 2 diabetes)

Some symptoms and health problems, however, are more commonly present in people with newly diagnosed type 2 diabetes than they are in a person with newly onsetting type 1 diabetes. These symptoms and health problems include:

- **Atherosclerosis.** *Atherosclerosis* (hardening of the arteries) is a blockage in the arteries that leads to reduced blood flow (and, therefore, reduced oxygen delivery) to the affected organs. When it affects the arteries in the heart it is called *coronary artery disease* (often simply called *heart disease*) and can cause angina or a heart attack. When it affects the arteries that supply the brain it is called *cerebrovascular disease* and can lead to a stroke. And when it affects the arteries to the legs it is called *peripheral arterial disease* and can lead to calf pain or, if severe, amputations. If you have one of these conditions, we recommend you ask your doctor to test you to see if you have diabetes. (You will likely find your doctor has already done so.) We discuss these conditions in detail in Chapter 6.

- **Numbness of the feet:** Numbness of the feet can be due to many different causes, one of which is nerve damage ("peripheral neuropathy") due to diabetes. If you have had high blood glucose levels for a number of years, you may develop an uncomfortable burning or numbness in your feet. This can be the first clue alerting you to the fact that you not only have diabetes, but you've had it for quite some time. We discuss this further in Chapter 6.

- **Slow wound healing:** If you have high blood glucose levels, your body's ability to heal itself can be impaired and you may find that seemingly minor cuts don't heal as quickly as they used to.

- **Yeast infections of the vagina and penis:** High glucose levels make the genital areas of your body prone to yeast infections. In a woman, this may manifest as vaginal discharge, and in a man, as a reddish rash at the end of the penis (balanitis).

Investigating the causes of type 2 diabetes

Although finding the initial trigger leading to type 1 diabetes has proven elusive, medical science knows a lot more about why people develop type 2 diabetes.

When you were told you had type 2 diabetes, you may have thought of relatives of yours who shared the same problem. Indeed, you may have thought of *many* relatives who had diabetes. What you and your extended family have in common is, of course, more than being at risk for this disease. You have many genes in common, including those that make you prone to diabetes. Note that just because your father or mother or sister or brother may have diabetes does not guarantee that you, too, will get it. But it does increase your risk.

If you have a parent with type 2 diabetes, you have approximately a 15-percent risk of developing type 2 diabetes. This risk rises to about 50 percent if both your parents have type 2 diabetes. If you have a sibling with type 2 diabetes, your risk is only 10 percent, but — and this is startling — if your sibling is your identical twin, your risk of developing type 2 diabetes rises to 90 percent. However, before you throw your hands up in despair, please note one very, very large *but*.

The "but" is that getting type 2 diabetes involves more than family background. In addition to having relatives with diabetes, most (but not all) people who acquire type 2 diabetes are overweight and sedentary. And recent scientific studies show overwhelming evidence that you can reduce your risk of developing type 2 diabetes drastically by making appropriate lifestyle changes. In other words, you can influence your destiny.

In the early stages of type 2 diabetes, you have lots of insulin in your body (unlike people with type 1 diabetes), but the insulin isn't working effectively. As we discuss in more detail in Chapter 3, insulin is like a key that opens up the cells (especially your fat and muscle cells) to allow glucose to enter. In type 2 diabetes, this key is malfunctioning. This is called *insulin resistance*.

Although the initial problem with type 2 diabetes is that your insulin isn't working properly, as time passes, the pancreas also runs into difficulties and eventually can't make enough insulin. That's one of the main reasons that so many people with type 2 diabetes end up requiring insulin as time goes by. If you have type 2 diabetes and you require insulin to keep your blood glucose levels under control, this doesn't mean *you* have failed; it simply means that *your pancreas* has failed. And that is not your fault!

People often think that consuming sugar causes type 2 diabetes, but in fact, it doesn't. Ingesting excessive amounts of sugar may bring out the disease by making you overweight, but that's quite different from saying sugar *causes* diabetes.

Screening for type 2 diabetes

The Canadian Diabetes Association recommends that *everyone* 40 years of age and older be screened (that is, tested) for type 2 diabetes every three years. However, if you have one or more risk factors (see the following list) for type 2 diabetes, then being tested starting at a younger age *and* more frequently than every three years is prudent. The idea is to detect diabetes *early* in the process; *before* it has damaged your body.

These are some risk factors for type 2 diabetes:

- **Having a biological first-degree relative with type 2 diabetes:** A first-degree relative is a parent, sibling, or child.

- **Being a member of a high-risk population:** This includes people of Aboriginal, African, Asian, Hispanic, or South Asian descent.

- **Having a history of prediabetes:** We discuss prediabetes later in this chapter.

- **Having a history of gestational diabetes:** We discuss gestational diabetes in Chapter 7.

- **Having delivered a large baby:** The scientific term for this is *macrosomia*. We discuss this in Chapter 7.

- **Having evidence of complications associated with diabetes:** Examples include *retinopathy* (eye damage), *neuropathy* (nerve damage), *nephropathy* (kidney damage), vascular disease affecting the heart (*coronary artery disease*), brain (*cerebrovascular disease*), or legs (*peripheral arterial disease*). We discuss these conditions in detail in Chapters 6.

- **Having risk factors for vascular disease such as abnormal lipid levels, high blood pressure, overweight, or abdominal obesity:** We discuss vascular disease, abnormal lipid levels, and high blood pressure in detail in Chapter 6.

- **Having a disease associated with an increased risk of diabetes:** Examples of such a disease include polycystic ovary syndrome, acanthosis nigricans, obstructive sleep apnea, certain types of psychiatric disease (bipolar disorder, depression, schizophrenia), and HIV infection.

> ✔ **Using drugs associated with an increased risk of diabetes:** Examples of such drugs are prednisone, certain types of psychiatric medicines, and certain types of drugs used to treat HIV/AIDS.

As you can see, the list is long and indicates that a great many people are at increased risk of developing type 2 diabetes.

Screening should be performed with a fasting blood glucose (drawn at a laboratory on a blood sample taken from a vein) or A1C. If your fasting blood glucose is 6.1 mmol/L up to and including 6.9 mmol/L or your A1C is 6.0 percent up to and including 6.4 percent, you should have further screening with a two-hour glucose tolerance test. (If you have risk factors for diabetes, your doctor may recommend you have a two hour glucose tolerance test if your fasting blood glucose is 5.6 up to and including 6.0 and/or your A1C is 5.5 up to and including 5.9.)

The Public Health Agency of Canada has an online "risk calculator" (called Canadian Diabetes Risk Questionnaire, or CANRISK) to help you determine your risk of having type 2 diabetes (or prediabetes). You can find this on their website at www.phac-aspc.gc.ca. (See the "Chronic Diseases" section and choose "Diabetes.")

Screening for diabetes is done to diagnose diabetes in someone who *does not have symptoms*. If you have symptoms of diabetes (which we discuss earlier in this chapter) then you need to be tested as soon as possible.

Preventing type 2 diabetes

Unlike type 1 diabetes, type 2 diabetes can often be prevented, or at the very least delayed.

Type 2 diabetes typically occurs in people who are overweight and sedentary. (Like anything in life, exceptions exist, but over 90 percent of the time this is the case.) However, by losing weight and exercising regularly, you can reduce your risk of developing type 2 diabetes by over 50 percent. If you already have type 2 diabetes, then do your loved ones a favour and share this information with them so they can start making the necessary lifestyle changes to help them avoid getting (or at least delaying the onset of) type 2 diabetes.

To achieve this huge reduction in risk, all you need to do is lose 5 percent of your body weight and exercise for 150 minutes per week (which is only about 21 minutes a day)! Regarding weight loss, if you weigh 100 kilograms (220 pounds) and you lose 5 kilograms (11 pounds), you drastically reduce your risk of diabetes. And you don't need to lose the weight overnight; you can do it over months and even years.

Research reveals that prevention is most likely to succeed with lifestyle therapy (that is, weight loss and exercise). But we know that lifestyle change is often the most difficult prescription of all. Studies also show that you can reduce your risk of developing type 2 diabetes by using certain medications. (We discuss these medicines in Chapter 12.) We believe that lifestyle therapy is a much, *much* better option for diabetes prevention than medication. However, if you've repeatedly tried yet not succeeded with lifestyle change, talk to your physician about using medication to prevent diabetes. (Of the various medications for preventing diabetes, we prefer metformin because it's effective, safe, and does not cause weight gain. Acarbose, however, is a reasonable alternative.)

The medical studies we're referencing looked at people who already had problems with elevated blood glucose levels. They had prediabetes, meaning their readings were higher than normal but not high enough to classify them as having diabetes. We talk more about this condition later in this chapter.

You can determine whether or not you are overweight in several ways, including the following:

✔ **Calculate your body mass index (BMI):** Calculating your BMI is the most commonly used technique to determine whether you're overweight. Basically, BMI is an indicator of whether you're the right weight for your height. (And no, we're afraid that the converse is not true: despite the best of wishful thinking, you can't be the wrong height for your weight!) Your BMI can be calculated — though nobody ever does it this way — by dividing your weight in kilograms by the square of your height in metres. Uh-huh. Realistically, do what doctors do and use an online calculator (many are available, including www.diabetes.ca/diabetes-and-you/nutrition/bmi). A normal BMI is 18.5 to 24.9. Note that the normal range for BMI does *not* apply to pregnant or breastfeeding women, infants, children, adolescents, or particularly muscular individuals.

✔ **Measure your waist circumference:** Another way to establish whether you're overweight is to measure your waist circumference. Your health risk goes up if your waist circumference is equal to or greater than 88 centimetres (35 inches) for women, 102 centimetres (40 inches) for men. (Other values may be more appropriate indicators of health risk depending on one's ethnicity.)

When considering your body fat, remember that not all fat is equal. If you have extra fat around your belly but not over other areas of your body, it puts you at much higher risk of getting type 2 diabetes than if you had extra weight distributed over all parts of your body. This is because fat over your midsection is more likely to cause insulin resistance (which we discuss earlier).

Knowledge is power. And now that you know the main risk factors leading to type 2 diabetes, you have the ability to modify your risk factors and lessen the likelihood of getting diabetes. And if you already have diabetes, reducing your BMI and your extra fat tissue can markedly improve your health anyhow. The point of finding out your BMI is not that you should get angry or frustrated with yourself. Rather, you know what the problem is and can now take steps (figurative and literal) to improve it.

Key Differences between Type 1 and Type 2 Diabetes

Type 1 and type 2 diabetes are similar in many ways; however, they also have some important differences. Table 4-1 highlights some of these differences. (This table lists the *usual* characteristics seen with type 1 and type 2 diabetes — but frequent exceptions exist. For example, although type 1 diabetes typically develops in young people, middle-aged or even older people can also develop it.)

Table 4-1	Differences between Type 1 and Type 2 Diabetes	
	Type 1 Diabetes	*Type 2 Diabetes*
Age at time of diagnosis	Under 20	Over 40
Length of time present before diagnosis	Months	Years
Weight status at time of diagnosis	Normal or underweight	Overweight
Most common symptoms at time of diagnosis	Thirst, frequent urination, weight loss	Thirst, frequent urination, visual blurring
Insulin defect	Insufficient insulin	Ineffective insulin (insulin resistance) and, with time, insufficient insulin
Antibodies present to insulin and/or islet cells	Yes	No
Family history of diabetes	Sometimes	Almost always
Initial therapy	Lifestyle & insulin	Lifestyle (with or without medication)

In most situations a physician can readily determine if your diabetes is type 1 or type 2 and can quickly get you started on the most appropriate therapy for the type of diabetes you have. The situation most likely to lead to a miscategorization of the type of diabetes (and the wrong therapy being prescribed) is when a person has the LADA form of type 1 diabetes (we discuss LADA earlier in this chapter).

Gestational and Pregestational Diabetes and You

If you're pregnant (yes, that excludes you men, but read on, gentlemen — you do have something to do with your partner's pregnancy) and you didn't have diabetes prior to your pregnancy, you could acquire a form of diabetes during pregnancy called *gestational diabetes*. If you already have diabetes when you become pregnant, that is called *pregestational diabetes*.

Gestational diabetes is usually simply treated, and typically the pregnancy goes quite uneventfully. Pregestational diabetes is a much more complex condition requiring more complicated monitoring and therapy.

If you've had gestational diabetes before or you already have diabetes, and you're considering snuggling up to your partner tonight with the most amorous of intentions, combine your *amore* with contraception unless you are absolutely sure that getting pregnant is safe for you. In fact, before you do any snuggling, we recommend you read Chapter 7, where we discuss pregnancy and diabetes in detail.

The Metabolic Syndrome and You

People who have insulin resistance (we discuss insulin resistance in Chapter 3) often also have other indicators which, taken together, put them at high risk of developing not only type 2 diabetes but heart disease also. When several of these indicators are present, you are said to have *metabolic syndrome.*

Metabolic syndrome is diagnosed if you have *three or more* of the following criteria:

- Fasting blood glucose of 5.6 mmol/L or higher
- Elevated blood pressure (systolic value 130 or higher and/or diastolic value 85 or higher; we explain the terms "systolic" and "diastolic" in Chapter 6)

✔ Triglycerides of 1.7 mmol/L or higher (*triglycerides* are one of the fats in the blood)

✔ HDL cholesterol (the good type of cholesterol) less than 1.0 mmol/L (for men) or less than 1.3 mmol/L (for women)

✔ Abdominal obesity (a waist circumference of 102 centimetres or more — about 40 inches — for men; 88 centimetres or more — about 35 inches — for women)

As you might have gleaned from looking over this list, a person can have both the metabolic syndrome *and* diabetes.

The importance of having the metabolic syndrome diagnosed is controversial. Some people say it is very important because if you have the syndrome it means you are at greatly increased risk of having a heart attack, and knowing about it means you can take appropriate preventive actions (such as modifying your diet, getting your cholesterol level in order, and so on). Naysayers would tell you that the metabolic syndrome is simply a label and, in any event, if you have high blood pressure or poor cholesterol, you *already* know that you have a problem that needs to be addressed.

Treating metabolic syndrome is, essentially, treating its individual components. So, for example, if you have elevated blood glucose or high blood pressure, you treat them with lifestyle measures and, if necessary, medication. Similarly, you treat abdominal obesity with lifestyle change (though we do discuss other treatment options in Chapter 10).

The bottom line: If you have metabolic syndrome, take that as a wakeup call that you need to make crucial lifestyle changes (and, when necessary, take helpful medications) to reduce the risk that the condition will deteriorate into diabetes, heart attacks, and other serious health issues. Your destiny is largely in your hands.

Prediabetes and You

Type 2 diabetes rarely appears suddenly. More commonly it's preceded by a period of time, which may last years, when your blood glucose levels are not high enough to say you have diabetes, but not low enough to say your levels are perfectly normal either. This blood glucose netherworld is called *prediabetes.* Note that having prediabetes is *not* the same as saying you have *borderline diabetes;* one can no more have borderline diabetes than one can be borderline pregnant.

Prediabetes is diagnosed if you have one or more of the following:

✔ **Impaired fasting glucose:** This means your blood glucose level before breakfast is higher than normal (but not as high as someone with diabetes); that is, 6.1 mmol/L up to and including 6.9 mmol/L.

✔ **Impaired glucose tolerance:** This means that your blood glucose level two hours after ingesting 75 grams of glucose as part of a glucose tolerance test (we discuss this test earlier in this chapter) is higher than normal, but not as high as someone with diabetes; that is, 7.8 mmol/L up to and including 11.0 mmol/L.

✔ An **A1C level of 6.0 percent up to and including 6.4 percent:** We discuss the A1C test earlier in this chapter and in detail in Chapter 9.

If you've been diagnosed with prediabetes based on a fasting blood glucose test result (of 6.1 to 6.9 mmol/L), it is important that your doctor send you for a glucose tolerance test to exclude the possibility that you actually have type 2 diabetes.

Prediabetes is important to know about for two main reasons. If you have prediabetes the following health risks apply to you:

✔ **High risk of developing type 2 diabetes:** Think of prediabetes as an early warning system that you're at high risk of getting type 2 diabetes. Indeed, the risk of prediabetes progressing to type 2 diabetes is as much as 10 percent in any year and about 50 percent over ten years (hence the reason for calling this condition prediabetes). Not good odds, eh? But despite the name, prediabetes not only doesn't have to progress to type 2 diabetes, with healthy lifestyle changes (and, when indicated, medication) one's blood glucose control can return entirely to normal (that is, prediabetes is no longer evident). Following the measures we outline in the section "Preventing type 2 diabetes," earlier in this chapter, will substantially improve your odds of avoiding — or, at the very least, delaying — diabetes.

✔ **High risk of heart attack and stroke:** Having prediabetes means you are at very high risk of developing hardening of the arteries (atherosclerosis), which can ultimately lead to heart attacks and strokes. However, this does not have to happen. Aggressive treatment of prediabetes and other risk factors for vascular disease can keep you healthy. This treatment involves paying attention to your diet, being physically active, achieving a healthy weight, making sure your blood pressure and lipids (cholesterol and triglycerides) are good, and, of course, not smoking.

The term *prediabetes* is apt in that it hammers home the message that if you have this condition you are at high risk for getting type 2 diabetes. But it misleads by implying that getting diabetes is inevitable. Just remember that prediabetes does not have to lead to diabetes.

Recognizing Other Types of Diabetes

The great majority of diabetes cases fall within the categories we discuss in this chapter (that is, type 1, type 2, and gestational diabetes). But dozens of other types of diabetes exist, including the following:

- **Diabetes from damage to the pancreas due to other diseases:** A number of diseases can damage the pancreas resulting in diabetes. Examples include *pancreatitis* (a condition of severe inflammation of the pancreas), *hemochromatosis* (a condition where excess iron accumulates in the body including the pancreas; because hemochromatosis leads to increased skin pigmentation, it is sometimes called *bronze diabetes*), and cystic fibrosis.

- **Diabetes due to genetic defects:** The most common of these is *maturity onset diabetes of the young* (MODY), which is the former name for a group of rare genetic diseases in which young, non-overweight people develop a condition similar to type 2 diabetes. We discuss this further in Chapter 14.

- **Drug-induced diabetes:** Some medicines can cause diabetes. Here are some examples. Prednisone (and similar drugs) is a type of steroid that is wonderful at treating some very serious diseases (such as asthma), but unfortunately has the potential to cause diabetes, especially if used in high doses for long periods of time. Some blood pressure medicines (for example, hydrochlorothiazide), some newer psychiatric medicines (for example, risperidone and clozapine), and niacin (a medication used to lower triglyceride levels) can occasionally do this also. Some evidence exists that statin medication can increase the risk of developing diabetes. That does not mean you shouldn't take these medicines. What it does mean, however, is that if you are taking one of these medicines and you have symptoms of diabetes (which we discuss earlier in this chapter), see your doctor to have your blood glucose level checked.

- **Hormonal disease-induced diabetes:** Other endocrine (that is, hormonal) diseases can cause diabetes. Examples include *acromegaly* (a pituitary gland disorder involving excess levels of growth hormone), *Cushing's syndrome* (a disease in which the body produces excess amounts of steroid hormones similar to prednisone), *hyperthyroidism* (a condition in which the thyroid gland produces excess quantities of thyroid hormone), and *pheochromocytoma* (an adrenal gland disorder in which too much adrenaline (or similar hormones) is made.

Breathing easy but experiencing drug-induced diabetes

Mohammed was a 55-year-old man with a long history of severe bronchitis. He came to the emergency department because he was having increasing difficulty catching his breath despite taking a number of different "puffers." The emergency room physician prescribed prednisone and advised Mohammed to follow up with his family doctor in three weeks.

Within a couple of days, Mohammed's breathing had started to improve and he was feeling very encouraged. A week later, however, he found himself having to get up during the night to go to the bathroom. Initially he blamed this on his prostate, but it kept getting worse and worse, and by the time he saw his doctor a week later, he had already lost 4.5 kilograms (10 pounds) and was feeling miserable.

Hearing Mohammed's story, his doctor immediately sent him to the laboratory, and the subsequent result confirmed his suspicion: Mohammed's blood glucose level was high — 25 mmol/L. Fortunately, by that time his breathing had improved and he was able to quickly come off the prednisone. Within two weeks his glucose level had returned to normal and his diabetes symptoms resolved. Mohammed's story is an example of drug-induced diabetes; in this case, due to prednisone.

Part II
How Diabetes Can Affect Your Body

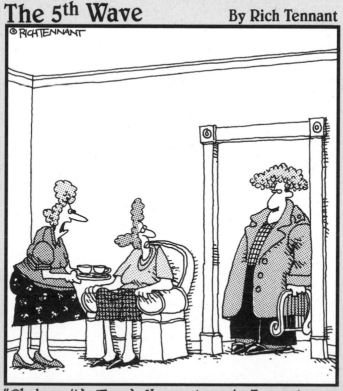

The 5th Wave · By Rich Tennant

"Oh dear, it's Troy's Harpo-glycemia. I can always tell — fatigue, confusion, the compulsion to play the harp in a trench coat and fright-wig...."

In this part . . .

This part explains how diabetes can affect your health and looks at the steps you can take to protect yourself from harm.

This part also looks at the special issues surrounding diabetes and pregnancy and discusses measures that will help you to have a healthy pregnancy and a healthy baby.

Chapter 5

Handling Low and High Blood Glucose Emergencies

• •

In This Chapter

▶ Recognizing when problems with blood glucose control become an emergency

▶ Dealing with low blood glucose emergencies

▶ Handling high blood glucose emergencies

• •

*I*f you have diabetes then you have a long-term goal of keeping your blood glucose control in check in order to feel well and to avoid diabetes damaging your body. Nonetheless, even with the best of efforts and the best of therapy, blood glucose emergencies can develop. In this chapter we look at these types of emergencies, how you can recognize them, how you can help avoid them, and what to do if they occur.

With the exception of mild-to-moderate hypoglycemia (low blood glucose that you can manage yourself), you should treat all the issues we look at in this chapter as medical emergencies. Don't try to treat these complications by yourself. Contact your health care team or, if necessary, call 9-1-1. In this chapter we discuss when and whom to call.

Understanding Hypoglycemia (Low Blood Glucose)

Hypoglycemia is a blood glucose level below normal. That much is straightforward. The problem is defining precisely how low a normal blood glucose can be. Sometimes this is said to be 3.3 mmol/L, and sometimes 3.9, and sometimes 4.0. Part of the reason for the varying definitions is that the lower limit of "normal" blood glucose depends on several factors including how the blood glucose is measured, on one's age, and if one is pregnant (in which case blood glucose levels can be as low as 3.5 mmol/L and still be considered normal).

The Canadian Diabetes Association Clinical Practice Guidelines — upon which this book is based — define hypoglycemia for non-pregnant individuals who are taking blood glucose-lowering medication to be a blood glucose level below 4.0 mmol/L. In this book we also use that definition.

Your body doesn't function well when you have too little glucose in your blood. Your brain needs glucose to allow you to think properly, and your muscles need the energy that glucose provides in much the same way that your car needs gasoline to run. As we discover in this chapter, diabetes in and of itself does not cause hypoglycemia; rather, certain *treatments* for diabetes can cause hypoglycemia.

Having diabetes isn't fair. It's unfair to get it. It's unfair to develop complications. And it's especially unfair that those people with diabetes who succeed in keeping their blood glucose levels as much in the normal range as possible are the most prone to getting hypoglycemia. If you have poorly controlled glucose levels with values running between 15 and 20 mmol/L, you may not feel great, but you are highly unlikely ever to run into significant problems with hypoglycemia. But if you look after yourself meticulously and keep your blood glucose levels in the 4.0 to 8.0 mmol/L range, you are at much greater risk of having hypoglycemia. Fortunately, you can have excellent control and, at the same time, minimize your risk of getting hypoglycemia. It ain't easy, but it is doable. We discuss how later in this section.

If you are on multiple daily doses of insulin, having two or three episodes of mild hypoglycemia per week is not uncommon; more than that is too many. If you aren't on insulin you should rarely, if ever, have lows.

Not every person develops symptoms of hypoglycemia at the same level of blood glucose. Some people notice it at blood glucose levels of 3.8, others only when their blood glucose level is between 2.0 and 3.0. Moreover, a person might notice it on one occasion when his or her blood glucose level is below 3.6, and that *same* person might not notice it on another occasion until it's below 3.2. You also need to remember that glucose meters aren't perfect. You may have already discovered that you can check your reading seconds apart and find discrepancies of 10 percent or even more. That doesn't mean your blood glucose level changed that much in that brief interval. It simply means the machines, though very good, aren't precision instruments.

Looking at the symptoms of hypoglycemia

Doctors traditionally divide the symptoms of hypoglycemia into two major categories:

- **Autonomic symptoms** are symptoms (such as tremors and palpitations, as we discuss later in this section) that are due to the effects of the hormones (especially epinephrine, also called adrenaline) that your body sends out to counter low blood glucose. They are called autonomic symptoms because they arise from the *autonomic* (automatic, in a sense) part of your nervous system.

- **Neuroglycopenic symptoms** are symptoms (such as confusion and disorientation, as we discuss later in this section) that are due to your brain not receiving enough glucose. *Neuroglycopenic* is derived from *neuro* (referring to the nervous system), *glyco* (glucose), and *penic* (insufficient).

The severity of hypoglycemia can be classified as

- **Mild:** Autonomic symptoms are present and you're able to treat yourself.

- **Moderate:** Autonomic and neuroglycopenic symptoms are present and you're able to treat yourself.

- **Severe:** Hypoglycemia is bad enough that you require someone else to assist you. Unconsciousness may occur. (With severe hypoglycemia, the blood glucose is typically less than 2.8 mmol/L.)

The main reason to know this classification is so that you and your health care providers are sure to be on the same page. Otherwise, a miscommunication could occur and you might get inappropriate advice. For example, if you are on insulin and you tell your doctor you had a "severe low," your doctor may interpret this as per the previous definition and give you advice — like substantially reducing your insulin dose — based on that. But if by "severe low" you *actually* meant you felt really, really crummy, but in fact your blood glucose was only slightly decreased (say, 3.6 mmol/L) and you were able to easily treat yourself by drinking a glass of pop, then you would likely receive very different advice from your doctor.

If you take medicines (such as insulin) that can cause hypoglycemia, for your own safety you should wear a medical alert bracelet or necklace. At the very least (though certainly not as good), carry some form of identification in your purse or wallet noting that you have diabetes. You may never need them, but being prepared is a good idea, just in case. We've had more than one patient who has received necessary emergency care (for hypoglycemia) that might not have been given if the person hadn't been wearing a medical alert.

John was a 42-year-old patient of Ian's. He worked very hard at maintaining excellent blood glucose control and as a result had remained free of diabetes complications despite having lived with type 1 diabetes for 20 years. One day he was rushing home from work and forgot to do his usual pre-driving blood glucose check. (We discuss driving issues in detail in Chapter 16.) His next recollection was being on the side of the highway with a paramedic at his side. The police had pulled him over for erratic driving and, finding him to be confused, thought he was drunk. They were about to handcuff and arrest him when they noticed his medical alert. It said he had diabetes. The police officer summoned a paramedic who measured John's blood glucose, found it be 2.3, gave him some glucose, and John quickly returned to normal. Wearing a medical alert had not only allowed for proper — and rapid — treatment of his severe hypoglycemia, it also spared him from being arrested!

Most people with diabetes go their entire lives without ever experiencing even a single episode of *severe* hypoglycemia. The vast majority of the time, if you are experiencing hypoglycemia, the early warning autonomic symptoms kick in and allow you to quickly rectify the problem.

Autonomic symptoms

Autonomic symptoms are your best friends. They're your warning system alerting you to a problem of low blood glucose and demanding that you attend to it before it progresses to the more dangerous neuroglycopenic stage (which we discuss shortly).

Autonomic symptoms include the following:

- Anxiety
- Hunger
- Palpitations (noticing a rapid or excessively forceful heartbeat)
- Sweating
- Trembling (shaking of your body, especially the hands)

As you look through the previous list, you may realize you've had some or all of these symptoms at various times in your life, even if you've never been on medicine that could cause low blood glucose. The reason: These symptoms can occur in *any* situation where epinephrine (adrenaline) levels are high, and that includes so-called fight-or-flight situations where you're under extreme stress. (Examples are if you're about to write a difficult exam, about to have a job interview, or are writing a book on diabetes and your editor calls you to let you know your manuscript is due . . . yesterday. Eeek.)

Because symptoms such as sweating or palpitations, which can indicate hypoglycemia, can also occur in situations of stress, where your blood glucose level may actually be perfectly normal, you should conclude that you have hypoglycemia only if you have demonstrated a low blood glucose level on your glucose meter.

Shortly after you begin therapy for high blood glucose, you may find that you're experiencing autonomic symptoms, suggesting you have hypoglycemia even though your blood glucose levels may not be low. This is perfectly normal — your body will take a few days to become accustomed to having normal blood glucose levels, at which point your symptoms will go away.

If you are on medications such as insulin or a *sulfonylurea* (medicines that help reduce blood glucose, as we discuss in Chapter 12), you may recall having had at least one episode where your hands started to shake, you became sweaty and hungry, and you recognized that something wasn't quite right. You probably reached for your glucose meter, checked your blood glucose level, and found it to be somewhere in the 3s. You likely took some sugar candies or a glass of juice or pop and felt better within a few minutes. Congratulations: You successfully diagnosed, treated, and cured your first patient.

Neuroglycopenic symptoms

Neuroglycopenic symptoms are much more of a problem than are autonomic symptoms. Neuroglycopenic symptoms are most definitely not your friends — quite the opposite. Whereas autonomic symptoms alert you to a problem, neuroglycopenic symptoms often interfere with your ability to recognize and deal with hypoglycemia. By the time these symptoms develop, your blood glucose level is usually profoundly low and has become a true emergency.

Neuroglycopenic symptoms include the following:

- Confusion
- Difficulty concentrating
- Difficulty speaking
- Dizziness
- Vision changes (such as double vision or loss of vision)
- Drowsiness
- Loss of consciousness (coma)
- Seizures

People lose their ability to think clearly when they become hypoglycemic; this is particularly a problem when blood glucose levels are very low. They make simple errors, and other people often assume that they're drunk. Fortunately, adult brains have an amazing capacity to put up with hypoglycemia, and long-term damage to the brain from low blood glucose almost never occurs. Because the brains of infants and young children are more sensitive to injury, however, avoiding severe hypoglycemia in this age group is especially important (we define severe hypoglycemia earlier in this section).

Considering the causes of hypoglycemia

Despite what many people (mistakenly) think, diabetes doesn't cause hypoglycemia. Certain medicines used to *treat* diabetes can cause hypoglycemia, but hypoglycemia is not caused by diabetes in and of itself. Indeed, if you have diabetes and are being treated purely with lifestyle measures (nutrition and exercise therapy), you will *never* experience hypoglycemia.

Hypoglycemia is always unintended. Ideally, your blood glucose levels would always be normal — never high, never low. Unfortunately, we seldom have that degree of success with our imperfect therapies. A number of the medicines we use to prevent blood glucose levels from being too high have the potential to drop them too low. The most important of these for you to be aware of are

- **Insulin:** Unlike insulin made by your pancreas, insulin you inject does not have the ability to turn itself off the instant you no longer need it. An injection of insulin will help to reduce your blood glucose level, but it also has the potential to drop your blood glucose level excessively. This drop is called an *insulin reaction.* (You may have heard the term *insulin shock* used in reference to particularly bad insulin reactions. Insulin shock is not a scientific term, however, and can be misleading. Indeed, we feel the term should never be used. Accordingly, we won't use it beyond this brief explanation.) We discuss insulin therapy in detail in Chapter 13.

- **Sulfonylurea medicine:** As we discuss further in Chapter 12, medicines from this family have the potential to cause low blood glucose. This is particularly true of glyburide.

- **Meglitinides (and d-phenylalanine derivatives):** Never do we, as diabetes specialists, consider ourselves luckier than when we attend conferences where these (and other new) medicines are discussed. Oh no, not just because they're important drugs to know about. No. We consider ourselves fortunate because at these conferences we learn how to pronounce them! Don't worry; no one uses these names anyhow. Doctors pretty well just use the trade names (GlucoNorm, Starlix) for drugs currently available within this group. These drugs, like sulfonylureas, make the pancreas release extra insulin and have the potential to cause hypoglycemia.

Although these medicines — especially insulin — can cause hypoglycemia, you can improve the odds that they won't by taking certain precautions. We discuss these precautions later in this chapter.

If you require blood glucose-lowering medications, ask your doctor if the prescribed medications have the potential to cause low blood glucose. If they do then ensure you have hypoglycemia treatment with you at all times (we discuss this next). This is especially important if you are using insulin.

Treating hypoglycemia

The vast majority of episodes of hypoglycemia are mild and you will be able to deal with them easily. Nonetheless — particularly if you have type 1 diabetes — severe episodes can and do occur, so it is best for you and your loved ones (and friends, workmates, and so on) to know what to do in the event that this happens to you. Inform people about your diabetes and about how to recognize hypoglycemia. Let them know where you store your emergency supplies (such as the dextrose tablets you use to treat hypoglycemia). Don't keep your diabetes a secret. The people close to you will be glad — and relieved — to know how to help you.

Treating mild and moderate hypoglycemia

If you find that your blood glucose level is low, then you must ingest some sugar to restore your level to normal. The Canadian Diabetes Association (CDA) recommends, for adults with diabetes, that if you have mild to moderate hypoglycemia (that is, you are still awake and aware enough to take things by mouth), you should take the following steps:

✔ **Step One:** Eat or drink 15 grams of a fast-acting carbohydrate such as

- Four 4-gram tablets of Dex4 tablets (this works out to 16 grams of glucose but that's close enough to 15 grams that the effect will be virtually the same)

- 175 mL (¾ cup) of juice or regular (*not* diet or sugar-free) pop (but see the tip following this list)

- 15 mL (1 tbsp.) honey

- 15 mL (1 tbsp.) table sugar dissolved in water

- Six jelly beans or six Lifesavers candies

- Rocket-type candies. Remember these from childhood? Yummy. How many you take will depend on the type you buy. Remember, you want to take the amount that will give you about 15 grams of carbohydrate. These candies are tasty, convenient, portable, cheap, and available at most convenience stores.

✔ **Step Two:** Wait 15 minutes, and then retest your blood. If your blood glucose level is still less than 4.0 mmol/L, ingest another 15 grams of carbohydrate.

✔ **Step Three:** If your next meal is more than one hour away, or you are going to be physically active, eat a snack, such as half a sandwich or cheese and crackers. The snack should contain 15 grams of carbohydrate and a source of protein.

Despite what most people think (and do), orange juice (or milk or, especially, glucose gel) is not as effective as products like Dex4 tablets because it raises glucose levels and relieves you of symptoms more slowly. Nonetheless, if you have some orange juice and it's handier than an alternative, it will work. Also, be sure to keep treatment for hypoglycemia on your bedside table. You do not want to risk falling and hurting yourself prowling the halls or using the stairs in search of treatment if you are hypoglycemic in the middle of the night.

Because acarbose (Glucobay) — see Chapter 12 — slows down absorption of sucrose, if you are taking this medicine and you develop hypoglycemia, you should be treated with glucose (such as Dex4), not sucrose (such as fruit juice).

If you are hypoglycemic and you're about to eat a meal, you should *first* treat your hypoglycemia with a fast-acting carbohydrate as described in the preceding steps. This will ensure that your blood glucose is brought up rapidly. More than one person with hypoglycemia, mealtime approaching, has ended up unconscious because they treated their low blood glucose by simply eating their meal (which only slowly raises blood glucose) rather than taking a fast-acting carbohydrate.

Because the symptoms of hypoglycemia are so unpleasant and because hypoglycemia is understandably scary, you may find yourself taking candy after candy until you feel better without actually giving time for the first treatment to take effect. Then, when all that sugar you have just ingested gets absorbed into your system, you may find that your glucose level is up into the teens. Be sure to give the first treatment time (as described earlier in Step 2) to work before you take another.

Dealing with severe hypoglycemia

If you experience hypoglycemia severe enough that you are unconscious (or nearly so) you will be unable to swallow properly. In this circumstance, people should *not* try to put sugar, honey, or anything else in your mouth because you could choke. Instead, your helper should call 9-1-1 and, if your helper can, also administer glucagon (see the "Using glucagon" section) to you.

If, however, you experience hypoglycemia where you are somewhat confused and unable to obtain an appropriate sugar source on your own, but are still alert and able to safely swallow, then your helper simply needs to find treatment for you and help you to ingest it. In this situation, use the same protocol listed in the immediately preceding section (see "Treating mild and moderate hypoglycemia") with the exception that in Step 1 consume 20 grams rather than 15 grams of carbohydrate.

Using glucagon

Glucagon is available by prescription in a package called a glucagon kit. You can see an example of what a glucagon kit looks like in Figure 5-1. The kit includes a syringe pre-filled with a sterile liquid and a vial containing 1 mg of glucagon (one of the major hormones that raises glucose). The glucagon is in powder form. Your helper needs to mix the glucagon with the liquid and then inject the syringe's contents inject into your leg muscle (the buttock and arm can also be used). The injection of glucagon raises the blood glucose, and within 15 to 20 minutes you will likely become fully alert. (Children 5 years of age or less are treated with half of the adult dose; that is, a child is given 0.5 mg of glucagon.)

You can find detailed instructions on how to administer glucagon by going to www.lilly.ca, then clicking "Our Medicines" and scrolling down the page until you come to "Glucagon."

People are much more likely to respond properly to an emergency situation if they are prepared for the eventuality. For that reason, it is important that those individuals who are most likely to be the ones giving you glucagon be very familiar both with the contents of a glucagon kit and what to do with them. Trying to learn how to use this at the time of the emergency is far from ideal to say the least. When you pick up the glucagon kit from the pharmacy, the person(s) who is most likely to be giving it should go with you. The pharmacist must explain to both of you how to use the glucagon kit.

Some people are, understandably, just too nervous or intimidated to take it upon themselves to administer glucagon. In that case, they should just call 9-1-1.

If you have just experienced a severe episode of hypoglycemia and you required an injection of glucagon, when you have fully come around and are able to swallow properly, you should consume a snack that includes 15 grams of carbohydrate (and a protein source) to help prevent redeveloping hypoglycemia as the glucagon wears off.

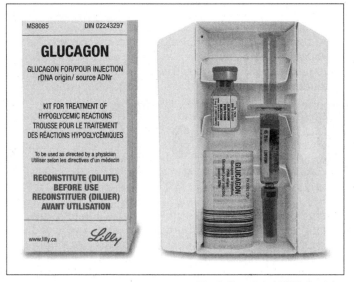

Figure 5-1:
A glucagon emergency kit from Eli Lilly Canada Inc.

Printed with permission of Eli Lilly Canada Inc.

Like most medicines, glucagon has an expiration date after which it may not work sufficiently well. For this reason, when you pick up your glucagon kit, find out when it will expire and mark a reminder on your calendar to pick up a new kit a few weeks ahead of time.

If you live, work, or play in an area where emergency health care services are more than just minutes away, having a glucagon kit is especially important for you. Do you snowmobile? Hunt? Hike? Boat? Do you live in a remote area? Does your job take you into the bush? All of these situations would warrant having a supply of glucagon readily available. Keep in mind the Boy Scouts' motto: Be prepared.

If you are the parent of a young child, you likely know all too well the phrases "I'm not hungry" or "I don't want to eat." These typically relatively harmless situations, however, take on a potentially much more serious meaning if your child has diabetes and is receiving insulin therapy. In this case, without food, your child will be at risk of hypoglycemia. If your child is receiving insulin, refuses food, and then develops mild hypoglycemia (or is about to), you can give her mini-doses of glucagon. The glucagon will help ward off or reverse hypoglycemia. We recommend you speak to your child's diabetes specialist or diabetes educator to find out more information on when you would use glucagon and the doses to administer.

Notifying your health team

If you have experienced severe hypoglycemia — even if you quickly recovered — notifying your family physician, your diabetes specialist, or your diabetes educator(s) is crucial, so that they can make appropriate adjustments to your therapy to lessen the likelihood of you having another episode. If you're feeling well and have fully recovered from the episode, you don't have to call your health care team right away, but be sure to get in touch with them within a day or two.

Preventing hypoglycemia

Not everyone with diabetes experiences hypoglycemia. As we discuss earlier in this chapter, if your treatment is lifestyle therapy alone (or lifestyle therapy in conjunction with certain types of oral medication such as metformin), you won't have low blood glucose. If, however, your treatment includes using medicines that have the potential to cause low blood glucose, then you can take certain measures to lower the likelihood you will experience hypoglycemia.

If you are using insulin then, as wonderful as this medication is, you are almost certainly going to have at least occasional episodes of low blood glucose. (You are particularly at risk of hypoglycemia if you have type 1 diabetes, but anyone on insulin therapy has this risk.) Therefore, if you are using insulin therapy, you must be aware of — and follow — the advice in this section.

These are ways you can help avoid experiencing episodes of hypoglycemia:

> ✔ **Don't miss or delay meals.** Because blood glucose-lowering medications do not have the good sense to know exactly when to stop working, like the famous battery-operated bunny, they sometimes tend to keep going and going. That can be a problem if your blood glucose level is normal, as it may be when your meal is due. If your meal is unduly delayed, depending on the type of blood glucose-lowering medication you're taking, it may pull your glucose level down too low. Options to deal with this are to not miss or delay a meal, or, if this is not realistic for you, speak to your physician about the preferred drugs to help you avoid hypoglycemia in these circumstances. (We discuss blood glucose-lowering drugs in Chapters 12 and 13.)

✔ **Plan your exercise.** Exercise is an essential component of your diabetes therapy (particularly if you have type 2 diabetes). If, however, you are taking certain medications to lower your blood glucose (insulin in particular), exercising could potentially cause your blood glucose level to go too low. By all means *do* exercise; however, if you know from experience that when you perform a certain type or amount of exercise you develop hypoglycemia, speak to your diabetes educator or physician about how to adjust your medicines or diet to reduce the risk of developing low blood glucose. Often the solution is something as simple as taking less insulin or having a small snack before (or even while) you work out. The worst thing is to have hypoglycemia every time you exercise; we can't imagine a stronger disincentive to exercising than that!

✔ **Have a bedtime snack.** Eating a bedtime snack is *not* necessary for most people with diabetes unless you're taking evening doses of NPH insulin, premixed insulin, or regular insulin and your bedtime blood glucose level is less than 7.0 mmol/L. In that case eating a bedtime snack containing at least 15 grams of carbohydrate and 15 grams of protein will help you avoid having a low reading overnight. An even better solution is to change to a different insulin (see the next bullet). Also, if you are on insulin therapy we recommend periodically testing your blood glucose level at about 3 a.m. to make sure it is not going low overnight without you knowing.

✔ **Change the type of insulin you are taking.** NPH insulin, premixed insulin, and regular insulin are more likely to cause hypoglycemia than are certain other types of insulin. If you are taking NPH, premixed, or regular insulin, and you are experiencing hypoglycemia, speak to your doctor about switching to a different insulin (we discuss insulin therapy in detail in Chapter 13).

✔ **Change the type of oral blood glucose-lowering medication you are taking.** As we discuss in detail in Chapter 12, some oral diabetes medications are much more likely than others to cause hypoglycemia (and some oral medications never causes hypoglycemia at all). If you are taking oral medication to lower your blood glucose and you are experiencing hypoglycemia, speak to your physician about switching to a different medicine. (Glyburide, in particular, is a notorious cause of hypoglycemia.)

✔ **Pay close attention to your symptoms of hypoglycemia.** By knowing what symptoms you typically get when you have hypoglycemia, you will be able to recognize hypoglycemia faster and treat it earlier.

✔ **Avoid overusing alcohol.** Alcohol is not forbidden if you have diabetes. However, taking insulin or oral medication that can cause hypoglycemia and drinking alcohol to excess — especially in the late evening — increases your risk of having hypoglycemia, particularly overnight. Avoid having more than one or two drinks. And if you do, make sure that you let your drinking mates know what to do if you might be low (as we discuss earlier in this chapter).

✔ **Review your non-diabetes medications with your physician.** Certain types of non-diabetes prescription medications (such as beta blockers) can make you more likely to experience hypoglycemia if you are also taking insulin or some types of oral blood glucose-lowering medications. Most of the time taking beta blockers is safe and uneventful, but if you're taking one and also having episodes of low blood glucose then speak to your doctor about whether or not to keep taking your beta blocker. (If you're unsure if you are taking a beta blocker, ask your pharmacist or other health care provider. Or look up the term "beta blocker" online. We could recommend you learn more about beta blockers in Ian's co-written book, *Understanding Prescription Drugs For Canadians For Dummies,* but that would be a shameless plug. So we won't. Oops, maybe we just did.)

✔ **Set higher blood glucose targets.** For some people, despite their best efforts and those of their diabetes team, recurring hypoglycemia is still a problem. (This is rarely the case unless you have longstanding type 1 diabetes.) In this situation, you may need to set blood glucose goals somewhat higher than the CDA target (see Chapter 9). We recommend you discuss with your doctor and your diabetes educator what your specific targets should be.

✔ **Wear a continuous glucose monitoring system (CGMS).** These devices continuously measure your (interstitial fluid) glucose level and alert you if your level is heading too low. They are particularly well suited to people with type 1 diabetes who are on insulin pump therapy. We discuss continuous glucose monitoring in detail in Chapter 9.

If you take insulin several times per day or are using an insulin pump (see Chapter 13), episodes of hypoglycemia are inevitable. Ian has found that, as a very rough rule of thumb, to achieve excellent overall blood glucose control in these circumstances, you can expect to have *mild* hypoglycemia about two to three times per week. Contrariwise, if you take insulin several times per day or you are using an insulin pump and you *never* experience episodes of hypoglycemia, your average blood glucose level is probably too high.

If you take insulin several times per day or are using pump, then once a week review your blood glucose readings in your log book or your blood glucose meter's memory and count how many times in the preceding seven days you've had a blood glucose less than 4 mmol/L. If you're blood glucose is less than 4 mmol/L more than two to three times per week, that is likely too often and will increase your risk of severe hypoglycemia. In this case, contact your physician or diabetes educator to see what changes should be made to your therapy to reduce the frequency of your hypoglycemia.

We discuss additional tips for people on insulin therapy in Chapter 13. We discuss issues surrounding driving and hypoglycemia in Chapter 16.

Coping with hypoglycemia unawareness

Hypoglycemia unawareness is a condition in which you lose your ability to recognize when your blood glucose level has fallen below normal. Samantha, one of Ian's patients, had this condition.

Samantha was 28 years old. She had developed diabetes when she was only 5 years of age. Samantha was a highly motivated patient and was monitoring her blood glucose levels many times per day. With aggressive use of insulin, nutrition therapy, and exercise, she was able to keep her glucose readings generally between 3.8 and 7.6. Recently, while she was at work, her boss found her staring vacantly into space. He was able to help her to drink some juice and she quickly came around, but the next day the same thing happened. Two days later, her husband awoke to find Samantha soaking wet in bed beside him. He couldn't wake her. He tested her blood glucose level and found it to be 1.8. He gave her an injection of glucagon (see discussion about glucagon earlier in this chapter) and over the next 15 minutes she gradually woke up. Later that day, she went to see Ian in the office, her therapy was adjusted, and soon thereafter she was again able to recognize when her blood glucose levels were too low.

Hypoglycemia unawareness can occur for several reasons:

- **Repeated hypoglycemia:** If you have been experiencing frequent hypoglycemia (generally speaking, this would be more than 2 to 3 episodes per week) — even if mild — your autonomic warning system symptoms (such as sweating and palpitations; see the "Autonomic symptoms" section earlier in this chapter) may start to fail and the first clue that you have low blood glucose can be when you are confused and unable to look after yourself. The best way to correct this is, *under your diabetes specialist's guidance,* to somewhat reduce your insulin doses to avoid any and all hypoglycemia for a few weeks, at which point your doses can typically be increased again, and your hypoglycemia awareness restored.

- **Longstanding diabetes:** Occasionally, if you have had diabetes for a very long time (typically this would mean decades), your autonomic warning system may fail. Setting higher blood glucose targets may be required. Also, using continuous glucose monitoring (see the "Preventing hypoglycemia" section and Chapter 9) may be helpful.

✔ **Other drugs impairing your ability to recognize hypoglycemia:** Several drugs can interfere with your body's ability to produce autonomic symptoms. Such drugs include beta blockers (such as propranolol), which are often used to treat heart disease and high blood pressure. If a medication is responsible, your physician (in consultation with you) will need to determine if another medication may be substituted. Also, alcohol use cannot only make you more prone to episodes of hypoglycemia (we discuss this in the preceding section), but can blunt your ability to recognize when you're hypoglycemic. We discuss alcohol and diabetes in detail in Chapter 10.

Dealing with Ketoacidosis

If you have type 1 diabetes, you're at risk for developing a dangerous, temporary condition called *diabetic ketoacidosis* (typically just called ketoacidosis or DKA). This is when your blood glucose level is high (typically above 14.0 mmol/L) *and* you have excess quantities of a type of acid called *ketones* in the blood. High blood glucose *without* the presence of ketones does not indicate DKA.

Ketoacidosis requires urgent attention because, if severe, it can be life-threatening.

Occasionally, the first clue that you have type 1 diabetes is when you become ill with ketoacidosis. More commonly, DKA occurs after you already know that you have the disease.

Exploring how ketoacidosis develops

If you have type 1 diabetes, you lack the ability to produce insulin and you need to give it to yourself by injection. But what happens if your body requires more insulin than you are giving?

Most of the time, so long as you are giving nearly enough insulin, the only thing that will happen is that your blood glucose levels run a bit too high. This is not good in the long term, but has little short-term danger. If, however, you are giving yourself far less insulin than you require, not only will your blood glucose levels be high, but your body will start to break down fat tissue. As fat tissue breaks down, it releases acids (ketones) into the bloodstream. This is called ketoacidosis.

Investigating the symptoms of ketoacidosis

These are the symptoms of ketoacidosis:

- ✔ **Extreme tiredness and drowsiness:** If your DKA is mild, your tiredness may also be mild, but as your DKA worsens you will feel increasingly drowsy, and if your DKA becomes severe you can lose consciousness.

- ✔ **Fruity breath:** The presence of ketones in your system gives your breath a fruity, not unpleasant, odour. Most people with DKA do not notice it, even though it might be apparent to bystanders.

- ✔ **Nausea, vomiting, and abdominal pain:** Many people with diabetes — and many doctors also — mistakenly attribute nausea, vomiting, and abdominal pain in a person with type 1 diabetes to "stomach flu" (*gastroenteritis*) when they actually are due to DKA. Never, ever assume you "simply have the flu" to explain these symptoms unless DKA has first been excluded. And don't let any doctor pass off these symptoms before first excluding DKA.

- ✔ **Rapid breathing:** You experience rapid breathing when your blood is so acidic that your body tries to compensate by ridding itself of acids through the lungs.

The CDA recommends that people with type 1 diabetes test for ketones in the following instances:

- ✔ During periods of acute illness when elevated blood glucose readings are present

- ✔ When before-meal blood glucose readings are above 14.0 mmol/L

- ✔ When symptoms of DKA (see previous section) are present

If you have type 1 diabetes we recommend you obtain a blood ketone tester and test strips. These products are available at your pharmacy.

Ketoacidosis occurs rarely in people with type 2 diabetes. Nonetheless, if you have type 2 diabetes and you develop typical symptoms of DKA, let your physician know.

If you notice that you have symptoms of ketoacidosis and when you test your blood ketone level you find it to be elevated (0.6 mmol/L or higher), in nearly all cases the safest and best thing to do is to go to the closest emergency department. However, if your symptoms are mild, your blood ketone level is only slightly elevated, and you are fortunate enough to be working with a diabetes educator who is trained and empowered to deal with DKA (and who is immediately available), you can contact your diabetes educator first for detailed advice.

Understanding the causes of ketoacidosis

Ketoacidosis is caused by a *relative* lack of insulin. When we say *relative* lack of insulin, we mean that the amount of insulin in your body — no matter how much — is not enough for your body's needs. It follows, then, that DKA will develop in one of a few general circumstances:

- ✔ **You are missing insulin doses.** If you have type 1 diabetes, your pancreas is unable to manufacture insulin, so you must give yourself insulin. If you miss doses — especially of long-acting (basal) insulin — you will be at substantial risk for developing DKA.

- ✔ **You aren't taking high enough doses of insulin.** Day to day you may give yourself a fairly similar quantity of insulin and get along quite nicely, thank you very much. That's great. But if you come down with some additional illness — a kidney infection or pneumonia for example — your usual insulin doses will likely be insufficient for your needs and your blood glucose levels will go up. If you don't deal with this by giving higher doses (and, often, additional doses) of insulin you can develop DKA.

- ✔ **Your insulin is defective.** If your blood glucose is elevated and you are giving higher doses and extra doses of insulin to no avail, then your insulin may be defective. Perhaps your insulin was inadvertently exposed to excess heat by being left in a hot car on a sunny summer day. Or, if it's winter, maybe it was accidentally left in the car when you were at hockey practice and it froze. Both of these circumstances will make your insulin "go bad" and become ineffective.

- ✔ **Your insulin pump isn't delivering insulin effectively.** We love insulin pump therapy and think it's a great option for many people with insulin-treated diabetes. Nonetheless, certain problems can arise wherein an insulin pump fails to deliver the insulin you think it's delivering, and as a result your blood glucose levels can rise and DKA can develop. (We discuss insulin pump therapy in detail in Chapter 13.)

If you have type 1 diabetes, you depend on insulin injections not only to preserve your health, but to preserve your life. Even if you're feeling rotten and aren't eating anything, you *cannot* forgo taking your insulin. In fact, you may need to give yourself *more* insulin than usual. The sickest patients that diabetes specialists ever see are those people with diabetes who, unfortunately, either weren't given this advice or knew it but didn't follow it. If you have type 1 diabetes, please follow this advice. It may save your life.

Treating ketoacidosis

Ketoacidosis is a serious condition that requires very careful and very aggressive treatment. In almost all cases hospitalization is required.

In hospital you will be given intravenous fluids, insulin, and potassium. Your blood glucose and potassium levels will be checked very frequently. Also, the doctors looking after you will try to determine the cause of your ketoacidosis. Usually the cause is easily identified and straightforward, such as having omitted insulin doses. If, however, the reason for your having developed DKA is not apparent, you may require additional blood and urine tests, X-rays, and so on to try to determine what may have triggered the episode (pneumonia, for example).

Preventing ketoacidosis

DKA is almost always preventable by following these measures:

- ✔ **Monitor, monitor, monitor:** Often the earliest signs of developing DKA are rising blood glucose readings. If you're testing your blood glucose frequently, you will detect a problem before it gets out of hand. Also, as we discuss in the preceding section, if your blood glucose is above 14.0 mmol/L or so, check your blood for ketones. You should have no — or only tiny — quantities of ketones.

- ✔ **Take your insulin:** Whatever you do, don't fall into the trap of figuring that if you're feeling unwell and aren't eating or drinking properly, you don't need insulin. Trust us; you *do* require insulin (possibly more than usual).

- ✔ **Get some fresh insulin:** If you are giving your insulin the way you should yet your blood glucose levels are not coming down the way they normally would, get some fresh, unopened insulin from the extra supply you keep in your fridge. If that isn't helping to bring down your blood glucose, then get some new insulin from the pharmacy.

- ✔ **Determine if your insulin pump or infusion sets are malfunctioning:** As we discuss in more detail in Chapter 13, insulin pumps and infusion sets (that is, the tubing and catheters that most pumps require) are increasingly used by people with type 1 (and to a far lesser extent, type 2) diabetes. If the pump malfunctions or the tubing, catheters, or infusion sites have a problem, then the pump may not deliver insulin the way it should.

- ✔ **Seek timely medical attention:** If your blood glucose levels are elevated, but you feel reasonably well and don't have ketones, then contact your diabetes educator (if they are empowered to address this issue and they are immediately available). If, however, your blood glucose is up into the teens, you have ketones present, and you're feeling unwell, go to the hospital.

We see people all the time who come to us after they've recovered from an episode of DKA that put them in the hospital. They invariably express their surprise at having had DKA. Yet, when we go through the measures listed earlier that could have helped them avoid DKA, they almost always haven't followed one or more of those measures. This is such a shame. Do yourself a favour and do whatever you can to avoid this life-threatening condition by following the actions we just mentioned.

This is an example of the *wrong way* to avoid DKA. Bill was a 22-year-old student with type 1 diabetes. One day he felt a bit under the weather and lost his appetite. Figuring if he wasn't eating then he didn't need insulin, he stopped taking it. He seldom checked his blood glucose levels at the best of times and, feeling unwell and not eating, he figured his blood glucose levels couldn't possibly be high. Later that day his roommate found Bill semi-conscious in bed, his breathing rapid, and his breath fruity. He called 9-1-1 and Bill was taken to hospital with a blood glucose of 36.0 mmol/L. A diagnosis of DKA was made. Bill was admitted to the intensive care unit and, with intensive therapy, gradually came around. He was discharged from hospital after four days, but didn't feel 100 percent for another week.

This is an example of the *right way* to avoid DKA. Beth was a 13-year-old girl who had had type 1 diabetes for three years. She was treated with four injections of insulin per day and her total daily dose of insulin was generally about 20 units. She typically checked her blood glucose readings three to four times per day. While visiting a friend at a cottage, she came down with terrible diarrhea. She spent the better part of the day on the toilet, but with her mom's encouragement, she was able to drink lots of fluids. When she became ill, she started testing her blood glucose every two hours. She noticed her blood glucose level was climbing, and when it reached 15.0 mmol/L, she checked her blood for ketones and found they were present in very small amounts.

Beth contacted her diabetes educator, who told her to take extra rapid-acting insulin every two hours if her blood glucose level was elevated. Over the next 12 hours she ended up taking an extra 30 units. By the next day, Beth was feeling back to normal, her glucose levels were normal, she had no ketones in the blood, her insulin doses were back to usual, and she was out playing with her friends.

Hyperosmolar Hyperglycemic State

The name *hyperosmolar hyperglycemic state* (fortunately abbreviated as HHS) refers to a situation where someone with type 2 diabetes develops tremendously elevated blood glucose. *Hyper* means "larger than normal," *osmolar* has to do with concentrations of substances in the blood, and *glycemic* has to do with blood glucose. In other words, the blood is simply too concentrated with glucose. HHS is a medical emergency requiring immediate hospitalization.

Identifying the symptoms of the hyperosmolar hyperglycemic state

The symptoms of HHS arise in part from the effects on the body of very high blood glucose levels (levels can be as high as 100 mmol/L!) and in part from whatever condition (for example, a heart attack or pneumonia) triggered it. Symptoms may include the following:

- ✔ Frequent urination
- ✔ Excessive thirst
- ✔ Dry mouth
- ✔ Leg cramps
- ✔ Weakness and lethargy
- ✔ Confusion
- ✔ Unconsciousness

The diagnosis of HHS is actually quite straightforward. If a person with known type 2 diabetes develops extraordinarily elevated blood glucose levels with evidence of dehydration and without the typical blood chemistry picture of ketoacidosis, the diagnosis is readily made.

If you measure your blood glucose regularly — and more frequently if you are feeling unwell — you will probably never develop HHS. You'll notice if your blood glucose is getting high and you'll take corrective action before it reaches a critical level.

HHS requires immediate and skilled treatment at a hospital. If you think you may have it, go to the nearest emergency department. The great majority of the time, however, the affected person does not recognize the problem; rather, a loved one (or, in the case of nursing home residents, a nurse) detects something is wrong. The affected person is usually too sick to even know that they are unwell.

Not all elevations of blood glucose indicate HHS. If you're feeling well, you don't have the symptoms described earlier in this section, and your blood glucose level is only mildly to moderately elevated (as high as 25 mmol/L or so), you probably don't have HHS. It may mean, however, that you need to speak to your health care team about improving your overall glucose control.

Examining the causes of the hyperosmolar hyperglycemic state

The hyperosmolar hyperglycemic state (HHS) is most common among elderly people with diabetes, though it can occur in younger individuals. HHS is most likely to occur if you have some additional serious illness that has triggered it. This illness may be, for example, a stroke, a heart attack, or a severe infection such as pneumonia.

Typically, HHS develops in an infirm person whose diabetes is reasonably well controlled until some additional factor (like those just mentioned) develops. Whereas an otherwise healthy person with type 2 diabetes would recognize the presence of the additional problem and seek medical attention, an infirm individual may not know something is amiss or may not be able to deal with it. The person then becomes increasingly unwell from the additional illness, the worsening blood glucose levels, and dehydration.

Treating the hyperosmolar hyperglycemic state

HHS treatment includes administering fluids, insulin, and potassium intravenously. Frequent blood tests are performed to monitor blood glucose levels, potassium levels, and kidney function. Additional tests (such as blood and urine tests, X-rays, and heart tests) are done to determine the cause of the HHS and the underlying cause is treated.

Even with the best possible therapy, the death rate for HHS is high because most people who suffer from it are elderly and have other serious illnesses that trigger it and complicate treatment.

Preventing the hyperosmolar hyperglycemic state

Hyperosmolar hyperglycemic state can be prevented in two broad ways, depending on where you or your loved one lives:

✔ **In the community:** If you or a loved one has type 2 diabetes and lives in the community and you find your (or their) blood glucose levels are climbing, contact your health care team to see if your treatment program needs to be adjusted or if a new health issue has come up that has made things worse.

✔ **In nursing homes:** If you or your loved one has diabetes and lives in a nursing home, speak to the staff (or the physician) to ensure that blood glucose levels are being checked regularly and even more often when you or your loved one is not feeling well. That way, if the blood glucose level is progressively climbing, someone will pick up on it and deal with the problem before it spirals out of control.

Chapter 6

As Time Goes By: Handling Long-Term Complications

. . . .

In This Chapter

▶ Discovering how you can prevent long-term complications

▶ Exploring the different types of long-term complications

▶ Dealing with complications specific to men

▶ Looking at complications specific to women

. . . .

You might ask yourself "What is my reward for year after year of eating healthfully, exercising regularly, checking my blood glucose regularly, taking my medications, and doing all the other things I need to do to manage my diabetes?" The answer: "*Nothing.*" Yup, nothing. Gee, who wants a job like that? Tons of work and as a reward . . . *nothing*. Well, nothing that is except for a long and healthy life! And that's the most important thing you need to know about the information in this chapter on diabetes complications. If you look after yourself well and manage your diabetes — with all the work this entails — you may never, ever get any of the complications we discuss here.

This chapter looks at the long-term complications that diabetes can cause, the best ways to avoid them, how to recognize them, and how to deal with them if they are already present. (We deal with acute glucose problems in Chapter 5.)

Complications Aren't Inevitable

As you read through this chapter you will come across complications that you will deem, correctly, to be minor, and others that will scare the pants (if that is your chosen attire) off you. Please, please do yourself and us a favour and if you see something that frightens you, keep repeating to yourself the following mantra: Complications aren't inevitable, complications aren't inevitable . . .

Not only are most long-term complications avoidable, but if they do occur, they can take years to fully develop. For this reason, if complications are creeping up on you, you must ensure they're detected early and treated promptly to minimize the risk that they'll get worse.

Ian was invited to speak to parents of teens with diabetes. As Ian spoke to the parents, his social worker colleague, Jeff, spoke to their children. Ian remarked to the parents how, with the excellent therapies now available, we could do so much to keep their children healthy. Afterwards, Jeff mentioned to Ian that the children had, each and every one of them, told him that they figured they would go blind eventually, or have amputations, or need dialysis. Ian was aghast: These poor kids must have felt awful, and all based on misinformation. Complications are *not* inevitable. So if you've been under the same impression as those youngsters, we are ever so thankful you're reading this chapter to get fully informed.

Preventing and minimizing complications require you to invest lots of energy, but hey, you're worth it. By the way, if anyone who doesn't have diabetes has the nerve to tell you that living with diabetes is easy, ask them if they would like to try it, and see how many takers you get!

If you do develop complications from your diabetes, *never* feel guilty and don't ever let anyone point an accusing finger at you. First, although terrific diabetes therapies (starting with healthy living) can greatly reduce your risk of developing complications, *reducing* risk is not the same as *eliminating* risk altogether. Second, as anyone who has ever been in a fender-bender knows, life happens and sometimes one's best efforts are confounded.

Categorizing Long-Term Complications

Many of the problems we discuss in this chapter can be lumped into two broad categories:

- ✔ **Organ damage due to narrowing or blockage of small blood vessels:** This is *called microvascular disease* or *microvascular complications*. Microvascular complications include damage to the eyes (retinopathy), kidneys (nephropathy), and nerve endings (neuropathy). Microvascular disease is primarily the result of inadequate blood glucose control. (We look further at this problem later in this section.)

- ✔ **Organ damage due to narrowing or blockage of large blood vessels:** This is called *macrovascular disease* or *macrovascular complications*. Macrovascular complications include damage to the brain (for example, stroke), heart (for example, heart attack), and legs (for example, amputations). Macrovascular disease is particularly likely to occur if you smoke or inadequately control your blood pressure and cholesterol. The relationship of high blood glucose to macrovascular disease is contro-versial. (We discuss this in the sidebar "Does reducing high blood glu-cose prevent macrovascular complications?")

The bad news: Macrovascular disease is the cause of death of the major-ity of people with diabetes. The good news: Macrovascular disease is often preventable and always treatable.

If you have been diagnosed recently as having type 2 diabetes, you may have already had it for a number of years without knowing it and, as such, you poten-tially already may have developed complications that you had no idea were present. For that reason, your physician must carefully check to determine if you have any evidence of damage to your body — even if you were diagnosed yesterday. This chapter details what you and your doctor should look for.

Familiarizing yourself with the following (often confusing!) terms — or at least knowing you can refer back to these definitions as you come across these terms in this chapter — will help you master the information in this section:

- **Coronary artery disease:** Typically, when physicians and lay people alike use the term *heart disease* they are actually referring to *coronary artery disease* (CAD) — or *coronary heart disease* — which is a specific form of heart disease involving blockages of the *coronary arteries* by a buildup of *plaque*. Plaque is a mixture of cholesterol, fat, and cal-cium. The presence of plaque in blood vessels is called *atherosclerosis*. Because the blood vessels become very stiff from all this scarring, ath-erosclerosis is commonly referred to as *hardening of the arteries*. CAD can lead to a heart attack (*myocardial infarction*).

- **Cerebrovascular disease**: This problem occurs when the arteries that carry oxygen to the brain become blocked. Cerebrovascular disease can lead to a stroke.

- **Peripheral arterial disease (PAD):** This problem occurs when the arter-ies that carry oxygen to your legs and feet become blocked. Severe PAD can lead to an amputation.

- **Cardiovascular disease:** This term encompasses all of the preceding terms (that is, it includes coronary artery disease, cerebrovascular dis-ease, and peripheral arterial disease).

If you are speaking about blood circulation issues with your physician or other health care provider, or reading about the topic on the Web or else-where, you need to be crystal clear if what you are being told (or are reading) concerns *arterial* circulation (that is, blood flow in the arteries) or *venous* circulation (that is, blood flow in the veins). With diabetes, *arterial* circulation is the main concern. (Problems with venous circulation are, if present, usually limited to causing swollen ankles.) In this chapter when we talk about circula-tory disease, we are talking about *arterial* circulatory disease.

Does reducing high blood glucose prevent macrovascular complications?

Studies have proven that reducing high blood glucose hugely lowers the risk of *microvascular* complications such as retinopathy, nephropathy, and neuropathy. Whether reducing high blood glucose similarly reduces the risk of *macrovascular* complications, like heart attack and stroke, is controversial.

Two very large and compelling studies found that people with *recently diagnosed* type 1 or type 2 diabetes had their risk of heart attack and stroke substantially reduced by good blood glucose control, but other studies looking at people with more long-standing diabetes (many of whom already had macrovascular complications) did not find similar results. These studies, taken together, strongly suggest that good blood glucose control is, indeed, important in preventing heart attack and stroke, but you must strive for it (and achieve it) early on after you've developed diabetes. Also, while you're striving for good blood glucose control, follow other proven protective measures such as keeping your blood pressure and cholesterol in check, following a healthy diet, exercising regularly, not smoking, and so on. We discuss these key measures in this chapter and throughout this book.

Coronary Artery Disease and Cerebrovascular Disease

Together, coronary artery disease (by causing heart attacks) and cerebrovascular disease (by causing strokes) account for the death of up to 80 percent of people with diabetes. This is a terrifying statistic. So in this section we detail the various ways you can help avoid these diseases and, if you have them already, how to keep them under control.

The heart is, essentially, a pump. An amazing, complex, wonderful pump (when was the last time you went to the hardware store and bought a pump that was likely to last for 80-plus years?), but a pump nonetheless.

The most common symptoms of coronary artery disease are chest discomfort (*angina*) and shortness of breath. Other symptoms can include dizziness or fatigue. Symptoms of coronary artery disease are especially likely to occur if you are exerting yourself, such as walking up a hill or climbing a flight of stairs.

The most common symptoms of cerebrovascular disease are those of a stroke: weakness of an arm or leg on one side of the body, slurred speech, drooping of one side of the face, weakness, difficulty walking, confusion, and headache.

If ever you experience chest discomfort or shortness of breath that lasts more than a few minutes, or symptoms of stroke, you must call 9-1-1 for an ambulance to take you to the hospital. You should *never, ever* drive yourself to the hospital if you think you are experiencing a heart attack. (And don't get your loved one or next-door neighbours to drive you, either, unless of course they happen to be a couple of paramedics with an ambulance parked in the driveway!)

Having an EKG be done when you are diagnosed with diabetes is typically a good idea. It will serve as a "baseline" for future comparison purposes in case your EKG becomes abnormal in the future. (Doing this baseline EKG is typically not necessary if you are both young and have a low risk for heart disease). Having your EKG repeated routinely from time to time thereafter is prudent; especially if you are at high risk for cardiovascular disease.

Preventing a heart attack or stroke

Although, in general terms, having diabetes increases the risk of heart attack or stroke, this risk is not the same for all people with diabetes. For example, a 22-year-old who has had type 1 diabetes for only one year is at minimal risk, and a 65-year-old who has had diabetes for 30 years and is a smoker with high blood pressure and high LDL cholesterol is at very, very high risk. (We tell you more about smoking and cholesterol levels later in this chapter.) This is important to know because, although everyone with diabetes should do their best to be healthy, you must take extra precautions if you are at high risk of having a heart attack or stroke.

The Canadian Diabetes Association (CDA) recommends the following heart attack and stroke prevention strategies for *all* people with diabetes:

- ✔ **Follow a healthy lifestyle by eating healthfully, exercising regularly, and striving to achieve a healthy weight.** We discuss these issues in detail in Chapters 10 and 11.

- ✔ **If you smoke, quit. If you don't smoke, don't start.** We discuss this further right after this list.

- ✔ **Keep your blood pressure within target (less than 130/80).** We discuss this in more detail later in this chapter.

- ✔ **Keep your A1C within target (7.0 % or less).** Your A1C is an indicator of your overall blood glucose control. (Certain people — such as older people with limited life expectancy — have a higher target A1C. We discuss A1C in Chapter 9.)

The Canadian Diabetes Association recommends the following *additional* precautions:

✔ **Take ACE inhibitor or ARB medication if one or both of the following apply to you:**

- You are 55 years of age or older.

- You have evidence of organ damage associated with diabetes.

✔ **Take statin medication if one or more of the following apply to you:**

- You are 40 years of age or older.

- You have had diabetes for more than 15 years and you are more than 30 years of age.

- You have evidence of organ damage associated with diabetes.

Depending on your specific situation, taking a statin medication may also be warranted in other situations such as being less than 40 years of age and having a very high LDL cholesterol.

✔ **Take ASA if you are known to already have cardiovascular disease or have multiple risk factors for cardiovascular disease:** If you cannot tolerate ASA (81 to 325 mg daily) because, for example, it upsets your stomach, you can instead take 75 mg daily of clopidogrel (Plavix). Both ASA and clopidogrel prevent blood clots by interfering with the clotting action of small particles in the blood called *platelets*. The CDA advises that ASA or clopidogrel "should not be routinely used" if diabetes is your only risk factor for heart disease and you are not known to have cardiovascular disease, but you may take it if you have multiple cardio-vascular risk factors.

Quitting smoking

Although many things about diabetes are unknown or uncertain, one thing that is absolutely, positively proven is that smoking and diabetes do not go together. Having diabetes puts you at increased risk of stroke, heart attack, amputations, and, for men, erectile dysfunction. These — and many other complications (including worsening of diabetes eye damage) — are much more likely to develop if you smoke. Do yourself the biggest favour in the world: If you have diabetes and you smoke, do everything humanly possible to quit. Do it for yourself, do it for your loved ones, and if you are Ian's patient, do it because that is the only way you are going to get him off your back! (Ian has this thing about keeping his patients healthy. Geesh, imagine that.)

Quitting cold turkey is the best option for some people. For others, using a nicotine patch (available over-the-counter) or a prescription medication like Zyban (bupropion) or Champix (varenicline) is helpful. You can also use sup-port services, such as help lines, available across the country. If you've tried quitting but have gone back to smoking, then try again the next day. And if that doesn't work, try again the next day. The key to success is not giving up. Ignore your failures and start your efforts afresh each day. Ultimately you can and will succeed.

Peripheral Arterial Disease

Diabetes can do many scary things. For most people, high up on this intimidating list are perfectly justified fears about poor arterial circulation leading to amputations. Poor arterial circulation to the legs is called *peripheral arterial disease* (PAD). (Sometimes peripheral arterial disease is referred to as peripheral vascular disease, or PVD, however this term is less precise.) PAD is due to atherosclerosis obstructing the flow of blood. It is caused by the same factors that lead to coronary artery disease and cerebrovascular disease. Similarly, you can avoid it by following the measures that we describe earlier in this chapter.

Far and away the most common symptom of PAD is an aching discomfort in your calves as you walk. This is called *intermittent claudication* (usually abbreviated to *claudication*). Generally speaking, the sooner the discomfort occurs when you walk, the worse are the blockages in the arteries.

If PAD is very severe, it can lead to changes in the feet, including the following:

- ✔ Pale appearance
- ✔ Hair loss
- ✔ Constant pain in the toes
- ✔ Small, usually red or black spots on the tips of the toes
- ✔ Open sores or ulcers on the bottom or sides of the feet

 If you have developed any of these symptoms, let your family physician or diabetes specialist know; however, if you have developed an open sore or ulcer on your foot, you may have an infection and you need to seek *immediate* medical attention.

Peripheral arterial disease is difficult to treat, but helpful therapies are available including medications and, in some cases, surgery to open or bypass a blocked artery. You must not smoke and must control your cholesterol and blood pressure. Your physician can also discuss certain helpful types of exercises that you can perform, or, alternatively, can refer you to a specialist in this field.

Numerous reasons not to smoke exist, but we want to make special mention of the influence of smoking on PAD. Smoking will make you much more prone to PAD. Even more important, if you continue to smoke when you *already have* PAD, your circulation problems will certainly get worse and you will be at enormous risk of developing foot ulcerations, gangrene, and, ultimately, amputations.

We talk more about foot care later in this chapter (see "Foot Disease in Diabetes").

The Lowdown on High Blood Pressure

High blood pressure is a common health problem whether or not you have diabetes. It is, however, especially common among people with diabetes. Not that diabetes *causes* high blood pressure; it's just *associated* with it.

The medical term for high blood pressure is *hypertension*. You may have noticed that your doctor refers to your blood pressure as being *something over something* (140 over 90, for example). The first number represents the *systolic* value and the second number the *diastolic* value. The systolic value is the amount of force exerted by the heart when it contracts to push blood around the body. The diastolic value is the pressure in the large arteries in-between heart contractions.

Keeping your blood pressure *normal* is essential. High blood pressure can lead to all sorts of problems — particularly if you have diabetes — including the following:

- ✔ Heart attack
- ✔ Kidney failure
- ✔ Stroke
- ✔ Worsening of retinopathy

Now, we didn't design this list to depress you. We want to alert you to the importance of the issue, because with proper therapy you can help avoid these problems. Indeed, modern medicine has very, very effective therapy for high blood pressure.

What exactly is normal blood pressure? This should be such a simple question to answer, but in fact it isn't. It seems that each year some new study comes out showing that we should be aiming lower. Suffice it to say, if you have diabetes, your target blood pressure is less than 130 over 80 (written as 130/80).

Never let your doctor (including us!) or any other health care provider simply report to you that your blood pressure is *good* or *fine* or *okay*, or some other equally vague and ultimately meaningless term. If he doesn't volunteer what your measurement is, ask. Furthermore, if your blood pressure is above target (remember, target is less than 130/80), ask your doctor how to improve it. Do not settle for second-rate blood pressure control. We're talking your health here!

The CDA recommends that you have your blood pressure measured every time you see your doctor for a diabetes-related visit (since diabetes can affect pretty well all your body, that would mean almost every visit).

The following are treatments for high blood pressure:

- ✔ Diet (limiting salt and alcohol)
- ✔ Exercise
- ✔ Weight control
- ✔ Medicines (An ACE inhibitor or ARB medication is a particularly good choice; however, often a combination of two, three, or even four different medicines is required.)

Some medicines used to treat hypertension can have an effect on your blood glucose control. For example, hydrochlorothiazide (HCT) could make blood glucose levels go up, and beta blockers can reduce your awareness of low blood glucose. This doesn't mean these drugs are bad or shouldn't be used, but pay especially close attention to your blood glucose levels if you are prescribed these drugs. (If HCT is going to make your readings rise, it will most likely happen shortly after you first start taking it.)

Abnormal Cholesterol and Triglyceride Levels (Dyslipidemia)

As we discuss in detail in a moment, cholesterol and triglycerides are types of lipids. Having abnormal cholesterol levels (in particular, having a high LDL cholesterol level) increases your risk of cardiovascular disease. Fortunately excellent therapy is available that allows almost everyone to have healthy lipid levels.

Many types of lipids exist. Far and away the most important one for you to be aware of — and to have within target — is your LDL cholesterol; however, there are other lipid levels that are also measured. These are lipid tests for you to be aware of:

- **LDL:** This stands for *low density lipoprotein*. LDL is thought of as the *bad* cholesterol. You want your LDL to be low. To remember this, think of "LDL is **l**ousy and should be **l**ow."

- **HDL:** This stands for *high density lipoprotein*. HDL is thought of as the *good* cholesterol. You want your HDL to be high because it helps protect your blood vessels (by removing cholesterol from the walls of your arteries). You can remember this by the phrase "A **h**igh HDL keeps you **h**ealthy."

- **Total cholesterol:** This is the total level of all the different types of cholesterol in your blood.

- **Non-HDL cholesterol:** This is your total cholesterol minus your HDL cholesterol. The lower the number, the better.

- **Total cholesterol/HDL ratio:** Just as it sounds, this is a ratio of total cholesterol to HDL cholesterol and is used by your doctor to help decide if you require treatment. The lower the ratio, the better.

- **Apolipoprotein B ("apo B"):** This is a component of LDL cholesterol.

- **Triglycerides:** These are the main fats in the blood. Their role in the development of atherosclerosis is not quite as proven as LDL and HDL; however, keeping your triglycerides in the normal range is wise (see proceeding section).

The CDA recommends that you have your lipid levels checked at the time your diabetes is diagnosed and then yearly (more frequently if treatment has been initiated or changed).

Traditionally, people are asked to fast when their blood is taken to measure their lipids because the results are more precise, but even on a non-fasting blood sample a very good idea of a person's lipid levels can be determined. (Apo B and non-HDL testing does not require fasting.) Also not to be ignored are the logistical difficulties in going for fasting blood work: getting up even earlier than usual in order to get to the lab, long lineups at the lab as you stand there beside dozens of other people that were also sent for fasting blood work, potentially being late for work, and, importantly, risking hypoglycemia if you are on certain blood glucose-lowering medications. Not surprisingly, many people end up not going for the blood test at all! And that serves nobody well. Therefore, feel free to ask your doctor, if they ask that you have a fasting blood test, if you may instead go for a nonfasting test.

If your doctor wants you to fast for your blood test, make sure he or she writes on the lab requisition precisely how long you should fast. If your doctor doesn't do this, the lab may tell you that you must be fasting for 14 hours before they will do the test. That can be dangerous if you are taking certain oral antihyperglycemic drugs (we discuss these in Chapter 12) or, especially, insulin (Chapter 13). If you are on these medicines, *never* fast for anywhere near 14 hours unless you have first checked with your doctor. In most cases, if fasting is required, an eight-hour fast is sufficient.

Looking at healthy cholesterol levels

Although cholesterol has a bad reputation, in fact, cholesterol is an essential substance required for maintaining healthy cells and manufacturing certain vitamins and hormones. Problems arise when too much cholesterol is in the blood or too much of the wrong type.

The CDA recommended LDL target is less than or equal to 2.0 mmol/L. Achieving this should be your and your doctor's main priority in terms of managing your lipids.

An alternative target is an apo B level less than or equal to 0.8 grams per litre. (An advantage of apo B testing, compared with LDL testing, is that fasting is not required although, as noted above, fasting may not necessarily be required when checking your other lipids either). Apo B testing isn't routinely available in all regions.

Your target non-HDL cholesterol level is less than or equal to 2.6 mmol/L.

Although the CDA guidelines do not have a specific treatment target for triglycerides, a level less than 1.5 mmol/L is considered optimal. (Keeping the level under 10 mmol/L is particularly important, because higher values are associated with an increased risk of developing *pancreatitis* — a serious condition where the pancreas becomes inflamed).

For people with diabetes, the most common problem is high LDL, low HDL, and high triglycerides.

Keeping your lipids under control

You can improve your lipids in these ways:

- ✔ Achieve and maintain a healthy weight (for more, see Chapters 10 and 11)
- ✔ Eat healthfully (see Chapter 10)
- ✔ Exercise regularly (see Chapter 11)
- ✔ Take medication (we discuss this next)

Your liver actually makes most of the cholesterol in your body. Although you may be able to limit your cholesterol intake, getting your liver to stop making cholesterol is quite different. The liver's tendency to make too much cholesterol is often genetic. Thus, lifestyle therapy (diet, exercise, weight control) may not be enough to bring your lipids in line — and medication becomes necessary.

A common mistake is when people stop taking their cholesterol medicine after their cholesterol level returns to normal, because they think they no longer need it. Stopping the medication only causes cholesterol levels to become abnormal again. Unless you change your genes (which we imagine is not very likely), you must continue taking the medicine.

The preferred medicine to get and keep your LDL cholesterol level in target is a *statin,* of which several exist, including the particularly widely prescribed atorvastatin (Lipitor) and rosuvastatin (Crestor). Statins have a long track record of safety and effectiveness. The most common side effect is muscle aching, which goes away promptly after discontinuing the medicine.

If a statin isn't working well enough, Ezetrol (ezetimibe) or a fibrate is often added. Less frequently used medicines to treat a high LDL are bile acid binding resins (cholestyramine and colesevelam).

If your main problem is very high triglycerides (greater than 10.0 mmol/L) you can lower these by improving your blood glucose control, losing excess weight, eating healthfully, not drinking alcohol to excess, and taking a fibrate or a drug called niacin.

Because statins lower your risk of a heart attack even if your lipids are within target in the first place, the Canadian Diabetes Association advises using statins — regardless of your LDL cholesterol level — if you are at sufficiently high risk of heart attack or stroke (we talk about cardiovascular disease earlier in this chapter).

Some medicines, like simvastatin, that are used to improve cholesterol levels work better if you take them in the evening, whereas others, like atorvastatin (Lipitor) and rosuvastatin (Crestor), work equally well no matter when you take them. If you are prescribed cholesterol-lowering pills, be sure to ask your doctor or pharmacist when to take them.

Eye Disease

Several types of eye problems can occur in people with diabetes. Some eye diseases, such as *glaucoma* (raised pressure within the fluid of the eye) and *cataracts* (cloudiness of the lens of the eye), also occur in people without diabetes, though you're more likely to get them if you have diabetes.

The eye disease of greatest potential danger to people with diabetes is *retinopathy* — damage to the back (retinal) surface of the eye — including *macular edema* (a form of retinopathy in which fluid leaks into the macula from adjacent blood vessels). Retinopathy is the leading cause of blindness in Canada.

Retinopathy

Diabetic retinopathy refers to several different types of injury to the back surface of the eye. This surface allows you to see the world around you. Retinopathy is divided into two broad categories:

- **Non-proliferative retinopathy:** In its earliest stages, tiny ballooning of small blood vessels, called *microaneurysms*, are present. In the next stage, small areas of bleeding (called *dot hemorrhages*) or slightly bigger ones (called *blot hemorrhages*) develop. These changes do not cause loss of vision.

- **Proliferative retinopathy:** This is the more severe category and could threaten your eyesight. With proliferative retinopathy, abnormal, fragile blood vessels form *(neovascularization)*, which have the potential to bleed and can both obscure vision and lead to a *retinal detachment*.

Macular edema, swelling of the *macula* (the area of the retina where light focuses and vision is sharpest), can also occur as part of diabetic retinopathy. It develops when the blood vessels lining the retina become so damaged that fluid leaks from these vessels into the macula.

Pregnancy can cause retinopathy to worsen rapidly. If you have diabetes and you are considering getting pregnant (see Chapter 7), you must see an eye doctor *before* you try to get pregnant, then regularly during your pregnancy. (This does not apply to gestational diabetes because retinopathy does not develop in this condition.)

If you look in the mirror one day and see that you have pinkeye or that you have a small area of bleeding in the whites of one of your eyes, you can rest assured that these are not features of diabetes eye damage. Diabetes damages the *inside* of the eyes, not the *outside*.

How you can prevent retinopathy

Always remind yourself of what we say at the beginning of this chapter: Damage to your body from diabetes — including serious eye disease — is *not inevitable*. By paying careful attention to your diabetes and working closely with health care professionals, you can minimize the likelihood of running into eye damage.

Here are the most important ways to protect your vision:

- ✔ Maintain excellent blood glucose control (see Chapter 9).
- ✔ Maintain excellent blood pressure (refer to the section "The Lowdown on High Blood Pressure," earlier in this chapter).
- ✔ Maintain excellent lipids (refer to the section "Abnormal Cholesterol and Triglyceride Levels (Dyslipidemia)," earlier in this chapter).
- ✔ Don't smoke (reason number 4,362, last time we checked).
- ✔ Get regular, expert eye care from a highly skilled optometrist or ophthalmologist.

As we discuss in Chapter 2, if your blood glucose levels are going through a major change (high to normal, or normal to high), you may develop temporary visual blurring. This is *not* a sign of retinopathy.

If you have had chronically poor blood glucose readings and are then placed on aggressive (as it should be!) treatment to improve things, retinopathy may initially worsen *if* you already have it. Ultimately, better blood glucose control will help protect your eyes, but because retinopathy could get worse at first, you must see an eye doctor shortly after starting aggressive blood-glucose-lowering treatment. Most doctors don't know this, so you may have to tell them. Feel free to show them this page. Don't worry about offending your doctor. No doctor in the world knows everything. (Just ask their kids.)

An optometrist or an ophthalmologist?

As you read this chapter you may be thinking, "Boy, I'd better make sure I see my eye doctor." You bet. But which one? Should you see an optometrist or an ophthalmologist? An optometrist is trained to detect eye disease and can prescribe glasses, but he or she is not a medical doctor and cannot perform eye surgery. An ophthalmologist is a medical doctor who is trained to detect and treat eye diseases — with medicines and, if necessary, surgery. An opti-cian, by the way, is someone who is trained to fit you with glasses but not to detect or treat eye disease.

If you do not have eye damage from your diabetes and simply need a routine eye exam and screening, you can see an optometrist or an ophthalmologist. If, however, you have diabetes eye damage — especially if it's severe — you should be referred to an ophthalmologist. Seeing a highly skilled eye specialist is key.

If your retinopathy is mild, no treatment is required (apart from all those measures we discuss earlier to prevent it from worsening). If your retinopathy is more advanced, an *ophthalmologist* (eye surgeon) may need to perform retinal laser surgery or inject special ("anti-VEGF") medications (such as Lucentis or Avastin) directly into the eye to slow down the growth of new blood vessels. Sometimes for severe cases, an ophthalmologist will perform an operation — called a *vitrectomy* — to remove fluid and blood from the back portion of the eyeball and replace it with a sterile solution. Recent medical research suggests that a drug (fenofibrate) used to treat dyslipidemia may also help prevent retinopathy from progressing. Fenofibrate is, however, not yet a routine part of retinopathy treatment.

Contrary to what is commonly thought, ASA (for example, aspirin) does *not* increase the risk of serious bleeding within the eye. If you need to take ASA (see the earlier section, Preventing a heart attack or stroke), having diabetic retinopathy should not prevent you from taking it unless your eye doctor has very specific concerns for your situation.

Screening for retinopathy

These are the Canadian Diabetes Association (CDA) recommendations for retinopathy screening:

> ✔ **If you have type 1 diabetes,** get assessed by an expert eye specialist annually beginning five years after the onset of diabetes if you are 15 years of age or older.

✔ **If you have type 2 diabetes,** get assessed by an expert eye specialist at the time of diagnosis then annually. (The CDA notes that if you have no or minimal retinopathy it may be possible for some people to have screening done every two years rather than every year. Ian, however, prefers to be extra cautious and advises *all* his patients to have their eyes checked *every* year.)

Nowadays, in addition to an eye exam, retinal photographs are often taken. These photographs are an excellent way of detecting and recording eye damage and providing a permanent record for future comparison. The charge for these pictures is typically between $30 and $60.

Before an eye exam (using an ophthalmoscope), your eye doctor will put eye drops in your eyes to *dilate* (widen) your pupils and see your retina. This will typically make your eyesight distorted (and very sensitive to light) for a few hours until the drops wear off. Until that time you won't be able to drive, so take someone with you to your eye appointment to give you a ride home.

Cataracts

A *cataract* is an opaque (cloudy) area of the lens of the eye that, if large enough, can lead to blurred vision. Cataracts tend to be more common in people with diabetes, even at a young age. Cataracts can be surgically removed by a fairly routine operation. The entire lens is removed, and an artificial lens is put in its place. This will not only get rid of the blurring the cataracts had caused, but for some people who previously required eye glasses, with their new, implanted artificial lens, eye glasses may no longer be necessary.

Glaucoma

Glaucoma is high pressure inside the eye. Untreated it can lead to damage to the optic nerve and, ultimately, blindness. Glaucoma is found more often in people with diabetes than in people without diabetes (but is common in both). Fortunately, medical treatment (typically with eye drops) can lower the eye pressure and save your eyesight. Eye doctors routinely check for glaucoma.

Resources to help you if you are blind or visually impaired

In the event you need them, many devices are available to assist you, including the following:

✔ **Glucose meters with speech capability:** Well, they talk to you, but don't bother talking back; not yet anyhow. We discuss glucose meters in Chapter 9.

✔ **Insulin pen devices that click as you dial them:** The clicking allows you to keep track of how much insulin you are about to give. Also, some insulin pens have a small magnifier attached to enlarge the display showing how many units of insulin are about to be given. We discuss insulin pen devices in Chapter 13.

Some excellent websites are available to assist you if you have vision impairment:

✔ **American Foundation for the Blind:** This site, www.afb.org, has resources, information, reports, talking books, and lots of facts and wisdom about dealing with visual impairment.

✔ **Blindness Resource Center:** This site, www.nyise.org/blind.htm, points you in the right direction for information on every aspect of blindness. It is a guide to other sites about visual impairment.

✔ **The Canadian Council of the Blind:** This site, www.ccbnational.net, is the online home of an advocacy group for visually impaired people, run by visually impaired people.

✔ **The Canadian National Institute for the Blind (CNIB):** The CNIB is a well-known organization that serves to assist people with visual impairment. The part of their website that deals specifically with diabetes-related eye troubles is www.cnib.ca/dr.

Kidney Disease

Think of your kidneys as filters. And what amazing filters they are! Not only can they rid your body of toxins that are produced as a normal by-product of metabolism, but they can maintain your salt and water balance, keep the level of acids in your body under control, and release hormones that regulate your body's production of blood. Practically the only thing these amazing filters can't do is help make coffee (though they do help you get rid of it!).

Unfortunately, diabetes can damage the kidneys. In fact, diabetes is the most common cause of kidney failure in Canada. Fortunately, this damage is largely preventable and is definitely treatable.

Diagnosing diabetes kidney damage

Diabetes takes years and years to cause kidney damage. That means you have lots of opportunities to prevent damage from occurring. A doctor's earliest clue that a problem exists typically is the discovery of excess levels of *albumin* (a type of protein) in your urine. This is called *microalbuminuria* and your doctor can detect it with a very simple urine test (a urine *albumin/ creatinine ratio;* abbreviated as *ACR*) that can be performed at any time of day. A normal ACR is less than 2 mg/mmol (milligrams per millimole). If damage progresses, it leads to larger quantities of protein in the urine and can cause your feet and legs to swell (edema). If things continue to worsen, your kidneys become unable to purify your blood of toxins. This last stage is called *kidney failure* and typically makes people feel unwell in many ways, including causing fatigue, weight loss, and malaise.

Kidney malfunction does not cause symptoms until it is very severe. You can't rely on having or not having symptoms to indicate kidney health. Only laboratory testing can determine if a problem is present. (Incidentally — and contrary to popular wisdom — kidney damage from diabetes does *not* cause back pain.)

Because the ACR can be temporarily elevated due to conditions *not* related to diabetes kidney damage (such as menstruation, recent heavy exercise, high blood glucose levels, very high blood pressure, heart failure, fever, or a kidney or bladder infection), your ACR should not be tested until these other conditions have passed. Additionally, if you have an elevated ACR, unless it is extraordinarily high, your doctor will need to retest your urine in order to confirm that you do, in fact, have a kidney problem.

If you have evidence, on blood or urine testing, of having more advanced kidney damage, your doctor may ask you to do a urine collection, which is basically what it sounds like: collecting your urine (for 24 hours) in a jug, which the lab will provide you. A urine collection measures your kidney function more precisely. Collecting one's urine for 24 hours is a hassle ("Hmm, I wonder if I properly labelled that yellow jug I put in the office fridge?"), so fortunately this test is not required for most people with diabetes and, even when a person needs to do it, it is done only occasionally.

Another important way that your doctor should assess your kidney function is with a blood test called the *creatinine level.* Your creatinine level is used to estimate your GFR (*glomerular filtration rate*; which, because it is being estimated, is abbreviated as eGFR where the letter "e" stands for "estimated"), which is a measure of how efficiently your kidneys can purify your blood. This test monitors your kidney function. A particularly important reason to do this test is that recent studies tell us that quite a few people will develop kidney damage without first having microalbuminuria. In other words, an abnormal creatinine (and GFR) may be the first clue that a problem exists. A normal eGFR is technically equal to or greater than 90 mL/min (millilitres per minute); however, laboratories, taking into account that people of different sizes and ethnicities can have different values and still be "normal," typically report a normal value to be equal to or greater than 60 mL/min.

The Canadian Diabetes Association recommends that adults with diabetes be screened for kidney damage by having their urine ACR, blood creatinine, and eGFR measured annually beginning at the time of diagnosis of type 2 diabetes, and beginning five years after the diagnosis of type 1 diabetes.

 People with diabetes can get the same non-diabetes health issues as anyone else, including kidney problems. Therefore, if you have diabetes and a lab test shows you have a low eGFR — especially if you do not have albumin in the urine — your doctor should consider the possibility that the cause is something other than your diabetes, for example, high blood pressure. If your doctor ever tells you that you have a kidney problem, ask if it might be due to something other than diabetes and, if so, if other tests might be required to sort this out.

Treating diabetes kidney damage

The most important factors leading to diabetes kidney disease are inadequate blood glucose control and elevated blood pressure. Other, unknown (perhaps genetic) factors must be present, too, because most people with diabetes never develop kidney malfunction. Because no one can predict whether you'll always have healthy kidneys, taking all possible precautions to protect these important organs is crucial.

With appropriate therapy, not only can you substantially reduce your risk of developing kidney damage, but if you already have it, you can help prevent it from worsening or, in some cases, undo some of the damage.

These are the ways to protect your kidneys from diabetes damage:

- Excellent blood glucose control.
- Excellent blood pressure control.
- Medication (either a member of the ACE inhibitor family or a member of the ARB family) if you have microalbuminuria. (We define microalbuminuria earlier in this section.)

ACE inhibitors and ARBs sometimes lead to potentially dangerous accumulation of potassium in the body and can, rarely, make kidney function worse, not better. For these reasons, if you are taking an ACE inhibitor or ARB, you should have your potassium and creatinine (this is a kidney test) blood levels checked at these times:

- ✔ One to two weeks after you start the medicine
- ✔ One to two weeks after the dose of the medicine is increased
- ✔ If you develop an acute illness (such as pneumonia or gastroenteritis or any other ailment which puts you at risk of dehydration)

Although the creatinine often goes up shortly after starting ACE inhibitor or ARB therapy, it shouldn't rise by more than 30 percent. If it does, that may signify worsening kidney function caused by the drug, and your doctor may tell you to stop taking the medicine.

The world of diabetes is complex, and not all doctors are familiar with the information in the preceding paragraph. So feel free to bring up with your doctor the need to monitor your potassium and creatinine if the circumstances apply to you.

If you have diabetes kidney damage, you're at high risk of cardiovascular damage and need to take protective action. We discuss these precautions in detail earlier in this chapter.

If, despite every effort, your kidneys have progressed to the point where they have almost completely stopped working, you'll require *dialysis* (a method of purifying the blood) or a kidney transplant. If you have type 1 diabetes and you have kidney failure severe enough that you will require a kidney transplant, ask your transplant specialist about the possibility of having a simultaneous pancreas transplant. A pancreas transplant would provide you with insulin-producing islet cells and would allow you to discontinue insulin injections. If this all sounds simple and straightforward, trust us, it is *neither* of these things. Your transplant specialist will provide you with all the details including the risks and benefits of both a kidney and a pancreas transplant.

Neuropathy (Nerve Damage)

Nerve damage from diabetes is a very common but very preventable problem. Many different types of nerve damage exist, and this topic alone could fill an entire book. Most forms are uncommon or downright obscure, however, so in this section we concentrate on the more frequent types of nerve damage that you should be aware of.

Think of the nervous system as a complex network of electrical circuitry with signals going in every direction as messages are relayed from one part of your body to another. Suffice it to say, no computer yet designed has even 1 percent of the complexity of the human nervous system. Shakespeare was right when he said, "What a piece of work is man."

The most important factor leading to neuropathy in people with diabetes is elevated blood glucose levels. Nonetheless, because other causes exist (such as certain types of vitamin deficiency, overuse of alcohol, and so on), your doctor will need to exclude these.

Many health care providers tend to automatically attribute all new health problems to a person's diabetes (which drives Ian around the bend!). And, true enough, if a person with diabetes has a new health problem — like neuropathy — it may well be due to the diabetes. But this should not be assumed and, like we just said, other causes unrelated to diabetes need to be considered. If ever you have a new health problem come up and your doctor immediately tells you it is due to your diabetes, ask if other causes might be responsible. Then ask if any tests may be required to determine this.

Peripheral neuropathy

The peripheral nervous system is made up of the nerves that travel from the spinal cord to the *periphery* of your body, including your arms and legs. *Peripheral neuropathy* is damage to the nerves that make up the peripheral nervous system.

Looking at the symptoms of peripheral neuropathy

The most common symptoms of peripheral neuropathy are abnormal sensations (the collective, though not technically accurate term is *dysesthesiae*) such as a burning or numbness in the toes (and, if more advanced, other areas of the feet also). Other sensations include throbbing; aching; prickling; sharp, shooting pains; or even a tickling. Sometimes, people say they feel like they are walking on marbles or as if their shoe was stuffed with tissue paper. If neuropathy progresses, it can lead to an in inability to perceive what should be a painful stimulus. Although being unable to perceive a painful stimulus is wonderful when a surgeon is using a scalpel on you during an operation, it's no good concerning your feet, because without being able to perceive what should be a painful stimulus you may not recognize when a sore or injury has developed.

Diagnosing peripheral neuropathy

Peripheral neuropathy is usually diagnosed on *clinical grounds,* which is a fancy way of saying that doctors generally make the diagnosis based on what symptoms you are having and what they find upon examining you. One very helpful and very easy test is to see if you can recognize the feel of a thin nylon rod *(a 10-gram monofilament)* when it is pressed against your foot (in particular, the big toe). We discuss additional issues in foot care later in this chapter.

The 10-gram monofilament test gives crucial information. If your test is abnormal, you're at much greater risk of developing a foot ulcer, which can lead to gangrene — and put you at risk for amputation. You can see an online demonstration of this test and you can order your own (free) monofilament at the LEAP (Lower Extremity Amputation Prevention) website. Go to www.hrsa. gov and type "leap" into the search box at the top of that page.

Treating peripheral neuropathy

Very helpful therapies are available to treat peripheral neuropathy due to diabetes, including the following:

- **Meticulous foot care:** Because peripheral neuropathy is a key factor in putting people at risk of amputation, you require meticulous foot care to protect yourself from this complication. We discuss this in detail later in this chapter.

- **Excellent blood glucose control:** Keeping your blood glucose levels under excellent control is a key measure both to help prevent further nerve damage and, if your neuropathy is very mild, to reverse existing damage. Yet another reason (we must be up to a hundred by now) for making sure your blood glucose control is as good as possible.

- **Medications that act on nerves:** The most commonly used of these medicines are amitriptyline, gabapentin (Neurontin), pregabalin (Lyrica), and duloxetine (Cymbalta). If the area of discomfort is very small, you can try applying a topical medicine called capsaicin. (Because capsaicin is derived from chili peppers, you might think that it could really sting if it got in your eyes. And you would be right! After you apply the capsaicin to your feet, make sure you wash your hands really well before you touch *anything* else.)

- **Analgesics (pain relievers):** For mild symptoms, acetaminophen (Tylenol and many other brands) is helpful. If your symptoms are more severe or not sufficiently responding to the other therapies we mention here, using narcotic-containing analgesics such as codeine (often in combination with acetaminophen) or tramadol can be very helpful.

You may come across heavily marketed (by the manufacturer) non-prescription drug therapies to ease the pain of diabetic peripheral neuropathy. Unfortunately, minimal scientific data supports using them for this condition. We look forward to properly done studies of these drugs and cross our fingers they will show benefit. Until these studies are available, we'll remain sceptical.

Autonomic neuropathy

The *autonomic* (automatic) nervous system works behind the scenes, regulating many body functions, such as stomach function, that a person doesn't directly control. Autonomic neuropathy is nerve damage to the autonomic nervous system. This occurs only if you've had diabetes for a long time. Often the symptoms are (incorrectly) assumed to be caused by something else. Some of the most common problems include the following:

- **Sexual dysfunction:** We discuss this later on in this chapter.

- **Disorders of the stomach and large intestine:** We discuss these in the next section.

- **Bladder difficulties:** You may lose your ability to recognize an urge to empty your bladder even when it is full (*neurogenic* bladder). This leads you to retain urine within the bladder, and can make you more prone to urinary tract infections and, in the most severe cases, kidney malfunction. The most common symptom alerting you that bladder malfunction is developing is repeatedly passing only tiny quantities of urine (basically a problem with overflow, akin to water dripping down the sides of an over-filled glass).

- **Abnormal heart rate:** Your heart normally has the ability to slow down and speed up to match your body's needs. If you develop damage to the part of the autonomic nervous system that helps regulate your heart rate, your heart may end up beating too fast.

- **Low blood pressure when standing:** When a person stands up the blood pressure normally drops by a very small amount (less than 10 millimetres of mercury on a blood pressure machine). Some people with autonomic neuropathy have a greater drop in blood pressure (called *orthostatic* (or *postural*) *hypotension*); this can lead to feeling lightheaded or faint.

- **Sweating problems:** Excess sweating can occur. One very unusual problem is sweating over your forehead as you start to eat your food. This is called *gustatory* sweating.

Other types of neuropathy

These are some other, important forms of neuropathy to be aware of:

- **Carpal tunnel syndrome:** Carpal tunnel syndrome causes certain fingers in the hand to become numb due to compression of a nerve in the wrist. We discuss this condition later in this chapter, in the section, "Musculoskeletal Problems (Muscles, Joints, and Such)."

✓ **Extra-ocular muscle palsy:** In this condition one of the muscles that controls eye movement becomes damaged, which typically leads to double vision. Fortunately, this problem spontaneously corrects, but that can take a number of weeks or even months.

✓ **Lateral femoral cutaneous nerve syndrome:** In this condition (also known as *lateral femoral cutaneous nerve entrapment* or more lyrically as *meralgia paresthetica*) the lateral femoral cutaneous nerve, which is located on the side of the thigh, is damaged, causing numbness in this region. This problem typically spontaneously resolves with time.

Hearing loss is also more common amongst people living with diabetes. The reasons for this aren't yet fully clear, but it could be that nerve damage within the ear is a main factor.

Having diabetes and reading about the various neuropathies that can occur may make you feel discouraged or alarmed or both. Although that makes perfect sense, remind yourself that most of these complications are avoidable by having the best possible blood glucose control. Ultimately, we hope the closest you'll ever get to a nerve problem will be when you try to get a date with that cute neighbour of yours.

Preventing Pneumonia

Having diabetes places you at increased risk of developing pneumonia. You can reduce your risk of developing two potentially dangerous types of pneumonia by being vaccinated against them.

For people living with diabetes, the CDA recommends the following vaccinations:

✓ *Influenza vaccination* (a "flu shot") annually to reduce your likelihood of acquiring *influenza,* a type of viral infection.

✓ *Pneumococcal vaccination* to protect you against *pneumococcal* pneumonia. This is a type of bacterial infection. Unlike influenza vaccination, pneumoccoal vaccination is not given annually. It is given when you are 18 years of age or older with a one-time revaccination if you are older than 65 and your initial vaccination was administered when you were less than 65 with at least five years between administrations.

Mental Health Problems

Over the past few years physicians have become increasingly aware of how commonly mental health problems affect people with diabetes. We discuss these here.

Depression

If you have diabetes, you're more likely to develop depression, and, conversely, if you have depression, you are more likely to develop (type 2) diabetes. The first of these seems, at first glance, to be readily explained given the hassles — both physical and mental — that diabetes poses. But that's only a partial explanation because many people with diabetes, despite handling these stresses just fine thank you very much, still develop depression. The reason for this is unclear. It is similarly unclear why people with depression are more likely to develop diabetes. Researchers have looked at factors such as whether depression could lead to diabetes because people who are depressed may be less likely to eat healthfully, less likely to exercise, and so on, but these factors do not give a full explanation.

(In yet another example of what's new is old, Thomas Willis, a famous British physician of yesteryear, observed in 1674 that "diabetes is caused by sadness or long sorrow.")

Suffice it to say, if you have diabetes and are feeling blue, don't ignore it. Dealing with depression is of paramount importance, both for its own sake and also because if you're depressed you are much less likely to pay attention to your diabetes. We discuss coping with diabetes and depression further in Chapter 1.

Dementia

For uncertain reasons, having diabetes increases one's risk of developing dementia. This higher likelihood may be related in part to higher rates of cerebrovascular disease and stroke, but other unknown factors are likely also present seeing as Alzheimer's disease is also more common in people living with diabetes. Until more is known about the relationship between diabetes and dementia (and likely even when it is), we recommend following the key measures of good diabetes care we espouse throughout this book — particularly, striving for excellent blood glucose levels, blood pressure, and lipid control.

Digestive Disorders: Problems of the Stomach, Intestines, and Liver

Think of your gut as a long, hollow tube extending from your mouth to your anus. Stretched end to end it would reach over 8 metres (26 feet); once again, please do *not* try this at home! Diabetes can affect the gut in a variety of ways. We discuss these in this section.

Gastroparesis

Gastroparesis is a condition in which your stomach becomes less efficient at propelling food into your small intestine. As a consequence, you may find that you get full very quickly as you eat. Additionally, because nutrients don't get absorbed as efficiently (nutrients get absorbed almost exclusively from the small bowel, not the stomach), your blood glucose control may become erratic.

Doctors treat gastroparesis with medicines (such as metoclopramide and domperidone) that enhance stomach emptying. Also, if you are taking rapid-acting insulin with meals, your doctor may recommend you take this insulin *after* your meal instead of before. (We discuss this further in Chapter 13.)

Diarrhea

Diarrhea can occur for one of several reasons, including damage to the nerves that control intestinal function and excess numbers of bacteria (bacterial overgrowth) within the bowel. Depending on the specific nature of the problem, your doctor may prescribe either antibiotics or medicine to slow down bowel function.

Celiac disease

Although not caused by diabetes, *celiac disease* is a common intestinal disease in people who have type 1 diabetes. (Studies show that about 5 percent of people with type 1 diabetes have celiac disease; however, often it is undiagnosed.) Celiac disease is a condition in which the lining of the small intestine in certain individuals becomes damaged when exposed to *gluten* (this is a protein found in wheat, rye, and barley). This damage leads to your body not absorbing food's nutrients consistently and, as a result, may lead to erratic blood glucose control. Symptoms include indigestion, bloating, diarrhea, and weight loss, although pretty well any gastrointestinal symptom can occur. Fortunately, if you stop consuming foods or any other nutrients that contain gluten, the bowel will be able to heal. However, you need to keep that up for the rest of your life. Celiac disease is diagnosed with a blood test and an *endoscopy*, in which a flexible fibre-optic tube is swallowed and passed through the stomach into the small intestine to get a biopsy.

Because celiac disease is common in people with type 1 diabetes (and is often undiagnosed or misdiagnosed), we recommend testing for it if your doctor has even the slightest suspicion that you may suffer from it. In particular, if you have type 1 diabetes and you have either persisting gastrointestinal symptoms (as described in the preceding paragraph) or erratic blood glucose control, ask your doctor to test you for celiac disease.

You can learn more about celiac disease in *Celiac Disease For Dummies* (Wiley); a book Ian co-wrote with the wonderful gastroenterologist, Dr. Sheila Crowe.

Liver disease

If you have diabetes — particularly if your blood glucose control isn't very good — your liver may accumulate excessive quantities of fat, a condition unimaginatively but straightforwardly called *fatty liver* (or, more fully, *non-alcoholic fatty liver disease*). It was long thought this was a pretty harmless condition, however, recent evidence suggests it may lead to the development of a much more serious condition: *cirrhosis of the liver.*

The first clue your doctor may have that you are developing liver damage is often the finding, on routine blood tests, of an elevated liver enzyme level (such as an *ALT*). Key aspects of treating fatty liver are weight control, exercise, optimizing blood glucose and lipid levels, and avoiding alcohol. Evidence also suggests that metformin and thiazolidinedione (TZD) medication may help (we discuss these drugs in detail in Chapter 12).

Foot Disease in Diabetes

The most serious threat to your foot is an ulcer, because this can lead to infection, gangrene, and, ultimately, the need for amputation. (This sequence of events is often triggered by seemingly minor trauma.) For this reason, you need to keep your feet healthy and happy. You must develop an obsession with your feet. A veritable love affair with your feet. Indeed, you must develop a foot fetish!

In a sense, foot disease is really a combination of many of the different topics we cover in this chapter. Typically, a person with diabetes who runs into foot problems has a combination of peripheral neuropathy and peripheral arterial disease (PAD) and may have skin problems as well (which we discuss in the next section). Peripheral neuropathy and PAD are most common if you're older and, especially, if you've had diabetes for many years. As such, if you are young and have had diabetes for only a short period of time you are at low risk of developing diabetes foot complications whereas if you've had diabetes for a number of years and you've already got numbness or lack of sensation in your feet or if you're known to have impaired circulation in your legs then you're at much higher risk of foot problems and it is especially important that you follow the advice in this section.

Protecting your feet

In this section we look at measures you can undertake to protect your feet.

Inspect at your feet

Inspect your feet carefully at least once a day. Usually this is most convenient after you complete your shower or bath. Check your toes (including between your toes) and check your soles and the sides of your feet. You are looking for cuts, cracks, calluses, flaking skin (which may indicate a fungal infection called *athlete's foot*), dry skin, sores, blisters, and foreign bodies. (No, this doesn't refer to visiting dignitaries; it refers to things like splinters or even tacks, which, if you have significant nerve damage, could be imbedded in your foot without your even knowing it.) Most important, you are looking for openings in the skin, such as ulcerations (which appear as small holes in the skin surface), and areas of redness with heat and pus (which likely indicate an infection).

If you see an open sore on your foot — in particular if pus and/or surrounding redness is present — you *must* seek *immediate* medical attention because you likely have an infection. If you have a foot infection, time is of the essence. Every day that goes by without proper treatment increases your risk of the infection worsening, potentially leading to amputation. Tragically, Ian has seen dozens of people who had amputations that could have been avoided if only they had followed the simple advice contained in this section. (If, however, you have only a minor cut or scratch, clean it with soap and water and then cover it with a dry dressing. Be sure to change the dressing daily. And keep a close eye on it to make sure it remains minor and heals promptly.)

If you're unable to lift your feet up close enough to your eyes to inspect them, you can try using a mirror propped up against a wall (like you see in shoe stores) or you can buy a mirror with a long shaft and an angled handle.

Here's one other simple, effective, and very inexpensive way to have your feet inspected: Ask a loved one to check your feet for you. Don't worry about asking. Remember, if they love you, they love *all* of you.

If you choose to go online and discover what a diabetic foot ulcer looks like, be forewarned that websites invariably show only the most grisly, worst-case scenarios. Finding images of the early, mild, more common type of foot ulcer is much more difficult than finding these horrific cases.

Your doctor should inspect your feet regularly — at least annually and more often if you're known to have foot problems or are at high risk for them. Help your doctor help you: If your doctor hasn't checked your feet recently, while you sit in the examining room waiting for the doctor, take off your shoes and socks and, when the doctor joins you, ask her to have a look at your feet. (If she tells you it's not necessary, feel free to blame us and tell her we felt it *was* necessary.)

Determine if you have a lack of sensation

As we discuss in the section on peripheral neuropathy, diabetes can make your feet less able to feel stimuli, including unpleasant ones that should be causing you pain. This puts you at much higher risk of developing foot ulcers.

Touch different parts of your feet (with your finger or, even better, with a monofilament as we discuss earlier). Do you feel your fingers touching your feet as you should? Can you feel crumbs — assuming there are crumbs! — underfoot when walking barefoot (which, of course, you shouldn't) on the kitchen floor? Does the kitchen floor feel cold on your bare feet? If you answered "no" to any of these questions you may have peripheral neuropathy and be at increased risk of further foot problems.

If your feet have an impaired ability to feel things (and in fact even if they don't), you should avoid using a heating pad on your feet.

Wear your shoes on your hands before you wear them on your feet

Before you put on your shoes, look and feel inside them (with your fingers, not your toes) to make sure that they don't contain any errant pebbles, tacks, paper clips, or any other object that could damage your feet. And speaking of shoes . . .

Buy only very comfortable, well-fitting shoes

If you have new shoes, break them in by wearing them initially for no more than one to two hours at a time.

If you are prone to swollen feet, make sure the socks you use are not too tight, and, because swelling tends to be at its worst after you've been up on your feet all day, be sure to buy your shoes in the late afternoon (when your feet will be at their largest).

Long-term diabetes complications — including foot complications — are more likely to develop the longer you've had diabetes. So if you are an 18-year-old woman who's had diabetes for one year and you're wondering if it's okay to wear high heels to your high school prom, it is. Well, from a diabetes standpoint anyhow.

Keep your feet well groomed

Your toenails must be kept short (but not too short). Cut them straight across (use an emery board to smooth the edges). If you have impaired eyesight have someone else cut your toenails for you. If you don't have a loved one or friend who can do this for you, a foot care professional — including podiatrists, chiropodists, and specialized nurses — can help you out.

You want to keep:

- *The soles of your feet from getting overly dry.* If dryness is a problem for you, apply a good skin lotion in the morning and at bedtime.
- *The spaces between your toes from getting overly moist.* If excess moisture between your toes is a problem for you, apply liberal quantities of powder after you bathe.

Check your feet for calluses

These are often a trigger leading to foot ulceration. If you have calluses, corns, or warts, you should not treat them yourself; have a foot care professional deal with them.

Test the waters

You would never dive into unknown waters, right? Well, you should never *step* into unknown waters either, even in your own bathroom. Before you step into a bath, use your hand (or, even better, your elbow) to make sure the water is not too hot.

The only place your feet can be naked is in bed

It is, of course, none of our business whether you sleep in the buff or in a parka. But we will take the liberty of making it our business to recommend that the only place your feet can be safely naked is when you're in bed. Anytime you are up and around (even in the middle of the night), walking around your house, down the street, at the beach or anywhere else you should wear appropriate footwear. We have seen many people who developed foot ulcers and, in some cases, gangrene and subsequent amputations because they didn't follow this advice, stepped on something sharp, and injured their foot. (Again, like most of the recommendations in this section, this advice is particularly important if you've had diabetes for many years.)

Don't soak your feet

You may be surprised to read this, but soaking your feet is seldom a good idea because it can make the skin overly soft and fragile (think waterlogged) and actually increase your risk for getting a foot infection. If you really want to soak your feet, ensure the water is not too hot *and* limit your soaks to no more than 10 to 20 minutes.

Don't smoke

'Nuff said.

Skin Disease in Diabetes

You may already have discovered that to cope with diabetes, having a thick skin — in a manner of speaking — helps. (Refer to Chapter 1 for our discussion about dealing with well-meaning but irritating casual acquaintances who act like diabetes police and try to instruct you about what you can and cannot eat.) In this section we focus on the other, physical, thick skin that people with diabetes can get as well as other skin problems that are of special importance.

These are the skin conditions you should watch out for:

- **Lipohypertrophy:** This is a buildup of fatty tissue under the skin in areas of repeated insulin injection (especially if you are reusing your needles — which, by the way, we don't advocate). It appears as bumps and lumps — sometimes as large as tennis balls (or even cantaloupes!). It isn't a danger in and of itself, but it's of major importance in another way. Insulin absorption from areas of lipohypertrophy can be erratic and, not surprisingly, causes erratic blood glucose control. Also, for people concerned with appearances, these lumps may pose aesthetic issues.

  Never inject insulin into areas of lipohypertrophy. By avoiding injecting insulin into these affected areas, the lipohypertrophy will gradually shrink, but it can take years to see much improvement. (Many people with diabetes treated with insulin develop a favourite spot to inject and repeatedly use this same area; this is understandable but unfortunate as it is a sure-fire way of promoting lipohypertrophy.)

- **Sores on the feet:** Take *any* wound, ulcer, sore, or other form of skin breakdown on the feet very seriously. See the section "Foot Disease in Diabetes" earlier in this chapter for more information.

Some skin problems may raise worries but in fact are fairly harmless. These include the following:

- **Acanthosis nigricans:** This is a dark, velvety increase in pigmentation on the back of the neck and the armpits in some people with type 2 diabetes. (It can also occur without type 2 diabetes if you have insulin resistance.) It isn't dangerous and doesn't require treatment. Some people mistakenly think these areas are signs of poor hygiene. This is definitely not the case.

- **Bruising:** This may occur at insulin injection sites.

- **Nail infections:** The medical term for this is *onychomycoses*. People with diabetes commonly develop fungal infections of the toenails. The affected nails appear thickened and yellow-brown. The problem itself is not serious, but if you have a fungal nail infection, you should pay special attention to the health of the skin around the nail to make sure that your nail is not irritating it and making it red, abraded, or sore. Infected nails can be treated with anti-fungal medicine, but this is usually unnecessary and in any event the problem tends to recur. The nails can be quite difficult to cut, in which case we recommend that you have it done professionally (by a podiatrist or other foot professional).

✔ **Necrobiosis lipoidica diabeticorum:** Try saying that quickly three times (assuming you can pronounce it in the first place)! This mouthful of a disease (fortunately abbreviated as NLD) affects the legs and feet (rarely the upper limbs) and shows up as reddish-brown, shiny patches. The skin is often thinner in these areas. Only rarely does it lead to significant problems apart from its appearance. No particularly effective treatment exists, but corticosteroid medication injected into the affected area or applied topically is sometimes used. Typically, NLD fades with time.

✔ **Thickened skin:** As mentioned in the introduction to this section, people with diabetes can have thickening of the skin. This is felt as, well, thick skin. It is not important and will not make you unwell.

✔ **Vitiligo:** People with vitiligo lose normal skin pigmentation and look very pale. Vitiligo is not unique to diabetes, but type 1 (not type 2) diabetes does put you at increased risk of developing it. Vitiligo has cosmetic importance (especially for Black Canadians), but is not a threat to your health.

✔ **Xanthomata:** These are small, yellow marks that can occur in a variety of parts of the body, especially the eyelids (where they are called *xanthelasma*). Their importance is confined to the fact that they are often a clue that your lipids may be abnormal (see earlier in this chapter for a discussion about lipids).

Musculoskeletal Problems (Muscles, Joints, and Such)

The *musculoskeletal system* in your body is made up of your muscles, bones, joints, and connecting material (such as ligaments and tendons), all of which allow you to move and get around. When most people think diabetes, they usually don't think of musculoskeletal problems, but, for unknown reasons, these too (alas) can occur. The most important types are as follows:

✔ **Carpal tunnel syndrome:** In this condition the *median nerve* gets compressed as it travels through the wrist. It can cause a feeling of numbness in the hand (particularly the thumb, index, and middle fingers). Carpal tunnel syndrome can occur for many reasons, diabetes among them. Treatment is geared toward avoiding precipitating factors (such as *repetitive strain injury,* as can occur with prolonged typing) and, if necessary, may include splinting, medication, or even surgery.

- ✔ **Diabetic hand syndrome:** In this condition the hands feel stiff and sore. Treatment is with anti-inflammatory medication and physiotherapy. Sometimes, scar tissue forms in the tissues that surround tendons in the palm of the hand and restricts movement of a finger (a *Dupuytren's contracture*); severe cases are treated surgically.

- ✔ **Frozen shoulder:** Even during another muggy summer heat wave, you can run into problems with a frozen shoulder. *Frozen shoulder* is a condition where your shoulder joint becomes stiff (and sometimes a bit painful) as a result of inflammation in the capsule that surrounds the joint. Treatment options include physiotherapy, anti-inflammatory medication, steroid injections into the joint (this procedure is most often done by either a *rheumatologist* — that is, an arthritis doctor — or an orthopedic surgeon), and, in severe cases, surgery.

Thyroid Disease and Diabetes

The thyroid is a small endocrine gland that sits in the neck just in front of the trachea (the windpipe). The thyroid gland has one job: to make thyroid hormone. This hormone controls metabolism.

If you have type 1 diabetes you are at increased risk for developing thyroid disease — especially thyroid underfunctioning. (It is less clear if people living with type 2 diabetes are at increased risk — compared to someone without diabetes — of thyroid disease.)

Symptoms of thyroid underfunctioning (*hypothyroidism*) include weight gain, feeling cold, constipation, muscle aching, brittle hair, and slow thinking. Symptoms of thyroid overfunctioning (*hyperthyroidism*) include weight loss, tremors, palpitations, feeling hot, excess sweating, frequent bowel movements, and anxiety. (Think of hyperthyroidism symptoms as the hormonal equivalent to how you'd feel if you drank 30 cups of caffeinated coffee; think of hypothyroidism symptoms as how you might feel if you were in *realllllly lowwwww* gear.)

If you have diabetes and you develop hyperthyroidism, it can make your blood glucose levels go up. Conversely, if you have diabetes and you develop hypothyroidism, it can make your blood glucose levels go down.

If you develop symptoms like those we describe, ask your doctor to check your thyroid. This is readily done with a simple blood test (the TSH). Also, because thyroid disease is so common in people with type 1 diabetes, we recommend that everyone with type 1 diabetes have their TSH level measured from time to time.

Gum Disease in Diabetes

Elevated glucose levels within your mouth can promote the growth of bacteria. These germs can attack the gums, causing *gingivitis* (gum infection), which in turn can lead to problems with your teeth and, of greater concern, blood infections. Conversely, gingivitis, like other infections in your body, can make your blood glucose levels go up.

You can help prevent getting gum disease by doing what your mother (or father, of course) likely prescribed for you when you were a child: Brush your teeth twice a day, floss your teeth once a day, and see your dentist regularly. It's that simple.

Erectile Dysfunction Due to Diabetes

Up to 50 percent of men with diabetes have some form of sexual dysfunction; most commonly *erectile dysfunction,* the inability to have or sustain an erection sufficient for intercourse.

Another form of sexual dysfunction that can occur with long-standing diabetes is called *retrograde ejaculation,* wherein you are able to achieve a normal erection and experience a normal orgasm, but no semen emerges from the penis, but instead goes the reverse direction into the bladder. This is not a serious problem and requires treatment only if you wish to father a child.

Your doctor is there to help you — *all* of you! — so you should feel free to bring up *any* problems you are experiencing including those related to erectile dysfunction. Some men are hesitant to talk about these issues, as they're concerned the doctor will find the topic uncomfortable. Trust us when we tell you your doctor — male or female — will find it about as uncomfortable to discuss your erectile dysfunction as discussing your sore throat or your indigestion or, for that matter, the weather!

Why the spirit may be willing, but the penis isn't

Erectile dysfunction (ED) in a man with diabetes is usually due to poor blood supply and/or nerve damage to the penis. Nonetheless, you and your doctor must not fall into the all-too-common trap of assuming that if you have diabetes, every conceivable problem you might develop must be diabetes related. People with diabetes can encounter the same problems as everyone else. Or, as Henry Kissinger (or Golda Meir, some would argue) famously said, "Even paranoids have enemies." Some non-diabetes-related causes of erectile dysfunction include the following:

- **An adverse effect from medication:** This is particularly common with medicines such as beta blockers, thiazide diuretics, and some antidepressants.

- **Hormonal abnormalities:** Insufficient levels of the male hormone testosterone or excess levels of a pituitary hormone called prolactin can interfere with normal sexual function.

- **Psychological factors:** Problems such as stress and depression can interfere with normal sexual function.

- **Trauma and other physical abnormalities of the penis:** *Peyronie's disease*, for example, causes a curvature of the erect penis which, if severe, can make intercourse difficult.

Psychological factors — whether anxiety, stress, depression, or something else — leading to erectile dysfunction are, of course, no less important to address than any other cause, including diabetes. Your family physician can help determine whether a psychological factor is the cause of your sexual difficulties.

You can help protect yourself from developing erectile dysfunction due to diabetes by

- Maintaining good blood glucose

- Keeping your blood pressure under control

- Having excellent lipid levels

- Not smoking (Smoking leads to blockage of the arteries, including the arteries that supply blood to the penis.)

Erectile dysfunction in a man with diabetes is, as mentioned, usually due at least in part to problems with arterial circulation. If you have circulatory problems affecting your penis, you also may have circulatory problems elsewhere in your body including your heart. Therefore, if you have erectile dysfunction you and your doctor should look at and reduce your risk factors for circulatory disease (see "Preventing a heart attack or stroke" earlier in this chapter).

How to improve erectile dysfunction

Several forms of therapy are available to treat erectile dysfunction. Some treatments are geared toward correcting specific reversible causes (such as stopping a medicine if it is causing your problem). Other treatments include the following:

✓ **Oral medications (Cialis, Levitra, Viagra):** These are members of the PDE5 (phosphodiesterase type 5) inhibitor family of medicines. You would have a hard time missing the numerous (and typically very entertaining) ads for these drugs. Each of these drugs has somewhat different properties but they are more similar than dissimilar. Some people respond better to one of these drugs than another, so, if one doesn't work, ask your doctor about trying another. One potential advantage of Cialis, compared to Levitra or Viagra, is that it can routinely be taken daily rather than "as needed" so that less planning is required before intercourse. For most men with erectile dysfunction, PDE5 inhibitor drugs are the first therapy that is recommended. Although PDE5 inhibitor therapy usually works well at first, as time goes by it often loses some — or all — of its effectiveness and other types of treatment become necessary.

PDE5 inhibitors may have side effects. Some men experience headaches, facial flushing, or indigestion. These drugs can also cause a temporary colour tinge to one's vision as well as increased sensitivity to light and blurred vision. These side effects tend to decline with continued use of the medicines.

Men who have coronary artery disease (which we discuss earlier in this chapter) and take nitrate drugs (such as nitroglycerine) should not take PDE5 inhibitor medicine. The combination of a PDE5 inhibitor and nitrates may cause a severe and even life-threatening drop in blood pressure.

✓ **Injection into the penis:** Several types of medicine can be injected directly into the shaft of the penis to create an erection. (This is called *intracavernosal* or *intracorporeal* therapy.) Giving yourself a needle into your penis may sound pretty nasty, but if you can overcome the understandable fear, you'll find that the amount of discomfort is usually minimal and that this type of therapy is often very effective.

✓ **Suppository in the penis:** This form of therapy involves inserting a small amount of medicine directly into the urethral opening at the tip of the penis. The success rate is not as good as with the first two options.

✓ **Vacuum device:** This is a tube that fits directly over the penis and, with the use of a connected pump, allows for blood to fill the penis, at which point an erection is achieved and a rubber band is placed around the base of the penis to prevent the blood from escaping. Some men find the device cumbersome to use, but in general it is quite effective, and we feel that this is an under-used therapy.

✓ **Implanted penile prosthesis:** If none of the other measures in this list is helping, another option is to have a prosthesis surgically implanted directly into the penis. A variety of types are available, some of which create a permanent erection while others have an implanted pump (placed in the scrotum) that allows a man to create an erection on demand. This is generally a very successful — and underused — treatment.

Your family physician is almost always the person for you to see about your erectile dysfunction and to receive a prescription for a PDE5 inhibitor. The other therapies listed above are more within the purview of a urologist (they are specialists in this field). If you are not responding well enough to a PDE5 inhibitor, let your family physician or diabetes specialist know. They can refer you to a urologist. We see far too many men who, if a PDE5 inhibitor is not helping them, assume no other treatment options exist and never bring up the topic with their doctor again. If, after meeting with a urologist and trying one of the therapies we discuss earlier, you still have issues, tell the doctor. The doctor needs to know so you can try one of the other types of treatment.

Dealing with Female Sexual Problems Related to Diabetes

Sexual problems in women with diabetes have, regrettably, not received nearly the attention that male sexual difficulties have. Some types of female sexual dysfunction, though not unique to people with diabetes, are more common for them. Fortunately, treatment is available that will allow you to have an active and pleasurable sex life.

These are the most frequent issues you may encounter:

- **Vaginal dryness:** The most common causes are poor glucose control, nerve damage, impaired blood flow, or estrogen deficiency. Vaginal dryness makes intercourse more difficult and less pleasurable (lubrication increases vaginal sensitivity) — sometimes even painful. It can be treated with lubricants that are water-based (such as K-Y Jelly) or oil-based (such as vegetable oil). Water-based lubricants are easier to clean up. Oral stimulation by your partner may also assist in lubricating the vagina. If you are menopausal, lack of estrogen could be the main cause of your vaginal dryness, in which case vaginal estrogen preparations (which are much safer than oral estrogen) may be an option for you. To know if vaginal estrogen therapy is a suitable option for you, ask your doctor to review your specific situation.

- **Vaginal yeast infections:** Diabetes and, in particular, poor blood glucose control can make you prone to recurrent vaginal infections. Improving your glucose control and taking an antifungal medicine would be in order.

- **Vaginal thinning:** Menopause leads to lower levels of estrogen and this, in turn, can cause not only vaginal dryness (see the first item in this list) but can also cause the lining of the vagina to become thin. In this case vaginal estrogen therapy may be an option for you.

✓ **Decreased genital sensation:** Nerve damage can lead to reduced sensitivity around the genital area and this, in turn, can reduce sexual enjoyment. Treatment options include gentle stimulation by touch or by use of a hand-held vibrator gently applied to the clitoris.

✓ **Bladder problems:** If you have difficulty controlling your bladder, you may experience leakage during intercourse. Try to empty your bladder before intercourse. Other treatments, depending on the cause of the problem, include medication or surgery (bladder suspension).

✓ **Adverse effects from medications:** Some medicines — particularly some types of antidepressants — can interfere with sexual function. If you have recently started a new medicine only to find your sexual function is becoming impaired, speak to your doctor about possibly switching to a different medicine.

✓ **Psychological factors:** Many different psychological factors can influence your ability to enjoy sexual relations, including poor self-image if you don't like your appearance or if you are concerned about what your partner thinks of your appearance. As you work with nutrition therapy, weight loss (if you are overweight), and exercise to improve your glucose control, you may find you're seeing yourself (and your partner is seeing you) as more attractive, and that, in turn, may be the best therapy of all for your sexual dysfunction. If you're feeling anxious, stressed, or depressed, speak to your doctor to see what kind of help is available. In some cases your doctor may refer you to a specialist for therapy.

Chapter 7

Diabetes and Pregnancy

- -

In This Chapter
▶ Looking at gestational diabetes
▶ Preparing for and handling pregnancy when you have diabetes before pregnancy

- -

*1*an remembers way back when, years ago, he received from his editor the draft of this very chapter from the first edition of this book. "Ian," the editor said, "aren't you concerned that you're going to worry people with all the pregnancy dangers you write about?" "Absolutely," Ian agreed, "but I'd be much more concerned if I *didn't* worry them." And that's the thing about diabetes and pregnancy; yes, you have many potential hazards to be concerned about. But you can greatly lessen these dangers with the meticulous health care that you and your pregnancy deserve. In this chapter we show you how.

If you have diabetes, pregnancy does complicate matters; often quite a bit. Nonetheless, it can and will still be a period of joy, excitement, and anticipation. You will never have another time when the efforts you apply to your diabetes are so crucial, and you can be assured you'll have many people working with you all the way.

When we talk about diabetes and pregnancy, we distinguish temporary, pregnancy-related diabetes *(gestational diabetes)* from diabetes that was present before you got pregnant *(pregestational diabetes)*.

Technically, gestational diabetes refers to *any* form of diabetes discovered during pregnancy. However, in the overwhelming majority of cases, when diabetes is found during pregnancy, it is temporary, pregnancy-induced diabetes, not pregestational diabetes. The implications, risks, and treatment are very different for both of these types. We discuss both gestational diabetes and pregestational diabetes in detail in this chapter.

Gestational Diabetes

Gestational diabetes (often abbreviated as GDM which is short for *gestational diabetes mellitus*) occurs in women who had normal blood glucose levels before pregnancy, but who run into elevations of blood glucose *during* pregnancy. (If you had diabetes *before* you get pregnant then you have a different condition, called *pregestational diabetes*, which we discuss later in this chapter.) With gestational diabetes, the degree of glucose elevation is so mild that symptoms of hyperglycemia (see Chapter 2), such as increased thirst and visual blurring, do not develop and your A1C level (see Chapter 9) remains normal. (Of course you may develop a frequent urge to pass urine during your pregnancy, but that is not due to gestational diabetes; it is due to a growing future gymnast testing out his or her skills by doing flips on your bladder or, as Ian's wife used to say, doing "bladder dancing.")

Gestational diabetes is very common. Just how common, however, depends on how one defines the level of blood glucose above which gestational diabetes is diagnosed. Depending on how one diagnoses gestational diabetes, it occurs in anywhere from 4 to 18 percent of all pregnancies.

As we discover in this section, the main reason that gestational diabetes is a concern is that this condition puts you at increased risk of delivering a large infant. This is important because a large infant can be difficult to deliver and, as a result, the baby can run into complications during delivery. Fortunately, excellent treatment exists to improve the odds that your infant will be of normal size. Indeed, the great majority of women with gestational diabetes have uneventful deliveries and perfectly healthy babies.

Exploring the causes of gestational diabetes

As you might imagine, many hormonal changes take place during pregnancy, not the least of which is the release of hormones produced by the *placenta*. These placental hormones increase insulin resistance (see Chapter 3 for a discussion of insulin resistance). In a normal pregnancy, the pancreas can respond to this challenge by increasing the amount of insulin it makes so that your blood glucose control remains normal. If you develop gestational diabetes, your pancreas cannot respond sufficiently, so your blood glucose levels rise above normal.

Diagnosing gestational diabetes

One of the most controversial — indeed, heated — areas of diabetes management among diabetes specialists and obstetricians around the world is determining the best way to diagnose gestational diabetes. Some organizations recommend one approach, other organizations another. Ian recently participated in a debate on the topic and, suffice to say, is still recovering from his injuries. (We discuss *why* this is so controversial in the sidebar "Controversies in diagnosing gestational diabetes.") The Canadian Diabetes Association (CDA) 2013 Clinical Practice Guidelines, do note a "preferred" strategy, but recognize that *either* of the available strategies is appropriate. Your physician will, therefore, use the approach they feel is best. We discuss both strategies in this section.

Although controversy exists over the best way to *diagnose* gestational diabetes, far less controversy exists over how to *treat* gestational diabetes. We discuss this in the next section.

The Canadian Diabetes Association recommends *every* pregnant woman be tested for gestational diabetes using either a two-step approach or a one-step approach.

The two-step approach

This is the traditional approach to diagnosing gestational diabetes (and the one the CDA notes to be preferred), so we discuss this first. This approach has — you guessed it — two steps:

1. **When you reach 24 to 28 weeks into your pregnancy, your doctor (usually the obstetrician) will send you for a 50-gram challenge.** This requires you to drink a sweet drink containing 50 grams of carbohydrate. You don't have to be fasting for this test. One hour after you drink the fluid, the laboratory will draw a blood sample from your arm to check your glucose level. If your test result is

   - **Less than 7.8 mmol/L,** it is normal, you do *not* have gestational diabetes, and no further testing is required.

   - **7.8 mmol/L up to and including 11.0 mmol/L,** it is *not yet determined* if you have gestational diabetes and your doctor will need to send you for an additional test. This additional test is a 75-gram tolerance test (which we discuss next).

   - **11.1 mmol/L or higher,** you *have* gestational diabetes, and no further testing is required.

2. **If your 50-gram challenge result is 7.8 mmol/L up to and including 11.0 mmol/L your doctor will then send you for a two-hour, 75-gram glucose tolerance test (GTT).** For this test, after you fast for eight hours, a health care professional will draw blood from you before, and then one and two hours after drinking a sweet drink containing 75 grams of carbohydrate. You have gestational diabetes if you have *one or more* of the following results:

   - Fasting blood glucose 5.3 mmol/L or higher

   - One-hour blood glucose 10.6 mmol/L or higher

   - Two-hour blood glucose 9.0 mmol/L or higher

The one-step approach

This approach differs from the two-step approach in that it has, yup, just one step. What is removed from the one-step approach is the need for a 50-gram challenge. Instead, with the one-step approach all pregnant women are sent directly for a 75-gram glucose tolerance test when they are between 24 and 28 weeks pregnant. Using the one-step approach you have gestational diabetes if you have *one or more* of the following results:

- Fasting blood glucose 5.1 mmol/L or higher
- One-hour blood glucose 10.0 mmol/L or higher
- Two-hour blood glucose 8.5 mmol/L or higher

You may have noticed that the blood glucose levels at which gestational diabetes is diagnosed are lower with the one-step approach than with the two-step approach. And you may have (correctly) surmised that this will mean a lot more women are diagnosed with gestational diabetes with the one-step approach than with the two-step approach. (This is part of the controversy about diagnosing gestational diabetes as we discuss in the sidebar.)

If you are at high risk for gestational diabetes then you should be tested for it earlier than the usual 24 to 28 week timeframe. *How early* is determined on a case-by-case basis by your physician based on their assessment of your particular risk of gestational diabetes. (We look at this topic next.) If your test is normal and you are at high risk for gestational diabetes you should be retested at 24 to 28 weeks and then again later in the pregnancy depending on your particular situation.

Determining if you are at high risk for gestational diabetes

You are at high risk of gestational diabetes if one or more of the following applies to you:

- You have previously had gestational diabetes.
- You have prediabetes (see Chapter 4).
- You have previously delivered a large infant.
- You're a member of a high-risk population (that is; being of Aboriginal, African, Asian, Hispanic, or South Asian ancestry).
- You're 35 years of age or older.
- You have a BMI of 30 or greater. (We discuss how to calculate one's BMI in Chapter 4.)

✔ You have polycystic ovary syndrome (PCOS) or acanthosis nigricans.

✔ You use corticosteroid medication.

✔ Your fetus is thought to be large or you have excess amniotic fluid (poly-hydramnios).

Treating gestational diabetes

As with other forms of diabetes, the most important part of the treatment of gestational diabetes is what *you* do for you, not what others do for you, so you must be well educated about the condition. Your doctor should refer you to a diabetes education centre where you will meet with a dietitian and a diabetes nurse educator who will provide you with the knowledge you need to help you monitor and control your gestational diabetes. Your doctor should also refer you to a diabetes specialist. The diabetes specialist will typically coordinate your diabetes care, help teach you about your gestational diabetes, review your blood glucose readings, and prescribe blood glucose–lowering medications if necessary.

Controversies in diagnosing gestational diabetes

As we discuss in the section "Diagnosing gestational diabetes," two sets of criteria are being used to diagnose gestational diabetes on a glucose tolerance test: the traditional criteria, and the newer, more stringent criteria in which lower blood glucose levels (compared with the traditional criteria) establish a diagnosis. (Both establish a diagnosis of gestational diabetes with only one abnormal test. Previous criteria required two abnormalities.)

Why the stricter criteria? These arise from data obtained in the Hyperglycemia and Adverse Pregnancy Outcomes (HAPO) study which monitored 25,000 pregnant women. This study determined that the risk of adverse maternal, fetal, and newborn outcomes was increased even at levels of blood glucose that were previously thought to be harmless and, indeed, normal during pregnancy. A subsequent meeting of diabetes experts from around the world decided, based on the HAPO data, that gestational diabetes should be diagnosed — and treated — when

blood glucose levels were lower than had previously been considered normal. This all makes perfect sense.

The controversy lies in the fact that if lower blood glucose levels on a glucose tolerance test are used to diagnose gestational diabetes, this will lead to many, *many* more women being diagnosed and treated resulting in fewer overly large babies — which of course is good — but at the price of diagnosing (and treating) many, *many* women who would have had uneventful pregnancies and healthy babies even if they had never been diagnosed and treated. So it becomes a matter of how wide a net one should use. The new criteria cast a wide net indeed.

Be sure to note, as you reflect on the information in this sidebar, that the controversy is *not* over whether gestational diabetes is an important condition and should be tested for and treated when present. The controversy is over how to define an abnormal test.

Treating gestational diabetes with nutrition

Your dietitian will set you up with a healthy eating program. This program will be geared toward assisting with blood glucose control while allowing for appropriate weight gain and ensuring adequate nutrition. Your carbohydrate intake will be moderately reduced and distributed over three meals and three snacks (one of which will be at bedtime). Think of this as a therapeutic indulgence! Your target weight gain will be based, at least in part, on your pre-pregnancy weight.

Treating gestational diabetes with exercise

Because gestational diabetes is associated with insulin resistance, and because insulin resistance is improved (though not eliminated) by exercise, daily exercise can help control your blood glucose readings. We're not talking marathon running here; even just taking a daily walk can help. Your doctor or diabetes educator can recommend exercises based on your specific circumstances and stage of pregnancy.

Treating gestational diabetes with insulin

If your blood glucose readings are too high (we discuss blood glucose targets in the next section) despite two weeks of lifestyle therapy (that is, nutrition and exercise) then medication is required. Because of its proven safety and effectiveness in treating gestational diabetes, insulin is almost always the preferred drug. (We discuss insulin therapy in detail in Chapter 13.) The idea of having to give yourself insulin may not sound particularly pleasant, but bear in mind three things:

- ✔ Unlike taxes and Canadian winters, insulin won't be forever. The moment you deliver your baby, in nearly all cases you'll discontinue your insulin.

- ✔ Giving insulin is not difficult and is not painful. If you require insulin to treat gestational diabetes you will almost certainly find it surprisingly straightforward to administer.

- ✔ Your efforts during your pregnancy will help you have a healthy baby. What could possibly be a better reward than that?

The type of insulin you are prescribed will depend on what time of day your blood glucose levels are above target. It could be one of these two types:

- ✔ **NPH insulin** will be prescribed if your blood glucose level is above target before breakfast. You take this insulin at bedtime to help keep your before-breakfast blood glucose levels in the target range. (Levemir and Lantus insulin are also effective at controlling before-breakfast blood glucose values, but NPH insulin, which typically works equally well to treat gestational diabetes, because of its longer track record of safe use during pregnancy is typically preferred for treating gestational diabetes.)

✔ **Rapid-acting insulin (Humalog or NovoRapid)** will be prescribed if your blood glucose level is above target after meals. (Sometimes regular insulin is used, but rapid-acting insulins are better at controlling after-meal blood glucose values and are therefore preferred. Apidra insulin, which, like Humalog and NovoRapid, is a form of rapid-acting insulin, has not yet been proven safe for use during pregnancy and thus is not routinely used.) You need to take rapid-acting insulin only before those meals which had been causing your blood glucose level to rise too much. For example, if your blood glucose levels after breakfast and after lunch are *within* target, but your after-supper blood glucose level is *above* target, you will need to take rapid-acting insulin only once daily (before supper). As the pregnancy progresses taking rapid-acting insulin before all meals is typically necessary.

The Canadian Diabetes Association recommends oral medication (instead of insulin) only for women with gestational diabetes who either decline insulin therapy or are taking insulin but, basically, are missing so many doses that it's not doing much good. The only recommended oral medications are glyburide and metformin. (We discuss these drugs in Chapter 12.) In the future, if scientific evidence proves that oral medications are as safe and effective as insulin, using them will be more recommended.

If you take insulin, you'll find that your insulin requirements progressively increase as your pregnancy goes along. You will know when your insulin requirements are going up because you will be frequently checking your blood glucose (see the next section) and when the insulin dose that *was* keeping your blood glucose readings within target *no longer* keeps them within target you'll likely need to increase your insulin dose. This is not only expected, it is, if anything, a good sign because it means your placenta (and fetus) are maturing the way they should. (Having said that, if your insulin requirements do not go up, that is typically fine too.) Your diabetes educators and diabetes specialist will help you adjust your insulin doses (and, indeed, will teach you how to adjust them on your own).

Think of your increasing need for insulin, as your blood glucose levels rise, as chasing a moving target: Your blood glucose levels rise, you increase your insulin doses. It works for a while then your blood glucose levels rise again, and you increase your insulin doses again. This is typical. Unfortunately many women with gestational diabetes do not know this and end up needlessly worrying when their insulin requirements climb.

When you go in to deliver your baby, unless your blood glucose level is unexpectedly high, you likely won't need any more insulin. (Labouring burns up glucose and will help to keep your blood glucose levels in check.) Similarly, after you've delivered your baby you almost certainly will no longer require insulin therapy.

Monitoring gestational diabetes

For you and your health care team to know if your treatment program is successfully controlling your blood glucose, you will need to monitor your blood glucose levels using a blood glucose meter. (We discuss blood glucose meters in detail in Chapter 9.)

Most diabetes education centres (DECs) will be able to provide you, free of charge, with a blood glucose meter (though not necessarily the blood glucose test strips), and will show you how to use it.

These are the Canadian Diabetes Association target blood glucose readings for women with gestational diabetes:

- ✔ Before meals: Below 5.3 mmol/L
- ✔ One hour after meals: Below 7.8 mmol/L
- ✔ Two hours after meals: Below 6.7 mmol/L

The CDA guidelines don't specify if "after meals" is after the start, middle, or end of meals. For the sake of consistency we suggest you use the time from *the start* of your meal. Also, whether to test one hour or two hours after a meal is controversial; so long as you aim for the target level for that time, it probably doesn't matter. Your doctor will make his or her own recommendation for you.

If you have gestational diabetes and your blood glucose level is only occasionally elevated, you need not worry — the total amount of time that your fetus is exposed to slightly higher levels of blood glucose compared to the entire nine months of your pregnancy is minimal, and will not harm your fetus. (Having quite elevated blood glucose or elevated values occurring often is a different matter; if this is happening, notify your physician to change your treatment program.)

Another source of gestational diabetes controversy is whether or not you should test your urine for ketones. Ketones are a type of acid. We know that high levels of ketones in the blood along with elevated blood glucose levels in pregnant women with *type 1 diabetes* are hazardous to a fetus. But we don't yet know if small amounts of urine ketones in women with *gestational diabetes* is any threat to the fetus.

Most diabetes specialists in Canada advocate that women with gestational diabetes check their urine once daily, before breakfast, for ketones. If they are present in more than small amounts it may indicate that you are not eating as well as you could be. In this case speak to your dietitian for nutritional advice and support.

Understanding the potential complications for the mother

Most moms with gestational diabetes sail through their pregnancy with no complications and deliver perfectly healthy babies. Serious complications seldom occur.

During labour your target blood glucose level is 4.0 to 7.0 mmol/L. Keeping your readings in this range will minimize the risk your newborn will have low blood glucose. (We discuss low blood glucose in a newborn in more detail in the next section.) Most of the time the woman with gestational diabetes who is in labour does not require insulin therapy in order to achieve these blood glucose targets since labour is, well, *labour* in the truest sense of the word. . . meaning that it is hard work and like any exercise, will help to keep your blood glucose levels in check.

If you have gestational diabetes, you do face an increased likelihood of delivering by Caesarean section because you're at risk of having a big baby (see the next section), and your obstetrician may determine that it would be unsafe for you to deliver vaginally. (Although, having said that, some evidence from medical studies shows that when a woman has been diagnosed with gestational diabetes, doctors are *automatically* more likely to deliver the baby by Caesarean section, even if little evidence exists that the fetus is large. This may be human nature at play: that is, some obstetricians understandably being influenced by what *might* happen rather that what *is* happening. Labels — including the label of having gestational diabetes — carry an impact; sometimes favourable, sometimes not.)

If you are going to have a Caesarean section and are taking insulin — particularly bedtime NPH insulin — ask your obstetrician to book your Caesarean for first thing in the morning. This will make managing your gestational diabetes easier. Because you will have given yourself insulin the night before your procedure, your morning blood glucose will likely be normal. Then, very soon, you will deliver your baby and your gestational diabetes will be gone.

Having women with gestational diabetes deliver a couple of weeks earlier than term (that is, at about 38 weeks rather than at 40 weeks) used to be standard practice. Although early delivery is sometimes necessary (such as when the fetus is too big), most women go to full term just fine. If, however, you have not delivered by 40 weeks, the obstetrician will almost always schedule your delivery, rather than waiting much longer.

Considering the potential complications for the baby

Your baby will likely be completely fine. Your baby will *not* be born with diabetes and your baby will *not* be at greater risk of birth defects. However, here are two important possible complications of gestational diabetes:

- ✔ **Macrosomia:** This is the medical term for a large baby. There are various definitions of, what exactly is, a "large" baby, but it is generally considered to be a newborn weighing more than 4000 grams (8.8 pounds). Avoiding macrosomia is the main reason that doctors look for gestational diabetes and treat it if they find it. Elevated blood glucose levels put your infant at higher risk of being large. This is not just a matter of appearances. The concern is that a large infant can be more difficult to deliver and the baby's shoulders can get stuck in the birth canal (called *shoulder dystocia*). This is an urgent situation and harm can come to the baby (due to impaired blood flow and hence, oxygen delivery to the baby's brain) during delivering.

- ✔ **Hypoglycemia:** This is low blood glucose, and your baby may develop it very soon after being born. Hospital staff usually treat it easily by giving your baby sugar water to drink. It typically does not recur beyond the first few hours after being born. Hypoglycemia in a newborn is typically considered to be a blood glucose of less than 2.6 mmol/L.

If you have gestational diabetes and deliver a large baby, you may find the hospital staff (including, alas, some doctors) look at you reproachfully and suggest — or even directly say — to you that your baby is large because you didn't monitor your diabetes well enough and, in particular, didn't control your blood glucose. However, if you're like the overwhelming majority of women with gestational diabetes, you likely looked after your diabetes *wonderfully*. The fact that you delivered a large baby does *not* mean you did anything wrong. Maybe you were destined to have a big baby, pure and simple. Or maybe some other, unknown, unrelated factor led to your baby being big. In any event, you have two choices: You can either correct the staff on their misapprehension, or you can grin and bear it. Your call. But please do not feel guilty. You did nothing wrong and, indeed, likely did everything right!

Knowing what to do after you've had your baby

Now that you've had your baby, you no longer have gestational diabetes, but some very important things remain left to do (in addition to the million other responsibilities you now have!):

✔ **Breastfeed:** Breastfeeding has many benefits for both mom and infant, especially if you've had gestational diabetes. Evidence suggests that breastfeeding may reduce your risk *and* your child's risk of subsequently developing type 2 diabetes. It may also help prevent your child from becoming overweight.

✔ **Follow a healthy lifestyle:** If you have (or have previously had) gestational diabetes you are at very high risk of developing type 2 diabetes. You can, however, substantially reduce this risk by following a healthy lifestyle after you have your baby. Do your utmost to achieve and maintain a good weight. Try to gradually get down to a BMI under 25 (we discuss how you can figure out your BMI in Chapter 4). Eat healthfully. Exercise. After all, you've got a family to stay healthy for!

✔ **Get screened for type 2 diabetes:** Because having had gestational diabetes means you are at high risk of subsequently developing type 2 diabetes, you need to be screened from time to time. The Canadian Diabetes Association recommends the following:

- Between six weeks and six months after delivery, have a 75-gram glucose tolerance test (GTT).

  Many women never end up having their glucose tolerance performed after they've delivered. To avoid missing this important test, we recommend that you and the doctor (likely your diabetes specialist) who helped you with your gestational diabetes organize the post-pregnancy GTT *before* you deliver. Doing so may be as simple as getting a lab requisition toward the end of your pregnancy and noting on your calendar when to go for your test. (And don't forget to be in touch with your doctor a few days after you've performed the test to get the results and find out what to do if it's abnormal.)

- Have ongoing periodic screening for type 2 diabetes.

- Be screened for type 2 diabetes *prior to* any future pregnancies. This is very important because if you have developed type 2 diabetes and then get pregnant, the implications are far, far greater than was the case when you had gestational diabetes. We discuss this in detail later in this chapter (see the heading "Pregestational diabetes").

✔ **Watch for symptoms of hyperglycemia:** If you start having symptoms of high blood glucose (we talk about how high blood glucose makes you feel in Chapter 2), promptly see your doctor to have your blood glucose level checked.

After you've delivered your baby you will not likely need to do any more finger prick blood glucose tests. The exception is if your doctor suspects you may have pre-existing type 2 diabetes, which just happened to be discovered during pregnancy. (Your doctor might suspect this, for example, if your blood glucose levels on the gestational diabetes GTT were far higher than normal.) In this case your doctor may recommend that you check your blood glucose daily for a few days after you deliver then, depending on your situation, from time to time thereafter.

If you used insulin during pregnancy, you probably won't have any further use for your insulin after having your baby. Rather than wasting it, if you have any unopened, unexpired insulin (or blood glucose testing supplies), consider donating it to the charity Insulin for Life (www.insulinforlifecanada.org). They will send your insulin to people in developing nations who don't have access to insulin and may get sick or even die without it.

Pregestational Diabetes (Pregnancy in Women with Type 1 or Type 2 Diabetes)

Pregestational diabetes is diabetes that you had *before* you became pregnant (and will still have after you deliver), whereas *gestational* diabetes (which we discuss earlier in this chapter) is diabetes acquired during pregnancy that goes away after your baby is born. If you have type 1 or type 2 diabetes and you get pregnant, then you have pregestational diabetes. Whenever we use the term *diabetes* in this section we are referring to *pregestational*, not gestational diabetes.

If you have diabetes and get pregnant, you have an excellent chance that everything will go well and, nine months down the road, you'll hold a beautiful, bouncing, healthy baby. You are, perhaps, waiting for a "but." If so, then you're right. Everything *can* go well, *but* to have a healthy, successful pregnancy you have tons of work to do and must look after your diabetes meticulously — indeed, obsessively — and be more careful than at any other time in your life.

How do we know that women with pregestational diabetes can have safe, healthy pregnancies and beautiful healthy babies? Well, medical studies show this and, moreover, we see it all the time! Ian has helped hundreds upon hundreds of women with pregestational diabetes navigate their way through successful pregnancies. Nothing brings greater joy to Ian's job than to have a new mom come to see him with a healthy baby in her arms. (Note to Ian's patients: please bring your baby to your appointments with him!)

Your pregnancy must be planned. Don't stop using contraception until you and your diabetes specialist have determined that getting pregnant is safe for you. This will allow you, along with your health care team, to take all necessary precautions to give you the best chance of a healthy pregnancy and a healthy baby.

Stopping your contraception (or not using any to begin with) is the same thing as *trying* to get pregnant — as many, many women (often to their great dismay) have discovered over the years.

Ian hates to sound like a disciplinarian, but as you can tell from the last two "warnings," he feels strongly — *really* strongly — about pregestational diabetes and your health. In this section we give you the straight facts. You may find this information intimidating and even scary. But it's essential reading and, well, you need to know it. So here we go . . .

Knowing what can happen to the mom

Most pregnant woman with pregestational diabetes don't run into serious problems, but they have an increased risk of the following:

✔ **High blood pressure and toxemia:** High blood pressure by itself can be successfully controlled with oral medications. If, however, you have high blood pressure with *toxemia* this is far more serious and requires hospitalization and, typically, early delivery. Toxemia is a condition of raised blood pressure, protein in the urine, and fluid retention leading to swelling and, at times, more serious complications including seizures.

✔ **Worsening of retinopathy:** If you have retinopathy before you get pregnant it can worsen during pregnancy. Usually the degree of worsening is small, but it can be substantial to the point of requiring retinal laser surgery. (If you have no retinopathy whatsoever prior to pregnancy, you likely won't develop it during your pregnancy.) We discuss diabetes eye disease in more detail in Chapter 6.

✔ **Worsening of kidney function:** If you have impaired kidney function *before* you get pregnant it can worsen during pregnancy:

- If prior to pregnancy your only kidney problem was that you had protein in the urine, then this may increase during pregnancy. This is not serious and will typically improve after you deliver.

- If prior to pregnancy your kidneys had a reduced ability to purify your blood (as reflected by a reduced eGFR; see Chapter 6), your kidney function may significantly — and potentially irreversibly — worsen during pregnancy.

- If you have no kidney damage prior to pregnancy, kidney malfunction is unlikely to start during your pregnancy.

✔ **More frequent insulin reactions (and an increased risk of severe insulin reactions):** Because you will be keeping your blood glucose levels under exceptionally tight control, you will experience more frequent hypoglycemia than ever before. You will also be more prone to hypoglycemia unawareness and, as a result, severe hypoglycemia (particularly toward the end of your first trimester). We discuss hypoglycemia unawareness and severe hypoglycemia in more detail in Chapter 5.

We discuss blood glucose testing and blood glucose control in more detail later in this section.

Knowing what can happen to the fetus and baby

Most of the time the fetus and baby are perfectly healthy, but an increased risk of the following exists:

- ✔ **Miscarriage:** Miscarriages are more common if your blood glucose control is poor in the early stages of pregnancy. If your control is excellent in early pregnancy, your risk of a miscarriage is much less.

- ✔ **Birth defects:** The medical term for birth defect is *congenital anomaly*. This is a dreaded complication, but fortunately it's largely preventable. If your blood glucose control at the time you get pregnant and for the first 12 weeks or so (when your baby's organs are forming) is *excellent*, your risk of having a baby with a congenital anomaly is about the same as if you never had diabetes (about 3 percent). But if your blood glucose control is poor during this critical period of time, your risk is as high as 30 percent. An astounding difference, indeed. And one that you can influence directly.

- ✔ **Other health problems:** These include difficulty breathing, prematurity, small or large size, and disorders of body chemistry such as low blood glucose or low calcium. Your baby will *not* be born with diabetes.

Reviewing things to do before you get pregnant

To maximize your likelihood of having a healthy pregnancy and a healthy baby, you must do many things *before* you get pregnant.

Find out how you will know it is safe for you to stop using contraception

Meet with your diabetes specialist and discuss when you can safely stop using contraception and try to conceive. Make sure you know how your specialist will determine this. Safety is based largely on the other factors in this section, especially your blood glucose control as determined by your A1C level as we discuss later in this section.

Meet with and ask questions of your health care team

Nothing in your life will ever be as important as your quest to have a healthy baby. If you have questions about the impact of your diabetes on your pregnancy, *ask*. Ask your family doctor, ask your diabetes specialist (*especially* your diabetes specialist), ask your dietitian, ask your diabetes educator, ask your obstetrician — ask *anyone* who is a part of your health care team. As well, make sure your partner is involved. Your partner needs to know what you're going to be dealing with and their support will be hugely helpful. We discuss the members of the health care team and their roles in Chapter 8.

Achieve excellent blood glucose control

The single greatest factor in helping you to have a healthy baby is how good your blood glucose control (especially as reflected by your A1C level) is at the time of conception and during the first few weeks as the fetus's organs are being formed. You should aim for the following targets:

✔ **A1C 7.0 or less (ideally less than 6.0):** Your A1C level (this is measured on a blood sample) reflects your overall blood glucose control for approximately the last three months. Having an excellent A1C at the time of conception and for the first few months of pregnancy will dramatically lower your risk of miscarrying or having a baby with a birth defect. You should strive to achieve an A1C of under 7.0 and, ideally, as close to normal (that is, less than 6.0) *as safely possible*. Achieving an A1C of under 7.0 can be very difficult; in part because the lower the A1C, the more frequent are episodes of hypoglycemia. Therefore, the ultimate goal is to get your A1C as close to this target as you can, but *safely* (that is, without experiencing overly frequent hypoglycemia). We discuss A1C in detail in Chapter 9.

✔ **Blood glucose levels as close to normal as can be safely achieved:** You should aim for your blood glucose levels to be as close to normal as you can safely achieve. Strive for these blood glucose levels:

- Before meals: Below 5.3 mmol/L

- One hour after meals: Below 7.8 mmol/L

- Two hours after meals: Below 6.7 mmol/L

The CDA guidelines don't specify if "after meals" is after the start, middle, or end of meals. For the sake of consistency we suggest you use the time from *the start* of your meal. You don't need to test both one hour *and* two hours after the start of meals; discuss with your diabetes specialist which of these tests is best for you.

If you happen to have read Chapter 9 (where we discuss target blood glucose readings for non-pregnant individuals) before this section, you may notice that target blood glucose levels when trying to conceive (and when pregnant) are lower than those for individuals who are not pregnant. This reflects the importance of blood glucose readings as close to normal as possible on helping the fetus to develop normally.

See your eye specialist

Because retinopathy (we discuss retinopathy in Chapter 6) can rapidly progress during pregnancy, having your eye doctor assess the health of your eyes *before* you get pregnant is crucial.

Be tested

Have certain tests done before you stop using your contraception:

- **Have your kidneys tested.** Because kidney malfunction can significantly worsen during pregnancy, you need to have your kidneys tested before you get pregnant. This will provide a baseline for comparison and also will help determine the risk of your kidney function worsening during your pregnancy. Your doctor can assess your kidneys through very simple blood and urine tests (as we discuss in Chapter 6).

- **Have your blood pressure tested.** Having high blood pressure before you get pregnant puts you at much higher risk of running into more severe blood pressure problems during your pregnancy. If your blood pressure is elevated, your doctor will need to work with you to bring it under control before you stop using contraception.

- **Have your thyroid tested.** Women with type 1 diabetes (and, possibly, women with type 2 diabetes) are at increased risk of thyroid malfunction — particularly hypothyroidism (that is, thyroid underfunctioning). Untreated thyroid dysfunction in the mom can harm the fetus. A simple blood test (the TSH) can easily determine your thyroid function.

Have your diabetes medications reviewed

If you have type 2 diabetes treated with non-insulin antihyperglycemic medications (see Chapter 12), you will need to stop taking them and start on insulin well before you try to get pregnant. (The exception is if you have infertility related to a condition called polycystic ovary syndrome or PCOS, in which case your obstetrician may advise you to take metformin to help you get pregnant and, typically, to discontinue it after you do.)

If you have type 2 diabetes treated with metformin or glyburide at the time you conceive, do *not* stop these medications until you are started on insulin. (Stopping your oral medication prior to starting insulin will result in your blood glucose levels going up, putting your fetus at risk.)

If you have type 1 diabetes or insulin-treated type 2 diabetes, speak to your diabetes specialist to ensure you are on the best possible insulin treatment program. In all cases of type 1 diabetes and in nearly all cases of type 2 diabetes this means taking either:

- Rapid-acting insulin (see the next paragraph) before meals and a longer acting insulin (NPH, Levemir, or Lantus) once or twice daily or

- Using an insulin pump (which we discuss in detail in Chapter 13).

If you and your health care providers feel you should go on an insulin pump, make the switch to this from your current insulin therapy well in advance of pregnancy.

The rapid-acting insulins Humalog and NovoRapid are proven safe for pregnant women. Studies are underway to determine if Apidra is similarly safe. If you are taking Apidra, speak to your health care providers about switching to Humalog or NovoRapid before trying to conceive.

Have your non-diabetes medicines reviewed

Your doctor will need to review any medicines you are taking, and if they're unsafe to take during pregnancy (as is true, for example, of ACE inhibitors, ARBs, and, likely, cholesterol-lowering statin medicines; we list these in Appendix C), you will need to stop taking them. If you are on medication for high blood pressure, depending on what type of pills you're taking these may need to be changed. (Some blood pressure medications are safer than others during pregnancy.)

Quit smoking

Smoking increases the risk of complications during pregnancy. Having diabetes you are already at increased risk of problems during pregnancy, so why aggravate the situation? You want to quit anyway, so here's the greatest of incentives to take your intention and turn it into reality.

Take a multivitamin and folic acid

Taking folic acid supplements is important to help prevent your fetus from developing spinal cord defects. Take 5 mg per day starting three months *before* you get pregnant and continuing until you are 12 weeks pregnant. Then reduce the dose to 0.4 to 1 mg per day, and continue until you finish breastfeeding. Also, take a multivitamin starting three months before you get pregnant and continue until you finish breastfeeding.

Many over-the-counter (that is, non-prescription) multivitamin preparations contain folic acid, typically in a dose of 1 mg per pill. If you require 5 mg of folic acid daily you will likely require a prescription for this from your doctor.

Managing your health while you are pregnant

Congratulations. You have done everything you had to, and you are now an excited, though perhaps apprehensive, mother-to-be. So what next? These are the things that you will need to do during your pregnancy:

 ✔ **If you drive, get a rewards card for your favourite gas station.** You'll be spending a lot of time in your car, what with visits to the diabetes educator, the dietitian, your doctors, and so on. (Ian advises his patients with pregestational diabetes to expect to see health care providers more than 50 times during the pregnancy.) So when you fill up, look at the bright side: You're earning points toward that holiday you will so richly deserve (even if you have to delay taking it).

✔ **Have your diet adjusted.** Your dietitian will work with you to devise an appropriate meal plan designed to ensure adequate nutrition while assisting with blood glucose control and appropriate weight gain. Your carbohydrate intake will be moderately restricted, and you will be advised to eat three meals and three snacks per day (one of which will be a bedtime snack).

✔ **Keep your blood glucose levels as close to normal as possible.** Test your blood glucose a *minimum* of seven times per day: before and after every meal, and at bedtime. Testing occasionally overnight is also advised. Your targets are the same as they were prior to conceiving:

   • Before meals: Below 5.3 mmol/L

   • One hour after the start of meals: Below 7.8 mmol/L

   • Two hours after the start of meals: Below 6.7 mmol/L

You don't need to test both one hour *and* two hours after the start of meals; discuss with your diabetes specialist which of these tests is best for you.

Do not expect perfect blood glucose control. Perfect blood glucose levels are simply not possible given the complexities of diabetes and the imperfection of existing therapies. Indeed, as Ian likes to say, the words "perfect" and "diabetes" should never be used in the same sentence! Expecting — or anticipating — perfection will simply make you frustrated. Fortunately, occasional mild hyperglycemia will not harm your fetus. Equally fortunately, when you experience hypoglycemia it will not hurt your baby.

✔ **Have your A1C checked regularly.** Just like when you were working at optimizing your blood glucose control before you stopped using contraception (as we discuss earlier in this chapter), strive to maintain your A1C under 7.0 and, ideally, as close to normal (that is, less than 6.0) *as safely possible* (that is, without overly frequent — or *any* severe — hypoglycemia). Ian recommends having the A1C checked monthly during pregnancy.

✔ **Adjust your insulin.** Because the placenta releases hormones that increase insulin resistance (refer to Chapter 3), your insulin requirements will rise substantially during most of your pregnancy. (Two exceptions exist: Insulin requirements may transiently fall toward the end of the first trimester and then again in the last few weeks of pregnancy.) By the time you deliver, you will likely be on three (or more) times the amount of insulin you were taking before you got pregnant. Every time you visit your diabetes specialist or diabetes educator, be sure to bring your logbook because they will need to review your readings and insulin doses. They will help you adjust your insulin; however, in almost all cases *you* also need to be making changes to your doses in-between visits to your health care provider.

Waiting to make a necessary change to your insulin doses until you see your doctor or diabetes educator is simply lost opportunity. If you determine, based on your blood glucose readings, that a change to your insulin doses is required — and if you know how to make the change — then, like the commercial says, *just do it*. If, however, you're unsure if a change is needed or how to make the change, then call your doctor or educator; they'll be pleased to help you make the change and also to teach you how to make future changes.

- ✔ **Test for urine ketones.** You typically test for urine ketones daily, first thing in the morning. You should have hardly any ketones in your urine. (If you have type 1 diabetes, then you're likely familiar with the importance of testing your blood for ketones when DKA is suspected. We discuss blood ketone testing in Chapter 5.)

- ✔ **See your eye doctor regularly.** The CDA recommends that women with pregestational diabetes see an eye specialist "before conception, during the first trimester, as needed during the pregnancy, and within the first year postpartum." Because seemingly minor eye damage can progress rapidly during pregnancy, Ian likes to err on the side of great caution and recommends that *all* his patients with pregestational diabetes — even those with no observed retinopathy — meet with the eye specialist not only before conception and during the first trimester, but routinely *every* trimester and then again *three months* after delivering. Better one eye exam too many than one too few!

- ✔ **Visit a geneticist.** If you reside in a community with access to genetics counselling, your doctor may refer you to this service. A geneticist will review your situation to assess your risk of having a fetus with a problem and, moreover, will arrange sophisticated ultrasound and laboratory studies — including an ultrasound of the fetus's heart — to determine if the fetus is developing normally.

Knowing what to expect during labour and delivery

Congratulations once again. You've made it through nine months of pregnancy and you're ready to have your baby.

When you are brought into the hospital, if you have been giving yourself insulin injections, they'll likely be replaced by intravenous insulin, which allows for minute-to-minute fine tuning of the dose. If you have been using an insulin pump (we discuss this form of therapy in Chapter 13), Ian recommends that, unless something precludes it, you continue using your pump throughout your labour and delivery.

Until recently, insulin pump therapy was not commonplace and neither physicians (except for diabetes specialists) nor hospital staff were comfortable having their labouring patients (or patients undergoing a Caesarean section) use them. As a result, as soon as a woman on a pump went into hospital to deliver, the pump was discontinued and replaced with intravenous insulin, and the woman didn't start using the pump again until a few days post-delivery. Fortunately, this is changing and most women using pump therapy continue it during their labour and delivery. Speak to your obstetrician well in advance of your delivery about this option. Also, in case you are not up to the challenge of doing your own blood glucose testing and insulin pump adjustment during labour and right after delivering, ensure that your partner is pump-savvy and can assist you. (The odds are overwhelming that you — and possibly your partner — will know much more about pump therapy than most of the staff looking after you.)

During labour, your blood glucose level should be checked often — as often as hourly — and your insulin dose adjusted to keep your blood glucose levels between about 4.0 and 7.0 mmol/L.

As soon as you've delivered, your insulin requirements will plummet. If you have type 2 diabetes, and if you didn't require insulin before your pregnancy, you're not likely to require it after you've delivered. If you have type 1 diabetes, your insulin dose after you deliver will likely be, at first, significantly below your pre-pregnancy doses. (As a rule of thumb expect your insulin requirements immediately after you deliver to be about 30 percent less than your pre-pregnancy requirements.)

Unless you happen to remember what your insulin dose amounts were right before you became pregnant, as your due date is approaching (or earlier if you wish) ask your diabetes specialist to look this up in your file. Calculate what 70 percent of each (pre-pregnancy) dose works out to be. Write these down and take this information with you when you go to hospital to deliver. As soon as you've delivered start giving yourself these new doses. These doses will likely suffice for the first few days (or somewhat longer) after you've delivered. Then your insulin requirements will likely gradually climb back to where they were before your pregnancy. (Be aware, however, that some women require even less than 70 percent of their pre-pregnancy doses for the first few days after delivering.) If you use an insulin pump, pre-program your pump with a second pattern equivalent to 70 percent of your pre-pregnancy insulin doses and as soon as you've delivered switch your pump over to this second pattern. This is easier than entering all the changes into your pump in the hectic time right after having a baby.

Nine months of appointments — a lifetime of joy

When Leanne, a newly married woman with type 1 diabetes, asked Ian what would be involved if she were to get pregnant, she was expecting a simple answer. The answer she got, however, was complicated. Leanne was surprised to hear about all the things she would have to do leading up to and then during pregnancy, but she was sure she was up to the challenge and was willing to do "whatever it takes" to have a healthy baby.

During her subsequent pregnancy, what with visits to doctors, the diabetes educator, the dietitian, and so on, at times she felt as if she was "doing nothing but going to appointments," but she persevered. Although her nine months of pregnancy seemed to Leanne to "take forever," all recollection of the hassles she went through instantly disappeared the moment she first cradled her newborn infant lovingly in her arms. All she could think was "how lucky" she was to have experienced this joy.

Shortly after you deliver, the hospital staff will check your baby's blood glucose level. If it's low, the staff will give your baby some sugar water to drink. A pediatrician will thoroughly examine your baby to make sure everything is all right.

Handling your diabetes for the first few months after having your baby

Unless you are unable to do so, breastfeeding is far and away the preferred way to supply your newborn with nutrition. Because your body is providing your baby's nutritional requirements, you'll need to ingest an additional 300 calories or so per day.

If you have type 2 diabetes and were being treated with non-insulin antihyperglycemic medications prior to your pregnancy, when you have delivered, your doctor will likely advise you to resume these medications and discontinue your insulin. If, on the other hand, you were taking insulin prior to (and during) the pregnancy, you should expect to continue doing so. Metformin and glyburide are safe to take during breastfeeding. (We do not have studies to tell us if other types of non-insulin antihyperglycemic medications — which we discuss in Chapter 12 — are safe to take in this situation.)

By now, you're likely very familiar with all the reasons that excellent blood glucose control is so crucial to maintaining your good health. And in almost all cases you should be striving for optimal glucose control. Recall, however, that the (terribly unfair) price to be paid for so-called tight blood glucose control is a much higher risk of severe hypoglycemia (which we discuss in Chapter 5). Hypoglycemia is a bad enough problem to begin with, but it is even more of a concern if you are going to be home alone with your newborn. Ian advises "his moms" on insulin therapy to run their blood glucose control somewhat looser for the first few months after they've delivered. You're in no danger if you have blood glucose levels in the 5 to 10 range for a few months after you've delivered and this will provide an extra margin of safety (by reducing the risk of your having hypoglycemia) when you're home alone with your baby. Ian also recommends that moms on insulin therapy not bathe the baby unless another capable person is home to assist in the event that the mom experiences hypoglycemia.

Because, soon after delivering, women with type 1 diabetes are prone to a temporary form of thyroid disease called *postpartum thyroiditis,* the CDA recommends that women with type 1 diabetes have a thyroid blood test (called a TSH, short for thyroid stimulating hormone) done between six to eight weeks after giving birth. Very few doctors are aware of this, so we recommend bringing it up with your doctor. You can discover more about postpartum thyroiditis at Dr. Dan Drucker's excellent website, www.mythyroid.com/postpartum.html.

Part III
Rule Your Diabetes: Don't Let It Rule You

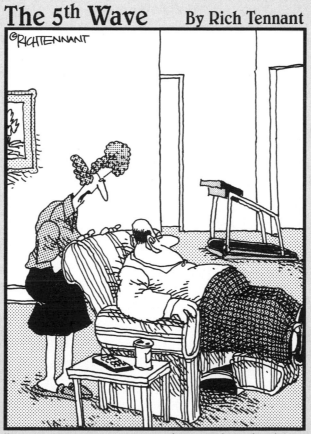

The 5th Wave   By Rich Tennant

"You know, anyone who wishes he had a remote control for his exercise equipment is missing the idea of exercise equipment."

In this part . . .

Y ou meet the members of your health care team and discover their roles. We also examine the ways in which nutrition, exercise, and medications can help you control your diabetes and keep you healthy.

Chapter 8

Meet Your Diabetes Team

. . . .

. . . .

*T*o the best of our knowledge, no hockey team has ever won a medal at the Olympics by sending only one player onto the ice. Nor do we know of any team that ever made it to the podium without having a coach, a general manager, and a slew of fans rooting along the way. And if an Olympic hockey team ever played without a trainer and an equipment manager, it surely must have been way back before Don Cherry put on his first red-checkered sport jacket (with matching lime-green tie, of course!). Heck, it must have been before Howie Morenz notched his first hat trick.

Now, you may never be the star on an Olympic hockey team, but you *can* be the star of *your own* team. Indeed, you *should be* the star of your own diabetes health care team, because for you to succeed with your diabetes, you must not only be the captain of the team, you must have all the other players working with you. Nothing's second rate about coming home from the Olympics with a silver or bronze, but regarding your health, you should always be after the top prize.

In this chapter we look at the different players on your health care team, starting with the first, second, and third star of each and every game. That would be — you guessed it — you.

You Are the Captain of the Team

You may not have wanted to be captain of the team; heck, you didn't want to be on a diabetes team to start with, but here you are, the star of the team. And as you might imagine, with stardom come certain responsibilities. Leadership, for example. This is where diabetes differs from almost any other illness. If you have appendicitis, it isn't very likely that you'll be the one to deliver the anesthetic, hold the scalpel, and put in the stitches. No, your role would be relatively passive as the experts around you tend to your needs. Diabetes is not like that.

When you have diabetes, *you* have to take charge. *You,* after all, live with you. Day and night. Night and day, too, we suspect. *You* are the one who ultimately decides what you will eat, when you will exercise, when you will test your blood glucose levels, when you will take your medicines, and so forth. Other people can offer advice, other people can prompt or even cajole you, but in the end, the decisions are yours. And with your keen and ongoing involvement in your health care, you'll be helping yourself to receive the best possible therapy to achieve and maintain good health.

Having so much responsibility on your shoulders may seem rather daunting. Indeed, it *is* daunting. But with time and support, you will grow into your role and become comfortable with it.

Here are your responsibilities as captain of your health care team. This list may seem intimidating, but you'll be surprised at how quickly these responsibilities can all become part of your normal day-to-day existence:

- ✔ **Follow your lifestyle treatment plan.** This means knowing what foods you should eat, how much, and how often; what exercises you should do and how often you should do them; how much weight — if any — you should lose and the best strategy to achieve this; how much alcohol you can safely drink; and if you smoke and want to quit, what cessation strategies are available to you. (Refer to Chapter 6 for more.)

- ✔ **Monitor your blood glucose and keep tabs on your A1C.** You should become familiar with how to test your blood glucose level, how often you should test, and what are your targets. You should also make sure that you have your A1C checked regularly and that you find out the result. (We discuss blood glucose and A1C testing in Chapter 9.) An additional responsibility that you really shouldn't have (because your doctor should be taking the initiative here), but, well, you do: If your blood glucose levels and A1C are above target, and your health care providers (in particular, your physician) don't recommend a strategy to help you improve things, *you need to ask them* how you are going to make things better.

- ✔ **Keep track of your blood pressure.** Anytime someone checks your blood pressure, ask what it is and write it down. Become familiar with what your target blood pressure is, and if your readings are too high, ask your doctor how he or she can help you reduce it. (We talk more about high blood pressure in Chapter 6.)

✔ **Keep track of your lipid levels.** Anytime someone tests your lipid levels (see Chapter 6 for a discussion on lipids), you should write them down or ask for a photocopy of the lab report. Also, find out from your doctor what your target levels are, and if you aren't within those targets, ask your doctor how he or she can help you meet those goals.

✔ **Determine if you are at high risk of heart attack and stroke.** Many people with diabetes are at high risk of heart attack and stroke, and need to take special precautions to avoid these diseases. In Chapter 6, we look at how you can avoid these problems.

✔ **Schedule visits to each member of your health care team.** How often you see each member of the team depends on many circumstances, including the state of your health.

Anytime you meet with your health care providers (be it your family doctor, diabetes specialist, eye specialist, diabetes educator, or other member of your health care team), ask them when they want you to return. Book the return appointment *before* you leave the office *and* enter the appointment as soon as possible into your calendar. (If you use a smart phone, enter the appointment into your phone before you leave the office.)

✔ **Know about your medicines.** If you see a diabetes specialist, every time you have an appointment bring *all* your medicines with you (both prescription and non-prescription). At the very least, bring a list of your medicines, making note of your drugs' names, dosages, and how many times per day you are taking them. Telling your doctor that you are "on a small blue pill once a day" and a "red capsule twice a day" tells your physician more about the state of your colour vision than the nature of your drugs. Indeed, Ian has seen more than one patient who became very ill because the drugs they *thought* (from memory) they were taking differed significantly from what they were *actually* taking. (Other health care professionals — especially other physician specialists such as kidney specialists, cardiologists, and so forth — may also want you to bring all your medicines with you to appointments with them. They will let you know if they do, or you can always ask.)

✔ **Ask questions.** To be an effective captain of your health care team, you must know how you're performing. And you can't know this without feedback from your teammates. So, before you leave an appointment, make sure you have a good understanding of what your health care provider has concluded. Don't accept vague phrases like "your blood pressure is okay" or "your cholesterol isn't bad" or "your sugars are reasonable." As diabetes specialists, we can tell you that these terms are meaningless. Meaning*ful* would be to hear that your blood pressure is 125/80, your LDL is 2.4, and your A1C is 7.3.

Your physician deals with many patients each day, and even the most conscientious, well-meaning doctor can easily forget some of the specific issues of your particular situation. Therefore, be sure to bring up any concerns or questions you have about your health. Tell your doctor if you're having a problem such as chest pain, shortness of breath, numbness in your feet, sexual dysfunction, and so forth. Otherwise, a potentially important problem may be overlooked.

Regarding your health care, never accept the old adage that no news is good news. Sometimes, no news means the lab lost your blood sample! If you have had tests done, follow up with your doctor (in person, by phone, by fax, by e-mail, or some other means) to obtain and discuss the results.

The remainder of this chapter looks at the responsibilities of the other members of your health care team. As you see what their roles are, you'll understand how you can help *them* help *you*. After all, as the old expression says, knowledge is power.

The Family Physician: Your Coach

Your family physician has a major role to play on your diabetes team; indeed, even if you have a diabetes specialist whom you see from time to time, if you have type 2 diabetes (and, possibly, if you have type 1 diabetes), your family doctor will still provide the great majority of your diabetes medical care. For this reason, if you're fortunate enough to live in one of the few communities in Canada where you can actually choose your doctor, find a family physician who has a particular interest in and expertise with diabetes. If you're unsure about this, simply ask him. If he doesn't feel that diabetes management is his forté, he may be able to recommend another doctor to help you.

Your family physician's responsibilities are far too numerous to list in their entirety (it would take many pages to itemize all the many tasks that these hard-working, dedicated doctors must do). But in terms of your diabetes, here are just some of the things your family doctor will do:

- **Review any symptoms you may have developed.** In most cases, your family doctor should be your first point of contact if you have developed symptoms (for example, such things as mood problems, vaginal discharge, diarrhea, or numbness in your feet).

- **Review your blood glucose control.** You should record your blood glucose readings in a logbook (see Chapter 9 for a detailed discussion of blood glucose record keeping) and review your numbers with your family doctor on a regular basis. If you don't keep a logbook then be sure to either download your readings from your meter and bring the printout to your appointment or, at the very least, bring your blood glucose meter itself.

✔ **Examine you.** Routine components of your physical examination should include checking your blood pressure and pulse, feeling your thyroid, listening to your heart and lungs, and examining your feet for problems with your skin, circulation, or nerve function (refer to Chapter 6 for a more detailed discussion on testing for nerve problems).

✔ **Order screening studies.** Your doctor should do a number of tests from time to time, including checking your A1C (see Chapter 9), cholesterol (refer to Chapter 6), eGFR and urine albumin/creatinine ratio (refer to Chapter 6).

✔ **Help organize your visits to other team members.** This includes things such as reviewing with you when you are due to see other team members — for example, your diabetes educators and your eye doctor — and, if necessary, arranging for visits to other providers, including your diabetes specialist and foot care specialist.

Please note again that this list is not meant to be exhaustive and does not include the numerous things your family doctor helps you with, independent of your diabetes.

The Diabetes Specialist: Your General Manager

Family physicians provide the great majority of diabetes care in Canada. Nonetheless, seeing a diabetes specialist from time to time is usually a good idea if you have type 2 diabetes (especially if you have known complications from your diabetes) and is essential if you have type 1 diabetes.

Defining the term *diabetes specialist* is exceedingly difficult. Sure, we can say it is a doctor who specializes in diabetes, and although that would be accurate, it would still be incomplete. We can arbitrarily classify diabetes specialists into three groups:

✔ **Endocrinologists** (such as Alan): These are doctors who, after medical school, trained in internal medicine and then did additional training in *endocrine* (hormone) disorders such as those affecting the pancreas (diabetes, for example), thyroid, and adrenal glands.

✔ **Internists** (such as Ian): These are doctors who, after medical school, trained in internal medicine and then usually tailored their practice to a particular area. In Ian's case this was diabetes. For other internal medicine specialists, it is, for example, heart disease or high blood pressure.

✔ **Family physicians:** This one may surprise you. Not many family physicians are diabetes specialists, but some are. These are doctors who, after medical school, trained in family medicine and then, because diabetes was a particular interest of theirs or because their community may not have had ready access to a diabetes specialist, or both, focused their practice on diabetes. We have given lectures to such family physicians and must admit we have felt that *they* could just as well have been the ones giving the talk. (Dr. Maureen Clement, who reviewed this manuscript, is an example of a family physician who is also a diabetes specialist, and a wonderful one at that.)

The main reason to see a diabetes specialist is the greater likelihood that they will be — by virtue of the time they devote to this one topic — "on top of the literature," that they will know about new research findings and new and innovative forms of therapy and how best to use them.

Your diabetes specialist can assess your diabetes-related issues and develop a treatment plan, and then share it with other members of your health care team.

Your specialist should send copies of her reports and your laboratory test results to your family physician. The great majority of specialists do this routinely, but some, alas, do not. Whenever you see your diabetes specialist, make a point of asking your specialist to do so. At the same time, ask the specialist to also send a copy of her reports to your diabetes educators, too. Otherwise, using our hockey analogy, you and your specialist will be the only players on your team handling the puck. And that will make your other teammates less effective.

The Diabetes Educator: Your Trainer

Dr. Christopher Saudek, a previous president of the American Diabetes Association once said, "Diabetes education is the single greatest advance ever made in diabetes care." (Ian loves him for having said it and quotes him widely.)

Although every member of your diabetes team is, in some way, an educator, a diabetes educator is typically the health care team member who provides the bulk of your initial and ongoing teaching. In Canada, diabetes educators generally have the initials *C.D.E.* (certified diabetes educator) after their names; however, many excellent educators do not have such certification. Diabetes educators are typically registered nurses (in which case they are referred to as *diabetes nurse educators* or, for short, *nurse educators*), dietitians, or, increasingly, other allied health care professionals such as pharmacists, who, after entering the workforce, do further training to teach people about diabetes.

A diabetes educator teaches you how to take your insulin or pills, how to test your blood glucose, and how to acquire many of the other skills you need. And that's just the beginning. They are invaluable resources, and if you haven't met with a diabetes educator, you're truly missing out.

If you haven't met with a diabetes educator, ask your doctor to refer you to one. If you haven't seen your educator for some time, call to arrange a follow-up visit. What health professionals know about diabetes keeps changing, so don't get left behind. Stay current; see your educator regularly. (If this sounds like a sales pitch, we offer no apologies. Diabetes education is paramount and the best place to get it is with a diabetes educator.)

The great majority of doctors are fully aware of the essential role that diabetes educators play and make a routine practice of referring their patients to them. (Trust us; sharing the work with other members of the health care team makes doctors' lives a lot easier!) Regrettably, there is the rare doctor who feels that diabetes educators are superfluous and, therefore, doesn't send patients to them. If you're placed in this unfortunate situation, ask your doctor to refer you anyhow. If he or she still declines, call your local diabetes education centre and ask if you can make an appointment — as is typically allowed — without a doctor's referral. (You can find your nearest diabetes education centre on the Canadian Diabetes Association website: Go to www.diabetes.ca, click on "Diabetes & You" and then "Locate a Diabetes Education Centre.")

The Dietitian: Your Energizer

Registered dietitians are pros at assisting you with your nutrition (hence, registered dietitians are sometimes referred to as nutritionists). To be called a registered dietitian in Canada, a person must have official certification establishing that he or she has the appropriate credentials. In Canada, the initials R.D. appear after the name of certified dietitians. Many registered dietitians are also certified diabetes educators. In this book, whenever we refer to dietitians we are referring to *registered* dietitians.

What you eat (and drink) is central to your success with your diabetes. Eat poorly, and you will render many of the medicines you're taking less effective. Your antihyperglycemic medications will be less useful. Your blood pressure pills won't work as well. Your cholesterol medicine will be fighting an uphill battle. And so on.

Your dietitian is the most knowledgeable person to advise you about what you should eat. It would be a terrible disservice to them — and, more important, to you — to think of the dietitian's role as simply putting you on a diet to lose weight. Sure, if you need to lose weight, dietitians can help you develop an appropriate nutrition plan, but they do so much more than that, too. Most importantly, they can help you determine the best choice and quantity of foods to help keep you healthy and your diabetes under control.

If you have diabetes and are on an *intensified insulin* program, your dietitian can teach you how to measure the number of grams of carbohydrates you consume with a meal and determine the amount of insulin that this will require you to take. This is called *carbohydrate counting* and is a highly effective means of achieving excellent blood glucose control; particularly if you have type 1 diabetes. We discuss intensified insulin therapy and carbohydrate counting in Chapter 13.

A good dietitian will help you to create a nutrition plan that is flexible, fits with your lifestyle, takes into account your ethnic and cultural background, and meets your religious requirements (if any).

The importance of tailoring a diet to fit the individual can be no better demonstrated than by the tale of two brothers that Ian met a few years ago. They were both teenagers and both had type 1 diabetes. Bob was athletic and was captain of his hockey team. David, a year younger than his brother, couldn't have been more different. David could dismantle (and reassemble!) a car or a computer, but the only red line he knew about was the one on the tachometer. For the sake of convenience, the first time they were to meet with their dietitian they went together. The advice they received and the meal plans they took home were as different from one another as night and day. But the plans worked. To each his own — diet, that is!

If you feel that the treatment plan your dietitian gives you is too rigid, is too out of keeping with your tastes, or is in some other way simply not realistic or practical, *do not* give up on the idea of proper nutrition therapy. Let your dietitian know of your concerns and he or she will be happy to work with you at creating a more appropriate meal plan.

The Eye Specialist: Your Cameraperson

An eye doctor has special expertise in detecting and treating eye disease. The two types of eye doctors are ophthalmologists and optometrists. In Chapter 6 we look at the differences between them and how often you should see one of them. We also look at the various types of eye disease for which you are at risk.

Eye damage from diabetes seldom causes symptoms until it's very advanced, so seeing an eye doctor routinely is *absolutely essential* — even if you have no problems with your sight!

Although your family doctor and your diabetes specialist may examine your eyes, an eye doctor has additional skills that you should take advantage of.

Although spending inordinate amounts of time in doctors' waiting rooms is the stuff of legend, eye doctors' offices are particularly famous for this. Make sure you bring something to read when you go. Hmm . . . how about *Diabetes For Canadians For Dummies?* And you had best plan on doing your day's reading prior to going into the examining room, because your eye specialist will typically dilate your pupils using eye drops. This can affect your vision for a few hours and may make reading difficult. More important, you won't be able to see well enough to drive yourself home from your appointment, so bring someone with you to drive you home.

The Pharmacist: Your Equipment Manager

If you have diabetes, you're likely taking (or are going to take) medications to assist with the ultimate goal of keeping healthy. And when you go to the pharmacy, your first thought may well be, "Oh heck, another errand." Okay, so going to a pharmacy isn't the highlight of your day (thankfully!). But your pharmacist is a great resource.

Pharmacists have expertise in medicines, so when you pick up your prescriptions, you have a golden opportunity to become an informed consumer. Here are some of the things that your pharmacist should review with you:

- The names of your medicines
- The dosages of your medicines
- How often you are to take your medicines
- What time you should take your medicines (for example, some cholesterol medicines work best if taken in the evening)
- Whether you should take your medicines with food or on an empty stomach
- Whether you can safely consume alcohol (Some people have bad reactions if they ingest alcohol while on sulfonylurea antihyperglycemic medications. We discuss these drugs further in Chapter 12.)

> ✔ What *adverse effects* (side effects) the medicines can cause and how likely they are to occur
>
> ✔ Whether any possible interactions between your different medicines exist. (For example, thyroid pills don't get absorbed as effectively if you take them at the same time as calcium or iron pills.)

You can also go online to check whether your medicines may potentially interact adversely with one another. Check out www.drugdigest.org.

A good pharmacist will not simply hand you your pills with a piece of paper (listing 50 potential side effects!) stapled to the bag and say goodbye. A good pharmacist will not only explain the items listed previously, but will put them in context. Without a pharmacist's help, as you read through the lengthy list of all the bad things that the medicines can do, you won't be truly informed. You'll simply be scared. And *that* is not effective counselling.

Increasing numbers of pharmacists are now also certified diabetes educators. This means that not only can they fulfill their traditional roles as pharmacists, but they can also provide you with other aspects of diabetes education.

If you're on several different medicines, ask your pharmacist to prepare a list of your medications that you can keep in your wallet or purse. This list should include the names, doses, and frequency of your drugs. Keeping track of when to take medicines can be very difficult. Your pharmacist can help you by packing your medicines in seven-day blister packs. Blister packs are a great way to help you avoid forgetting doses, and we wish that more people took advantage of them.

The Foot Doctor: Your Sole Mate

The foot doctor *(podiatrist* or *chiropodist)* is your best source of help with the minor and some of the major foot problems you may encounter. He or she can assist you with such problems as toenails that are hard to cut, bothersome corns and calluses, and difficulties with excessively dry or cracked skin. If areas of your feet undergo excessive pressure as you walk, a foot doctor can also help fit you with special insoles called *orthotics*, which more evenly distribute the forces upon your feet.

The longer we are in practice as diabetes specialists, the more we have come to rely on and use the expertise that foot doctors have to offer. They truly are the experts at helping you keep your feet healthy.

Not all foot care services are covered by provincial health care plans. Before you meet with your foot doctor, you might want to call ahead to find out what charges to expect. If there is a fee and if you have private health insurance, call your insurer to see if they will cover the cost of the appointment. Your insurer may also cover the cost of orthotics should you require them. (It's wonderful if they do seeing as orthotics are pricey.)

The Dentist: Your Opening Act

Okay, so we think it's great that hockey players these days wear mouth guards, but Ian admits to a soft spot for pictures of a young Bobby Clarke's very boyish, and very toothless smile. Well, times change, as they should. And with diabetes one thing that has changed is the increasingly recognized relationship between good oral health and good diabetes health.

If your diabetes is not well controlled you are at increased risk of oral health problems — particularly gum disease like *gingivitis*. Conversely, having gum disease can worsen your blood glucose control. Your dentist can help you maintain good oral health and, if problems exist, help correct them.

The bottom line: See your dentist regularly.

Your Family and Friends: Your Fans and Cheerleaders

Okay, so the 1985 Oilers likely would have done just fine, thank you very much, even if they didn't have a single fan in the stands. But they were the exceptions. The rest of us need people rooting for us as we deal with the trials and tribulations of life. And this is especially true if you are living with a health issue such as diabetes.

Your fans and cheerleaders are the people you live with, eat with, and play with. Your family and friends can be a tremendous source of support, but for them to help you, they will need your guidance. For example, you can teach them what to look for if you become hypoglycemic (refer to Chapter 5). And you can ask them to avoid eating indiscriminately in your presence. (Following your diet is challenging enough without your family exposing you to constant temptation.) Your family or friends can also become your exercise partners. Sticking to a program is a lot easier when a partner is counting on you to show up to work out.

Remembering the rest of the roster

In this chapter we look at the central players on your diabetes team, but many other teammates may be asked to take a faceoff from time to time. These include, among others, hospital emergency room staff, cardiologists, neurologists, gastroenterologists (stomach doctors), and mental health workers such as social workers, psychologists, and psychiatrists.

Have someone accompany you when you see a member of your health care team — especially if you're meeting the dietitian and you're not the main cook at home. You can expect to get a lot of information, and an extra set of ears is helpful.

If you plan to bring an extra set of ears to your doctor's appointment, be sure to ask your physician if they wish to first see you in private. On occasion, your doctor may want to discuss some issues with you alone before your friend or relative joins you. You likely wouldn't want to have important conversations with your doctor about, say, sexual dysfunction with your daughter or son in the room.

Let people who are important to you know about your diabetes. Showing them this chapter might be a good way to introduce them to their important supporting role.

Chapter 9

Monitoring and Understanding Your Blood Glucose Levels

- -

In This Chapter

▶ Understanding the whys and wherefores of blood glucose monitoring

▶ Knowing how to use a blood glucose meter

▶ Choosing a blood glucose meter

▶ Recording your blood glucose results

▶ Knowing your blood glucose targets

▶ Understanding what to do with your blood glucose results

▶ Assessing longer-term control with an A1C

▶ Looking at continuous glucose monitoring

- -

*I*n earlier chapters we discuss the bad things that can happen if you're exposed to elevated blood glucose. And because *bad* things can happen if your blood glucose levels are *bad,* you might suspect that *good* things can happen if your blood glucose levels are *good.* And you'd be exactly right. Many diabetes complications — such as blindness and kidney failure — are directly influenced by your blood glucose control. The better your blood glucose levels, the more likely you are to maintain your eyesight and avoid kidney failure. But how will you know if your blood glucose levels are good? Ah, we're so glad you asked. Because that is exactly what we look at in this chapter.

Understanding the Importance of Measuring Your Blood Glucose Levels

Have you ever gotten dressed in the dark only to find out as you were heading out the door that your socks were mismatched or the blue pants you put on were actually black or your red purse was actually brown? You probably either made a mad dash back inside to change, or you just headed out, hoping no one would notice. Well, not monitoring your blood glucose levels is like getting dressed in the dark every day.

If you are not testing your blood glucose, you will not know if your

- ✔ Nutrition (diet) plan (see Chapter 10) is helping your blood glucose control.

- ✔ Exercise program (see Chapter 11) is improving your blood glucose levels.

- ✔ Antihyperglycemic medications (see Chapter 12) — especially insulin doses (see Chapter 13) — need to be changed.

- ✔ Recent illness, such as a lung infection, is making your glucose readings dangerously high.

Basically, you'll be in the dark, without guidance and, equally important, without feedback.

We feel strongly that the great majority of people living with diabetes should be testing their blood glucose regularly. Note, however, that "great majority" is not the same as "everyone." If you have type 2 diabetes and your blood glucose control is consistently excellent — with lifestyle therapy alone or lifestyle and antihyperglycemic medications, like metformin, that don't cause hypoglycemia — regular blood glucose testing may not be necessary. Your doctor or diabetes educator can let you know if this applies to you. (Also, see "How often to test" later in this chapter.)

If you test your blood glucose regularly and find your readings are consistently elevated you may well start to question why you're testing. "Why do I want to be frustrated by always seeing crummy readings?" you might ask. And you would be perfectly justified in asking this — at least, if you couldn't improve your blood glucose control. But you can *always* improve it. If your readings aren't where they should be, meet with your diabetes educators to see if your lifestyle plan needs adjusting. And call your family doctor (or diabetes specialist if you're in regular contact with one) to have your antihyperglycemic medications reviewed.

Testing your blood, not you

Ian recalls his very first meeting with Bill, a 25-year-old man who had had type 1 diabetes for several years. When Ian asked Bill how his blood glucose readings were doing, Bill told him they were excellent and pulled out his blood glucose logbook (we discuss logbooks later in this chapter) which showed his past two months' readings — all of which were within target — consistently and neatly noted. "That's great," Ian said, "why don't I borrow your blood glucose meter for a moment so that we can download your values to keep a computerized record of them in the chart?"

"Ah," Bill replied, hesitantly, "actually, I don't have my meter with me today."

"No problem," Ian replied, "maybe you could drop it off tomorrow."

"Don't think so," Bill went on, "*I lost it months ago.*"

Bill expected recrimination, but got none. Instead, both Bill and Ian shared a knowing smile. Like having homework conveniently chewed by the household dog, people "losing" their blood glucose meter is very common. It's also common for people to make up blood glucose numbers. The reason? Because many people with diabetes have never been sufficiently taught that measuring and recording blood glucose levels are a guide — not a report card or, worse, a disciplinarian's rod. Similarly, many people with diabetes have never been sufficiently taught that their diabetes educators and doctors are there only to help, never to judge. As Ian tells his patients, "Think of me as your guidance counselor, not the school principal." Ian made sure Bill knew this, and from then on, like Little Bo Peep, when Bill came to his appointments, his blood glucose meter and logbook were sure to follow.

People with diabetes tend to look at a record of their glucose readings as a report card, keeping constant score and noting whether they have passed or failed. That is understandable, but terribly inappropriate. Your glucose readings aren't meant to judge you or your efforts. Your glucose readings may be good or bad, but that doesn't mean you as person are good or bad. Your numbers are just numbers! Your readings serve as an aid — a tool — to help you and your team know when changes to your therapy are in order. And if your readings are good, they serve as a nice source of positive feedback.

Determining if Your Blood Glucose Is in Control

You can know if your blood glucose control is where it should be through several different ways:

✔ **Test your blood glucose using your own blood glucose meter.** We discuss blood glucose meters in the next section (Testing with a blood glucose meter).

✔ **Have a blood glucose test performed at a laboratory.** The laboratory will draw blood from a vein in your arm.

✔ **Have your A1C tested.** This is typically done at a laboratory, but can also be measured at diabetes education centres if they happen to have "desktop" machines that do this. Also, you can buy disposable (but pricey) A1C test kits at pharmacies. (See "Testing for Longer-Term Blood Glucose Control with the A1C Test," later in this chapter, for more.)

✔ **Have your *fructosamine* level performed at a laboratory.** This is a seldom-required test that indicates what your average blood glucose level has been over the preceding two weeks.

✔ **Have your *1,5 anhydroglucitol* level performed at a laboratory.** This test indicates what your average blood glucose level has been over the preceding one to two weeks. The 1,5 anhydroglucitol test is not routinely available in Canada and is currently used primarily as part of research studies.

✔ **Use a continuous glucose monitoring system (CGMS).** See "Using a Continuous Glucose Monitoring System," later in this chapter, for more.

Of the various ways of determining your blood glucose control — and far and away the easiest, most convenient method — is for you to use a blood glucose meter. We look at this in detail in the next section.

Testing with a Blood Glucose Meter

Managing diabetes was revolutionized back in the 1980s with the advent of portable blood glucose meters. Before their invention people living with diabetes had to test their urine for glucose to get a sense of what kind of diabetes control they had; an imprecise and hassle-filled procedure at best. The original blood glucose meters cost one thousand dollars and each test took several minutes. Nowadays most meters are essentially free and each test takes just a few seconds. Now *that* is progress!

Reviewing the supplies you need

Just like any test, a blood glucose test requires some basic supplies:

✔ **Lancet:** If you're like us, the notion of intentionally wounding yourself is not your idea of a good time. Well, you need not despair because obtaining a blood sample is a nearly painless procedure. To prick yourself, you use a small, sharp, disposable *lancet*.

✔ **Lancet holder:** Your lancet fits into this spring-loaded holder, and when you push the release button, the lancet springs out and pokes your finger. Lancet holders are typically adjustable so that you can vary the depth the lancet will penetrate your skin. That way you can set it to the minimum depth necessary to get blood (and minimize discomfort).

✔ **Test strip:** This is the small disposable strip onto which you place your drop of blood.

✔ **Blood glucose meter:** This is the device that determines the glucose level in your blood sample. We talk more about meters in a moment.

✔ **"Sharps" container:** This is a small box into which you place your used lancets. You can pick up a sharps container from your drugstore. When the container is full, seal it and bring it back to the drugstore for proper disposal.

Performing a test with a blood glucose meter

Here's how you obtain a blood sample and perform a blood glucose test:

1. **Wash your hands (or at least your finger).** Although you do not need to prepare your site — or your psyche — with alcohol, you need to make sure your finger (or arm if you are using an alternate-site meter, which we discuss in the next section) is clean.

2. **Obtain a blood sample.** Insert a lancet into the lancet holder (or, if you're using a multi-test lancet holder, ensure it is loaded with a cylinder), press it against the *side* of your fingertip, and activate the trigger. In an instant, you will see a tiny drop of blood appear. It does not hurt much at all, but to make it hurt even less you can

   • Use a lancet holder that allows you to adjust the depth of penetration.

   • Avoid re-using your lancets because they dull quickly. (It's okay to use the same one a few times, but not more than that.)

   • Use the side — not the fleshy pad — of the end of your finger.

   • Change fingers often or — quite the opposite — stick to the side of the same finger and you will find that after you have built up a small callus it hurts less to draw blood from that site.

   • Take blood from an alternative site such as your forearm. (To do this you will need an alternative-site meter.)

3. **Apply the end of the glucose-measuring strip to the blood.** Only a tiny drop of blood is required, but it has to be sufficient to cover the marked area on the strip. Most strips are designed to draw up the blood in the same way a strip of paper towel, when dipped into water, draws up the water (a process called *capillary action,* in case you were wondering).

4. **Presto, you're done!** Your meter will display your result in a matter of seconds.

If you have difficulty obtaining a sufficient quantity of blood, try one or more of the following:

- ✔ Warm your finger with warm water.
- ✔ Let your arm hang down at your side for a minute before you test.
- ✔ Hold your finger about 1.5 centimetres (about half an inch) from the tip and squeeze — but only once, as repeated squeezing can interfere with the test's accuracy.

Because blood glucose test strips can be damaged (and thus, provide inaccurate results) if exposed to the elements, be sure to look after your unused strips according to the manufacturer's instructions. In particular, keep them stored in the airtight container that they came in.

If ever you find that your test result is far lower than you expect, you may have put insufficient blood on the strip (this can give falsely low readings). If your blood glucose meter tells you that your reading is, for example, 2.8 mmol/L and you had expected 12.8 mmol/L, retest yourself. Also, bear in mind that as accurate as blood glucose meters are (which is *very*), they are not perfect and results can be off by as much as 20 percent and still be "within specifications." So if you test your blood and it measures, say 8.6 mmol/L and you retest a moment later and it measures 9.1 mmol/L, that doesn't mean your machine is inaccurate or malfunctioning.

Incidentally, with lancing devices and used lancets, remember the old adage: Neither a borrower nor a lender be. To avoid the possibility of spreading blood-borne infections, your lancing device and used lancets should be yours and yours alone.

Knowing how often to test your blood glucose

How often you should test your blood glucose depends on several factors including the type of diabetes you have, the type of treatment you are using, and how stable are your blood glucose levels. As you can tell, this is not a one-size-fits-all issue. (We discuss *when* to test in the next section.)

If you have a diabetes specialist on your team, the specialist should advise you how often to test your blood glucose. If you don't have a diabetes specialist then ask your diabetes educator or family doctor how often you should test.

Ian observes that many people living with diabetes test their blood glucose *not nearly often enough* and many other people test *way too often*. Testing needs to be meaningful and done with a purpose. If you are testing your blood, but you and your health care providers are not doing anything with the results, then why bother testing? We discuss this further later in this chapter (see "Interpreting Your Blood Glucose Results").

If you have type 1 diabetes you should be testing your blood glucose level a *minimum* of 3 times per day; indeed, most people with type 1 diabetes should be testing more often than that.

If you have type 2 diabetes, although how often you test your blood glucose will depend on your specific situation (again, ask your health care providers what they recommend), the Canadian Diabetes Association provides some general recommendations. Tables 9-1 and 9-2, which are based upon (and modified from) CDA recommendations, provide some rules of thumb for how often testing should be done.

Table 9-1	Recommended Blood Glucose Testing Frequency for People with Type 2 Diabetes Not Being Treated with Insulin
If You . . .	*Then You Should Test . . .*
Have been diagnosed with type 2 diabetes *within the past 6 months*	1 or more times per day (at different times of the day) to learn the effects of various meals, exercise, and antihyperglycemic medication (if being taken) on blood glucose
Have excellent blood glucose control using lifestyle therapy alone (that is, you are not taking antihyperglycemic medication)	1 time per week (or less)
Have excellent blood glucose control using antihyperglycemic medications that *cannot* cause hypoglycemia (we discuss these medications in Chapter 12)	1 or 2 times per week
Do *not* have blood glucose levels consistently within target	2 or more times per day to assist you with the effects of lifestyle changes and/or to help you and your doctor determine if you need a change to your antihyperglycemic medication
Come down with a new illness (such as an infection) that can make your blood glucose levels go up	4 or more times per day
Start taking a medication (such as prednisone) that can make your blood glucose levels go up	2 or more times per day

If you are taking antihyperglycemic medications that can cause hypoglycemia and you develop symptoms of hypoglycemia (see Chapter 5), you should test your blood glucose at the time you experience these symptoms. That way you can verify whether or not your symptoms are due to low blood glucose.

If you've been having episodes of hypoglycemia at a certain time of day (or night) and your therapy is then changed to correct this problem, test your blood glucose for the first few days (at the same times that you'd been having your lows) after your medication adjustment. Doing so double-checks that you are no longer having lows at those times.

Table 9-2   Recommended Blood Glucose Testing Frequency for People with Type 2 Diabetes Being Treated with Insulin

If You Have Type 2 Diabetes and Are Using Insulin . . .	Then You Should Test . . .
1 time per day	At least 1 time per day
2 times per day	At least 2 times per day
3 times per day	At least 3 times per day
4 or more times per day or are using an insulin pump	At least 4 times per day

Never fall into the trap of assuming that if you feel well, your blood glucose levels *must* be good and you don't need to test. The truth is, your blood glucose level can be significantly higher than normal and you may not have a single symptom, even though your body is being irreversibly damaged.

As you can tell from the preceding two tables, the frequency of testing is directly related to how often you need the information to make decisions about your care. If you're being treated with lifestyle measures alone, for example, getting occasional feedback is usually enough to let you know if your treatment plan is effective. On the other end of the spectrum, if you're on several injections of insulin per day, you need to test much more often to know what insulin dose to administer.

Almost everyone has times when they get fed up with testing, testing, testing. Don't feel guilty if you feel this way; it's perfectly normal. And if you do happen to go through times when you aren't testing nearly as much as you should, don't berate yourself about it. Just grab hold of your meter and get back into the routine.

Mr. Pereira was a middle-aged man with insulin-treated type 2 diabetes who came to Ian's office for a consultation. Ian asked him how his blood glucose control was, and Mr. Pereira replied, "It was 7.4 today." Ian asked him if he had any other readings to share. "Sure. It was 9.3 last month so it's getting better." Ian explained to his patient that glucose control varies not only month to month, but day to day and even meal to meal, so knowing two readings taken a month apart tells us virtually nothing about how control is or what trend it's following. Hearing this explanation, Mr. Pereira, a math teacher, asked if he could borrow Ian's calculator, and, a moment later, announced, "Gee, Doctor, now I get it. I've told you what my readings were for a total of 2 minutes out of the past 43,200 minutes. That's not even five one-thousandths of 1 percent of my readings. *No wonder* that doesn't tell you much." Couldn't have said it better ourselves.

If you have prediabetes (refer to Chapter 4), then routine blood glucose monitoring with a blood glucose meter is not essential, so long as your physician sends you to have your blood glucose checked at a lab from time to time. Nonetheless, having a blood glucose meter may be helpful. It allows you to keep tabs on things by checking your blood once in a while and, especially, if you develop symptoms of high blood glucose (we discuss these in Chapter 4).

Looking at when you should test your blood glucose

In the preceding section we look at *how often* you should check your blood glucose. In this section we discuss *when* you should test. Later in this chapter we discuss how to *interpret* your test results (see "Interpreting Your Blood Glucose Results").

Determining the best times to test your blood glucose is directly related to what information you and your health care providers need. Remember: Testing has to have a purpose; otherwise testing is a waste of both your time and your money.

What times you should test depend on a number of factors including your type of diabetes, your overall blood glucose control, your diabetes medications, your exercise routine, whether you are experiencing hypoglycemia, and other factors. Therefore, discuss your particular needs with your own health care providers. Having said that, the following rules of thumb typically provide helpful information to guide you and your health care providers in managing your diabetes:

✔ **If your therapy *does not* include insulin:** Do most of your tests before breakfast, but be sure to also sometimes test before your other meals and two hours after the start of your meals.

✔ **If you are taking NPH, Lantus, or Levemir insulin once daily (and no other insulin injections):** Always test before breakfast, and sometimes test before your other meals, two hours after the start of your meals, and at bedtime.

✔ **If you are taking NPH, Lantus, or Levemir insulin *and* you are also taking meal-time insulin (Apidra, Humalog, NovoRapid, or regular insulin):** Always test before breakfast *and* before you give your meal-time insulin dose *and* sometimes two hours after the meal.

✔ **If you are taking premixed insulin:** Always test before your breakfast and before your supper. The other times to test depend on the type of premixed insulin you are taking (so check with your doctor or your diabetes educator). We discuss premixed insulin in Chapter 13.

If you are taking insulin, you should sometimes test your blood glucose level in the middle of the night.

Choosing a Blood Glucose Meter

It seems like not a day goes by without a new blood glucose meter making its way onto the scene. Indeed, with so many different meters and their many different sizes, shapes, and features (including colours) knowing which meter to buy can be terribly confusing. In this section we discuss factors to consider when purchasing a meter.

Ian's Preferred Testing Schedule

When Ian first meets a patient with type 2 diabetes who doesn't customarily do blood glucose testing — or hasn't tested in quite some time — he generally asks them to test their blood glucose twice a day for a few weeks: daily before breakfast and rotating the second measurement between a variety of times during the day as illustrated at the end of this sidebar. (In the figure, "after meals" is 2 hours after the start of meals.) This allows, within the short span of a few weeks, for a quick and quite comprehensive assessment of the person's blood glucose patterns, the impact of meals and exercise, how

their blood glucose-lowering medications are working, and so forth. After a few weeks of testing in this manner Ian then alters their testing schedule based on the CDA guidelines and the person's individual circumstances (especially the patient's treatment program).

When your doctor or diabetes educator asks you to begin testing (and recording) your blood glucose readings you may wish to discuss with your health care provider if they would like you to do so in similar fashion.

BLOOD GLUCOSE MEASUREMENT

DATE	BREAKFAST		LUNCH		DINNER		BEDTIME
	Before	After	Before	After	Before	After	
1	•	•					
2	•		•				
3	•			•			
4	•				•		
5	•					•	
6	•						•
7	•	•					
8	•		•				
9	•			•			
10	•				•		
11	•					•	
12	•						•
13	•	•					
14	•		•				
15	•			•			
16	•				•		
17	•					•	
18	•						•
19	•	•					
20	•		•				
21	•			•			
22	•				•		
23	•					•	
24	•						•
25	•	•					
26	•		•				
27	•			•			
28	•				•		
29	•					•	
30	•						•
31	•	•					

With rebates, promotions, and trade-ins, you'll find, with a few exceptions, almost every meter you look at is nearly free. Alas, although blood glucose meters are cheap, the test strips are anything but. Typically they are about a dollar per strip (ouch!), regardless of which meter you are using. If you shop around, however, you will find that some drugstores sell them for less than others.

To make sure your blood glucose meter is sufficiently accurate, once a year your doctor (or diabetes educator) should have you do a finger-prick test with your meter at the same time as the lab is testing your glucose by drawing blood from your arm. When the lab result is available, the two values should be compared. They should be similar (within 20 percent of each other).

Some provinces and territories will subsidize the cost of your blood glucose strips. For more information you can contact your provincial or territorial government or the CDA (visit their website at www.diabetes.ca and type "financial support" into the search box at the top of the page).

Many people ask Ian what the "best" blood glucose meter is, or what his "favourite" meter is. These questions are easy to answer because Ian has no favourite and no single meter is "best." Depending on your needs and preferences, the best meter for you may or may not be the best meter for someone else. So you need to look at the different features that the various meters provide and choose the meter that seems most suited to you and your needs. (Remember, however, that all meters basically do one thing — measure your blood glucose — and they all perform this function well. Everything else is, by comparison, less important.)

Consider these factors (in no particular order) when deciding which blood glucose meter to buy:

- **Esthetics and ergonomics:** Many of the newer devices have a nicer look and feel than older meters. Meters differ in a few ways:

  - **General appearance and esthetics:** Some meters come in a variety of colours.

  - **Feel:** Consider how comfortably they fit in the hand, how easy they are to grip and manipulate.

  - **Size:** Is the meter too big or too small for you?

  - **Simplicity:** Some meters are very simple to use, some are more complex. Some have basic button pushing you can master in a second, some have fancy features that require you to use a manual to figure out.

✔ **Display readability and features:**

- Some meters, like the VerioIQ, provide a vivid display and excellent contrast making reading the screens a pleasure. Some displays, however, are shades of grey that some people find difficult to read.

- Some meters have backlighting so you can use them in low light conditions.

- Some meters have screens that display many of your previous blood glucose readings at a glance; others are limited to displaying one value at a time. If you think you are more likely to review your readings on your meter than writing them down in a log or regularly downloading them, then this feature can be helpful. Particularly helpful are those screens that display your readings in a format similar to a logbook. (We discuss the best logbook format later in this chapter.)

  Making sense of the readings in your meter's memory, whether when scrolling through them on your meter or after you've downloaded them (see later in this list), is of far greater value if the date and time of the tests are recorded. Therefore, make sure you set the date and time on your meter (and periodically double-check these are correct; especially when switching to/from daylight savings time).

- If you have severe visual impairment and are unable to read the screen, you can purchase a meter, like the Prodigy Voice (`www.prodigymeter.com`), that says your blood glucose result aloud.

✔ **Calibration:** A few meters require you to calibrate them each time you open a new package of test strips. This is typically a fast and simple procedure, but if you think you might find it a hassle, obtain a meter that doesn't require this step. Most modern meters do not require calibration.

✔ **Ability to test from alternative sites:** If you want to test from alternative sites such as your palm, forearm, or thigh, buy a meter designed to allow this. (Alternative-site tests, however, should not be performed when your blood glucose level is rapidly rising or falling — such as after meals or when exercising — or if you suspect you're hypoglycemic.)

✔ **Ability to interpret blood glucose patterns:** The newest meters on the market provide some basic analysis of blood glucose levels and give basic feedback, such as advising you if your blood glucose level is consistently elevated at a certain time of day. This feature may be helpful for some people. (We look forward to far more sophisticated blood glucose pattern analysis from future meters.)

✔ **Helping to calculate your mealtime insulin dose:** If you perform carbohydrate counting (see Chapter 13) and find figuring out your insulin dose a challenge, a meter like the InsuLinx is designed to make performing the calculations easier.

✔ **iPhone compatibility:** A (tiny) blood glucose meter (the iBGStar) is available that can attach to an iPhone or iPod touch. (As the currently available iBGStar uses a 30 pin adapter, not the new "lightening" adapter it is therefore compatible with the iPhone 4S/4/3S/3, but not the iPhone 5.) The blood glucose result is displayed on the iPhone or iPod itself. Very cool. Ian finds this meter is particularly helpful for those iPhone users who are disinclined from keeping a written record of their readings and, especially, for those people who are disinclined from doing much testing. The convenience of using the iBGStar encourages people to test more often and it's nice iPhone display facilitates interpreting the blood glucose readings.

✔ **Blood ketone testing capability:** If you have type 1 diabetes you need to have a device that can test for ketones. (See Chapter 5 for more on ketones.) You might, therefore, wish to buy a meter that can test both for blood glucose and blood ketones. Alternatively, you can buy a blood glucose meter (based on the considerations in this list) *and* buy a separate blood ketone tester.

✔ **Ability to hold multiple test strips:** Most blood glucose meters require you to insert a single test strip each time you are going to test. Some blood glucose meters, however, contain a drum that holds many test strips and advances them one at a time whenever you need to do a test.

✔ **Download capabilities:** If you want to be able to download your readings onto your computer so you can graph (and print) them, buy a meter that has this capacity. You can buy a meter that plugs directly into your computer's USB port; most meters, however, require you to buy a connecting cable separately. (Having a blood glucose meter that can download readings for printing can be particularly important in certain circumstances; for example, if you are obliged to provide a record of your blood glucose readings to a ministry of transport to regain a driver's licence that was suspended after an episode of severe hypoglycemia. We discuss driving issues further in Chapter 16.)

You'll save much time, energy, and, potentially, aggravation by speaking to your diabetes educator before you buy a meter. Not only can your educator show you the latest meters and point out their pros and cons but, more importantly, your educator *knows you* and will able to help you select a meter that meets your needs. (Your pharmacist can also help you to choose a meter. But bear in mind that the pharmacist will, of course, be most familiar with the devices the pharmacy sells.)

If you would like to do some of your own research, you can find (far from impartial) information regarding meters by going to the different manufacturers' websites. Table 9-3 lists the main manufacturers in the Canadian market and their websites.

Table 9-3	Main Meter Manufacturers
Company	*Websites*
Abbott Diabetes Care	www.abbottdiabetescare.ca
Bayer Healthcare	www.bayerdiabetes.ca
Lifescan Canada	www.onetouch.ca
Roche Diagnostics	www.accu-chek.ca

Recording Your Results

As we discuss in detail later in this chapter (see "Interpreting Your Blood Glucose Results"), testing your blood glucose gives you two hugely important pieces of information:

- ✔ **Your current blood glucose level:** Your current level tells you if you are high, low, or in target and, for those people taking insulin, will help you determine the best dose to take. Your current blood glucose level appears on the screen every single time you test your blood with your meter.

- ✔ **Your blood glucose trends and patterns:** This allows you to know if your blood glucose levels are gradually climbing or gradually falling or are consistent; how often your values are within target; if your treatment program is gradually improving your control or losing its benefit; if your antihyperglycemic medications (including insulin) need changing; if your carbohydrate counting (see Chapter 13) ratio is satisfactory; if your exercise pattern or frequency or timing needs to change; and so forth. Alas, at present no blood glucose meter in existence provides anything remotely close to all this detail. But if you keep a log (be it written or electronic) of your readings *and then spend time analyzing it*, this information and more is all available to you whenever you want and whenever you need. And that is why keeping a log remains so invaluable despite all the bells and whistles of today's meters.

Although for most people living with diabetes, keeping a log is invaluable, it is not necessary for everyone. If you are not taking insulin and your blood glucose readings are consistently within target, then your blood glucose meter's memory is sufficient. If, however, you are taking insulin or your blood glucose readings are not consistently within target, then we recommend keeping a log. Your next step, then, is to determine how best to format your log.

Ian recalls going for a haircut a while back (when he used to have to go more often) only to find his barber profoundly upset. "What's the matter?" Ian asked, to which his barber replied that he could not find his scissors. "Why not just use somebody else's?" Ian innocently asked. His barber immediately stopped his searching and looked at Ian with disbelief. "Use somebody else's? Would you use somebody else's wife?" And that just about sums up how Ian feels about the way that blood glucose readings should be recorded. You can do it many different ways, but why not do it the *best* way, which, ahem, just happens to be Ian's way!

Logbooks are available (for free) from pharmacies, from diabetes education centres, at most diabetes specialists office, and other places. Alas, these logbooks seldom have a particularly good format. For that reason Ian created his own log sheet which you can download for free from his website (go to www.ourdiabetes.com then click on "Log Book").

We recommend each page in your logbook be laid out as shown in Figure 9-1. (Of course, if you're not on insulin you won't use the right-hand side of the page.)

	Blood Glucose Levels								Insulin Injections					Notes
Date	Breakfast		Lunch		Dinner		Bedtime	Other	Insulin Type	Units Taken				
	Before	After	Before	After	Before	After				Breakfast	Lunch	Dinner	Bedtime	

Figure 9-1: Preferred logbook format.

One shortcoming with this layout is, potentially, insufficient space for you to write in the Notes column (where you might want to write things such as "birthday party" or "missed snack" to remind you later of some past event that might explain a high or low reading). If you need more space, you can always create your own sheet on a piece of paper (which you could photocopy) or with a spreadsheet program such as Excel.

Using this layout enables you to quickly assess your overall blood glucose trends and patterns for a given time of day. To illustrate what we mean, have a look at two different ways of recording your readings.

Table 9-4 is the typical way a log is kept or a machine's memory displays results (although a machine would usually display the time of day, not the meal of the day). The readings in this table are before-meal values.

Table 9-4	Blood Glucose Readings Listed Chronologically
Time of Reading	*Blood Glucose Level*
Breakfast	12.6
Lunch	4.1
Dinner	14.7
Bedtime	5.6
Breakfast	11.7
Lunch	5.2
Dinner	12.1
Bedtime	7.0
Breakfast	10.0
Lunch	5.9
Dinner	11.9
Bedtime	4.0
Breakfast	9.9
Lunch	4.2
Dinner	14.4
Bedtime	4.4
Breakfast	11.1
Lunch	6.3
Dinner	12.2
Bedtime	5.1

If you were to record your readings like this, you would likely feel that your glucose values were all over the place (or, as Ian often hears, "My sugars are up and down like a toilet seat!") and you would likely be feeling frustrated by what you concluded were inconsistent values. Although your conclusion would be perfectly understandable, you might be surprised to see that if we look at your readings from a different perspective, they're actually remarkably consistent. Table 9-5 takes those same readings and charts them differently.

Table 9-5	Blood Glucose Reading Listed by Time of Day		
Breakfast	*Lunch*	*Dinner*	*Bedtime*
12.6	4.1	14.7	5.6
11.7	5.2	12.1	7.0
10.0	5.9	11.9	4.0
9.9	4.2	14.4	4.4
11.1	6.3	12.2	5.1

Now, scan the columns from top to bottom. Aha! Your readings at any given time of day are remarkably similar. You're consistently too high at breakfast, consistently normal at lunch, consistently too high at dinner, and consistently normal at bedtime.

Record keeping is important because when you have identified your blood glucose patterns and trends, you and your health care team can adjust your therapy accordingly. In the preceding example, if you were on long-acting insulin at bedtime, we would know that you need a higher dose in order to bring down your breakfast blood glucose; and if you were taking rapid-acting insulin at lunchtime the dose would need to be increased in order to reduce your suppertime readings (see Chapter 13 for a detailed discussion of insulin adjustment). We could have figured this out from Table 9-4, but it would have been much more difficult and time-consuming. We discuss how to interpret blood glucose log readings in the section "Interpreting Your Blood Glucose Results," later in this chapter.

A few blood glucose meters have the capability to either display or to present downloaded readings in the format Table 9-5 shows. Keeping a log is still preferred (and is essential if you are taking insulin so that you can write in your insulin doses). But if you are one of the great number of people for whom keeping a log "just isn't going to happen," then using a blood glucose meter that can is a good choice.

If you own a smart phone you can download apps that allow you to enter your blood glucose readings (and insulin doses). More of these apps are available all the time, but we haven't found one that we consider ideal — yet.

If you're using an insulin pump (see Chapter 13) you may need an even more detailed logbook; ask your diabetes educator for a recommendation.

Although bringing your logbook with you to every appointment with your diabetes educator and diabetes specialist is essential, your blood glucose testing and recording is primarily *for you*, not for your health care providers. Testing guides you day-to-day and tells you a lot: You get feedback on how your nutrition, exercise, and medications are working. You can notice worsening trends or overly frequent hypoglycemia. You know when you're on track (and should "stay the course") and you see when things have fallen off the rails and you need to make a change and/or seek advice from your health care providers.

Discovering Your Blood Glucose Targets

The Canadian Diabetes Association (CDA) guidelines recommend that most adults with type 1 or type 2 diabetes (we look at children's targets in Chapter 14 and targets for pregnant women in Chapter 7) aim for the following readings:

Before Meals	*Two Hours After Meals*
4 to 7 mmol/L	5 to 10 mmol/L

If you have achieved these blood glucose targets yet your A1C remains above 7.0 percent the CDA recommends aiming for a lower two-hour after-meal target of 5 to 8 mmol/L. (We discuss the A1C level later in this chapter in the section "Testing for Longer-Term Blood Glucose Control with the A1C Test.")

The CDA guidelines don't specify if "two hours after meals" is two hours after the start, middle, or end of meals. For the sake of consistency we suggest you measure the two hours from the start of your meal. (Mind you, for all too many of us as we wolf down our dinners to then rush out the door to get our kids to hockey practice, soccer, ballet and the like, the start, middle and end of a meal are often just minutes apart!)

Not everyone can safely achieve these targets. Here are some of the things that might make aiming for these levels unsafe or inappropriate for you:

- ✔ You have other health problems (such as severe coronary artery disease) that may put you at undue risk of harm if you experience hypoglycemia.

- ✔ You have *irreversible* problems with hypoglycemia unawareness (refer to Chapter 5).

- ✔ When you try to bring your blood glucose into this range, you experience excessively *frequent, unpredictable, and unavoidable* hypoglycemia.

- ✔ Your life expectancy is such that you're at low risk of developing diabetes-related, long-term complications.

No one with diabetes has glucose readings that are always within target. Indeed, having two-thirds of your readings within target is a wonderful accomplishment. Achieving and maintaining target readings requires a concerted and ongoing effort by you and your diabetes team.

Consistently achieving target blood glucose values can be very difficult and, for some people, it may simply not be possible. If you and your health care team have worked hard at reaching these goals but have not been able to achieve them, don't feel that all is lost. The reason for this is simple: Although optimal blood glucose readings are our goal, as we discuss in Chapter 6, *any* improvement in your blood glucose control will significantly reduce your risk of microvascular complications (such as blindness and kidney failure) and, possibly, macrovascular complications (such as heart attack and stroke).

Interpreting Your Blood Glucose Results

In the section "Understanding the Importance of Measuring Your Blood Glucose Levels" earlier in this chapter, we mention that testing your blood glucose (and recording your results) is only of value if you do something with the results. Otherwise, it's a waste of your time — and an expensive waste at that. And we don't want you to waste your time — or money — so in this section we look at how you can use your blood glucose results effectively. We do so by providing a few examples of common problematic blood glucose patterns and what you can do to make them better.

The first step in interpreting your blood glucose results is laying them out in front of you in a log that lends itself to interpretation. We illustrate the most helpful log format earlier in this chapter (refer to Figure 9-1 and Table 9-5).

Everyone living with diabetes requires mentoring to learn how to interpret their blood glucose patterns. This is a key aspect of the teaching that your diabetes educators and diabetes specialist provide. Having problems figuring out your blood glucose readings? Be sure to contact your health care providers for advice. Don't just ask them to "tell you" their interpretation, but have them explain to you how they came to their conclusion. Otherwise you will be in a quandary the next time problems arise. What you want to be (and need to be) is empowered so *you* can figure things out. After all, you live with your diabetes and will encounter this or some other blood glucose quandary from time to time. Living with diabetes a lot easier if you can identify and tackle blood glucose problems when they arise.

When your before-breakfast readings are high (and other readings good)

As we discover in Chapter 13, one particularly common scenario is for people with diabetes (regardless of their treatment) to have higher readings first thing in the morning than later in the day. A typical logbook might look like Figure 9-2.

Date	Breakfast		Lunch		Dinner		Bedtime
	Bef.	After	Bef.	After	Bef.	After	
	8.5	7.2					
	9.0		6.1				
	7.8			5.2			
	6.1				4.4		
	8.2					7.9	
	9.9						8.2

Figure 9-2: High before-breakfast (fasting) blood glucose readings.

The reason for this pattern is that overnight your liver produces and releases glucose into your blood (this is called the *dawn phenomenon*). Often, the best way to treat this increased before-breakfast glucose level is by taking a dose of insulin (NPH, Levemir, or Lantus) before you go to bed (sometimes these insulins are given at other times instead). Or, if you are already taking one of these insulins, by increasing the dose (under the guidance of your diabetes educator or physician).

When your after-meal readings are high (and other readings good)

You may observe that your readings are good before your meals but two hours after your meals your values have climbed. Your logbook might look something like Figure 9-3.

In this case, the first thing to do is to review your diet with your dietitian, because your choice of foods may be responsible. Alternatively, if you're taking non-insulin antihyperglycemic medications, you might benefit from using one (such as GlucoNorm) that specifically targets after-meal blood glucose spikes. Another very effective measure is to take rapid-acting insulin (Apidra, Humalog, or NovoRapid) before your meals. If you're having this blood glucose problem despite already taking one of these medicines, then your dose(s) may need to be adjusted. (We discuss insulin adjustment in greater detail in Chapter 13.)

Date	Breakfast		Lunch		Dinner		Bedtime
	Bef.	After	Bef.	After	Bef.	After	
	5.5	10.1					
	6.0		6.1				
	7.0			11.3			
	6.1				6.8		
	4.2					10.5	
	5.9						7.2

Figure 9-3: High two-hour after-meal blood glucose readings.

For many people, their only elevated after-meal value is the one following supper. Why? Most Canadians have supper as their biggest meal. In this situation, taking a rapid-acting insulin once daily, before supper, is often the best solution. (You could, of course, try to spread out your calories — and carbohydrates — more evenly over three meals per day. But Ian's adage is that unless you are doing something unhealthy, adjusting your diabetes therapy to suit your life is better than changing your life to suit your diabetes.)

When all your readings are elevated

Most people with diabetes periodically encounter situations where *all* their blood glucose levels are elevated to some degree, as Figure 9-4 illustrates.

If you encounter this situation, the first thing to do is to look back at readings for the days and weeks prior and analyze what your glucose trend has been:

- If your readings were excellently controlled then *suddenly* worsened, you (and your physician) need to determine if some new problem is the cause. Have you come down with a bug? Have you forgotten to renew a prescription for one of your antihyperglycemic medications? Has your insulin gone bad?

- If your readings have been *gradually* climbing over the preceding weeks and months, a more gradual change likely accounts for the worsening results. Have you gotten off track with your nutrition program or been exercising less? Have you been gaining weight? Or, if no obvious change has occurred, maybe (if you have type 2 diabetes) your pancreas's ability to make insulin has been progressively declining, and you need your doctor to prescribe some additional antihyperglycemic medication?

Date	Breakfast		Lunch		Dinner		Bedtime	Other
	Bef.	After	Bef.	After	Bef.	After		
	7.2		12.1					
		10.3					12.3	
	8.4			12.6				
		11.2						
				14.2				
	9.4					19.3		

Figure 9-4: High blood glucose at all times.

The point from these examples is not to cover all possible scenarios and their solutions; rather, the point is that if you keep track of your blood glucose levels *and* make a point of routinely looking at, reflecting upon, and analyzing your values, you will quickly know when something is amiss and can take rapid action to make things better. Sometimes this is simply getting on track with lifestyle improvement. Sometimes it is seeking treatment for a new ailment like an infection. And, not, uncommonly it means you need to contact your doctor to see if you need to make a change to your diabetes medication.

We discuss the issue of loss of blood glucose control in detail in Chapter 2.

When you are having too many lows

One less common blood glucose pattern that is especially important for you to know about is having too many episodes of hypoglycemia. Figure 9-5 illustrates this scenario, which seldom occurs unless you have type 1 diabetes.

As we discuss in Chapter 5, having occasional episodes of hypoglycemia is (the incredibly unfair) price many people with type 1 diabetes (and some people with insulin-treated type 2 diabetes) pay for having excellent blood glucose control. Having *frequent* lows, however, is never safe or acceptable and it *always* warrants a change to one's therapy. The problem, however, is that many people who are experiencing too many lows don't know it because they either don't keep a log, or they do keep a log but they don't analyze it. (In general, "too many" lows is more than 2 or 3 a week.)

Date	Breakfast		Lunch		Dinner		Bedtime	Other
	Bef.	After	Bef.	After	Bef.	After		
	5.2	3.6				6.4		
	2.9							
	6.5		3.4		4.3			
				4.3				
				3.5			7.2	
	3.2							

Figure 9-5: Overly frequent hypoglycemia.

You can help avoid running into problems with overly frequent hypoglycemia (and the risk of severe hypoglycemia) by always documenting an episode — *any* episode of *any* severity — of hypoglycemia in your logbook. And, at least once weekly, looking at your logbook and highlighting all your lows. If you are having too many (refer to Chapter 5 for a discussion on this), contact your physician to change your therapy as soon as possible.

When your readings have no pattern

Perhaps your blood glucose readings are inconsistent, and really have no discernable pattern at all. High then low, up then down — resembling (and making you feel like you're on) a roller coaster. Your logbook may look something like Figure 9-6.

Fortunately, some correctable or at least modifiable factor is almost always present that you can address to improve this situation.

If you're having wide and unpredictable swings in your glucose levels, get in touch with your diabetes specialist and your diabetes educators. They will be able to help sort out the reasons for the problem and help you improve it (though not necessarily totally eliminate it).

Date	Breakfast		Lunch		Dinner		Bedtime	Other
	Bef.	After	Bef.	After	Bef.	After		
	4.1	8.2						3.5
	12.5		4.2		19.9			7.7
	3.2			14.7				
	16.5				24.4	5.4		
	6.7		13.4			9.9		
	11.2			2.6			7.2	

Figure 9-6: Inconsistent blood glucose readings.

Highly variable blood glucose readings seldom occur in people who have had type 2 diabetes for only a few years; it is much more likely to be a problem in people with type 1 diabetes or, occasionally, very longstanding type 2 diabetes, when the pancreas has lost almost all its ability to make insulin.

These are possible causes of erratic blood glucose levels:

✔ **Your nutrition plan isn't optimal for you.** If your nutrition program isn't working out the way it should, visit the dietitian. Perhaps your food selection or amount might need to be changed, or maybe you would benefit from carbohydrate counting (see Chapter 13) or using lower glycemic index foods (see Chapter 10).

✔ **Your adherence to your nutrition plan needs some work.** Are you eating *in*consistently? Do you eat almost nothing all day and then consume the bulk of your calories at suppertime? Do you graze from the time you get home in the evening until you go to bed? All these patterns can adversely affect glucose control. Also, eating disorders are not uncommon for teenage girls and young women with diabetes and can wreck havoc on blood glucose control. We discuss this further in Chapter 10.

✔ **Your exercise pattern needs to be revised or your treatment needs to be changed to accommodate your exercise pattern.** Are you exercising intensively for 10 minutes one morning and then at a leisurely pace for 30 minutes the next evening and then 15 minutes intensively again the next afternoon? Exercising for consistent periods of time and at the same time of day is often helpful in maintaining consistent glucose control. Having said that, if you prefer to maintain your current, variable exercise pattern, that is okay too; just be sure to have your diabetes therapy adjusted to address this. (Remember: Don't adjust your life to suit your therapy; adjust your therapy to suit your life!)

✔ **You have gastroparesis or celiac disease.** (We discuss these conditions in Chapter 6.) These conditions cause erratic absorption of nutrients into the body and, as a result, can cause overly variable blood glucose readings.

✔ **You are stressed out.** Stress does not cause diabetes, but it can certainly influence it. Stress causes the release of certain hormones in your body, including cortisol and adrenaline, both of which can make glucose levels rise. If you're on an emotional roller coaster, your glucose readings may be too.

✔ **Your menstrual cycle is a factor.** For some women with diabetes, where they are in their cycle can influence their glucose control. Some women find their glucose readings are higher around the time of their period and some find their readings are lower. Most women don't find much difference. (Also, this would typically cause blood glucose levels to be higher, or lower on certain days of the month, not both high and low on a given day.)

✔ **Your work schedule changes often.** If you work a variable shift, you may find your readings are also variable. As most people with diabetes quickly find out, diabetes loves consistency. Nonetheless, working variable shifts does not make excellent glucose control impossible, just more difficult. If you work variable shifts and are on insulin therapy, we recommend basal-bolus therapy (see Chapter 13).

Another very important reason for inconsistent blood readings, as illustrated in Figure 9-6, is that your insulin therapy isn't working sufficiently well for you. You may need to do one of the following:

✔ **Change to a different type of insulin or a different insulin regimen.** Different insulins have different properties and, like the expression, "different strokes for different folks," you need to take the insulin that most closely matches your needs and works best for you. For example:

- If you're taking NPH insulin and have inconsistent blood glucose readings, switching to Lantus or Levemir may provide more consistent blood glucose control.

- If you have type 1 diabetes but are only on twice-daily insulin, your blood glucose control is almost guaranteed to be erratic, and switching to basal-bolus therapy (this is closer to normal insulin release from the pancreas; see Chapter 13) is recommended.

- If you're having erratic readings despite basal-bolus injection therapy, switching to insulin pump therapy may provide you with much more consistent blood glucose control.

✔ **Not miss insulin doses.** If you're missing insulin doses due to forgetfulness, set reminders for yourself when your insulin is due or ask others to remind you. If you are omitting insulin doses intentionally (as teenage girls sometimes do to help them lose weight), this is very, very dangerous and you must not do it. Speak to your diabetes educator or physician urgently to see what other, safer measures can help you keep your weight in check.

✔ **Better mix your insulin.** Cloudy insulins such as NPH need to be properly mixed before you inject them (see Chapter 13).

✔ **Make sure your insulin hasn't lost its potency.** If your insulin has been exposed to excessive cold or heat, or is beyond its expiry date, it will have lost its potency and you should not use it.

✔ **Change the place you are injecting your insulin because of problems with insulin absorption.** You may give yourself the same dose of insulin every day (something, by the way, that's seldom a good idea, as we discuss earlier in this chapter), but that doesn't mean that your bloodstream sees the same dose. Factors that can affect the rate of absorption of insulin from your injection sites include the following:

- Whether your injection sites have scar tissue. You shouldn't inject insulin into these areas.

- Whether your injection sites have fat buildup (*lipohypertrophy*; refer to Chapter 6). Insulin absorption varies considerably injection-to-injection if you inject it into these areas. Also, injecting into areas of lipohypertrophy makes the lipohypertrophy worse. You shouldn't inject insulin into these areas.

- Which part of your body you are injecting into (regular insulin will begin to work more quickly if injected into the abdomen than into the arms or legs). Speak to your diabetes educator about the best locations to inject your insulin and how often you should change the sites you use.

- Whether you exercise a certain part of your body after you inject there. If, for example, you inject regular insulin into your leg and then go for a run, the rate of insulin absorption will speed up. You should not inject insulin into a limb that you're about to exercise.

- Whether you're accidentally injecting into muscle. (This would cause the insulin to be absorbed faster.)

The list of possible causes of overly variable blood glucose readings is lengthy. One term, however, that is missing from the list is *brittle diabetes*. We consider this, in general, to be a four-letter word. *Brittle diabetes* can be defined as erratic and disabling blood glucose variability that happens for no known reason and cannot be improved. Although we often are referred patients with erratic blood glucose readings (some of whom have been labelled as having brittle diabetes), there is *almost always a cause* and *always a way to make it better*. For a doctor (or other health care provider or, indeed, for a person with diabetes) to simply attribute erratic blood glucose control to brittle diabetes without first carefully looking for (and treating) all possible causes is, in Ian's opinion, not only a shame, but a travesty. (Not that he feel strongly about this or anything.)

Testing for Longer-Term Blood Glucose Control with the A1C Test

Individual blood glucose tests are great for telling you how you're doing at a specific moment in time, but they don't give you the big picture. Frequent blood glucose measurements help, but even then, they only provide a series of snapshots of your glucose levels. So what you need is a test that gives an estimate of your *overall* control over a longer period of time. And that's precisely what a test called an A1C can determine. Your *A1C* is a measure of how much glucose has become attached to your red blood cells over the preceding three to four months.

You may come across other terms for A1C, including *hemoglobin A1C, glycosylated hemoglobin,* or *glycohemoglobin.* You may also come across it abbreviated as HbA1C or HgbA1C. These all mean the same thing. Also you may find an A1C written as a number (9, for example) or as a percentage (9 percent, for example); both are correct and mean the same thing. There is also a new way of reporting the A1C (as mmol/mol rather than as a percent) being used in Europe and, in the future, quite possibly in Canada too. We discuss this in the sidebar "New ways of reporting A1C."

Learning the importance of your A1C

Knowing your A1C is crucial because your likelihood of developing microvascular complications (that is, eye, kidney, and nerve damage, as we discuss in Chapter 6) is directly related to your A1C. A normal A1C reading is 6 or less. An A1C of 7 or less is very good indeed and puts you at quite low risk for microvascular damage. An A1C of 9 or higher is poor and puts you at much greater risk. An A1C that is too high is an alarm to you and your health care team that you need to improve your control. If you can drop your A1C by even 1 percent, you'll substantially decrease your risk of microvascular complications. One landmark study found that reducing the A1C by just 1 percent (equivalent to a reduction in average blood glucose of only 1.6 mmol/L) resulted in an astounding 37 percent lower risk of microvascular complications.

New ways of reporting A1C

On the horizon are two new ways of expressing the A1C:

1. Rather than the current method of reporting the A1C as a percent, increasingly often laboratories will report it in *mmol/mol.*(Oh heavens, can't anyone leave well enough alone?!)

2. In the future — and what Ian feels will be of more value compared to the aforementioned change — the A1C will also be reported as an "estimated average glucose." Estimated average glucose, as the name suggests, is the estimate of your average blood glucose, expressed in mmol/L, based on the A1, for approximately the preceding three months.

Here is a table that shows the A1C in percent and in mmol/mol; as well as the corresponding estimated average blood glucose. (You can find an online calculator to convert A1C from percent to mmol/mol at www.ngsp.org/convert1.asp. You can find an online calculator to convert A1C to estimated average glucose at http://professional.diabetes.org/glucosecalculator.aspx):

A1C (percent)	A1C (mmol/mol)	Estimated Average Glucose (mmol/L)
5.0	31	5.4
5.5	37	6.2
6.0	42	7.0
6.5	48	7.8
7.0	53	8.6
7.5	59	9.4
8.0	64	10.2
8.5	69	10.9
9.0	75	11.8
9.5	81	12.6
10.0	86	13.4
10.5	91	14.1
11.0	97	14.9
11.5	102	15.7
12.0	108	16.5

After you have had your A1C tested, contact your doctor (or diabetes educator) to find out the result. If your A1C is above target (we discuss targets later in this section), ask your diabetes educator, diabetes specialist, and/or family physician what steps you, working with your health care team, can take to improve your result.

The A1C test doesn't replace blood glucose meter testing; it's *complementary* to it. Because the A1C represents an overall estimate of your blood glucose control, it doesn't express how many highs and lows you may be having. Your average glucose level may be good even though half your readings are too low and the other half too high. It's sort of like having one foot in ice water and the other in boiling water and saying, "On average, I feel fine."

Understanding your A1C result

As we mention earlier in this section, your *A1C* is a measure of how much glucose has become attached to your red blood cells over the past few months. This tells us about the relationship between the A1C and average blood glucose readings. Table 9-6 shows what the average blood glucose levels are over the preceding three to four months for a given A1C (a more comprehensive table is illustrated in the sidebar "New ways of reporting A1C").

Table 9-6	A1C with Corresponding Average Blood Glucose Level
A1C (%)	*Average Blood Glucose (mmol/L)*
6	7.0
7	8.6
8	10.2
9	11.8
10	13.4
11	14.9

As the table demonstrates, the higher your A1C, the higher your blood glucose levels have been running. The lower your A1C, the lower your recent blood glucose levels.

As you can see, your A1C reading is *not* the same as your average blood glucose reading. This is commonly misunderstood. (For example, an A1C of 8.0 percent does *not* mean that your average blood glucose level is 8.0 mmol/L; it actually corresponds to average readings of 10.2 mmol/L.)

The Canadian Diabetes Association recommends that most adults with diabetes have their A1C tested every three months (up to every six months if your A1C is consistently within target).

These are the CDA-recommended A1C targets for adults (we discuss the target A1C for children in Chapter 14 and for pregnant women in Chapter 7):

- ✔ For most adults: 7 percent or less.

- ✔ For adults with limited life expectancy, extensive coronary artery disease, multiple serious health problems, hypoglycemia unawareness, recurrent severe hypoglycemia, or other health problems that make experiencing hypoglycemia potentially dangerous: 7.1 to 8.5 percent.

- ✔ For certain young individuals in good health: 6.5 percent or less. (This lower target may help to further reduce the risk of eye and kidney damage.)

Check with your physician to find out what is your specific A1C target. And always bear in mind what we said earlier in this section: Even if you are unable to reach your target, *any* reduction in A1C reduces your risk of diabetes complications.

Looking at why your A1C and your blood glucose readings don't fit

For most people, their A1C result will fit with what they anticipate from their blood glucose meter readings. Sometimes, however, people find their A1C to be high despite very good meter readings, or, conversely, their A1C may be excellent despite consistently high meter readings. (The former situation is much more common than the latter.) When this occurs, you and your health care team need to figure out why.

Far and away the most common reason for your A1C to be discrepant to your blood glucose readings is if your blood glucose levels are up (or down) when you're not testing. In this situation your A1C seems out of keeping with your blood glucose test results because you're not testing often enough or at sufficiently variable times and you are missing your high (or low) values. If your readings are discrepant to your A1C, test more often (especially after meals) and at times you haven't been testing (including overnight). If that doesn't sort things out, an excellent next step is to have continuous glucose monitoring performed (see later in this chapter).

John was a 45-year-old man with type 2 diabetes newly referred to Ian. John had faithfully been checking his blood glucose twice daily: before breakfast and before dinner. His values were consistently within target; indeed, they almost never were above 6.9 mmol/L. When Ian measured John's A1C it was 9.0 percent, indicating John's overall average blood glucose was 11.8 mmol/L.

Johns was disappointed and surprised to hear this. "My blood glucose tests are great," he said with frustration, "so why would my A1C be so out of whack?" Ian asked John to routinely test his blood glucose daily two hours after all his meals and every few nights in the middle of the night for two weeks when they had another appointment. After two weeks John came in and handed Ian his logbook. John had highlighted in yellow all his readings that were above target. The book was as yellow as the mid-day sun. "Well, I guess we have the answer," John said. "My readings are up after every meal, especially after dinner where they're routinely in the high teens. Guess I've screwed up, eh?" "Not at all," Ian replied. "You've not screwed up in the least. You've collected some great data and now we know how to change your therapy to correct the problem." John's medications were adjusted and he also reduced how much carbohydrate he was eating with his supper. A few months later John's A1C was down to 7.5 percent and closely fit with his blood glucose test results.

Typically, as John discovered, a readily identifiable reason explains why a person's A1C doesn't fit with one's blood glucose readings. Sometimes, however, finding the answer is more difficult and requires some detective work. Particularly important is to figure out if you have some other medical condition or factor that makes the A1C an unreliable test to assess your overall blood glucose control. We discuss this in the next two sections.

Many excellent, knowledgeable health care providers are unaware that in some circumstances the A1C level does not truly reflect a person's blood glucose control. If ever you find yourself in the situation where you have an unexpected and unexplained discrepancy between your A1C and your blood glucose meter readings, and if your health care provider is unable to determine why, bring this book with you to your next appointment and show them this section (or refer them to the website we mention right after the lists below). Reading this will make your health care provider aware of possible explanations for the discrepancy so he can investigate.

If you have a condition (as we discuss in the next two sections) that makes your A1C an unreliable indicator of your overall blood glucose control, then you need to rely primarily on your blood glucose meter readings to determine your blood glucose control. Additionally, your doctor can check your fructosamine level from time to time (we discuss the fructosamine test earlier in this chapter) and can also periodically have you perform continuous glucose monitoring (we discuss this later in this chapter).

Conditions causing an increased A1C not due to high blood glucose

These are some conditions that can make a person's A1C elevated due to factors apart from blood glucose control:

- ✔ Having iron deficiency
- ✔ Having vitamin B12 deficiency

✔ Having a reduced production of red blood cells

✔ Overusing alcohol

✔ Having undergone a *splenectomy* (that is, your spleen has been removed)

✔ Taking high doses of ASA (aspirin)

✔ Using narcotics (such as morphine) chronically

Chronic kidney failure and a blood disorder called a *hemoglobinopathy* (examples are sickle cell anemia or thalassemia) can also occasionally cause the A1C to be elevated, but more commonly cause the A1C to be reduced (see the next section).

Conditions causing a lower A1C not due to excellent blood glucose

These are some conditions that can make a person's A1C lower due to factors apart from blood glucose control:

✔ Taking iron supplements

✔ Taking supplements of vitamin B12, C, or E

✔ Taking certain types of prescription drugs (such as certain anti-viral medications)

✔ Having chronic liver disease

✔ Having chronic kidney disease

✔ Taking ASA

✔ Having a *hemoglobinopathy* (we define this in the preceding section).

✔ Having a large spleen

✔ Having rheumatoid arthritis

✔ Having high triglyceride levels

The preceding two lists are not exhaustive. For more information have a look at the Canadian Diabetes Association document "Use of Glycated Hemoglobin (A1C) in the Diagnosis of Type 2 Diabetes Mellitus in Adults," which you can find on the CDA website (www.diabetes.ca).

Apart from going to the lab to have them take blood from your arm, you can check your A1C in two other ways. Some diabetes centres have a desktop machine that can process a finger-prick sample in a few minutes, so that you (and they) know your result while you are there for your visit. The cost is usually about $10 per test. A disposable home test kit is also available, but it is expensive and isn't covered by most provincial or private health plans, and thus, isn't often used.

Using a Continuous Glucose Monitoring System

Continuous glucose monitoring (CGM), which is used as part of a continuous glucose monitoring system (CGMS), is one of the most important recent advances in the world of type 1 diabetes. Ian predicts it will ultimately revolutionize the way diabetes (of any form) is managed. He envisions the day when people will look back at managing diabetes in the pre-CGM era with the same "how did you possibly manage?" disbelief that we now feel about the days before blood glucose meters.

Continuous glucose monitoring is, as its name suggests, the continuous measuring of your glucose level. Two types of CGM exist:

- ✔ **Real-time CGM:** This type continuously measures and displays your glucose level, allowing you to make moment-to-moment changes to your therapy. Real-time CGM also allows you to set alarms if your glucose level is too high or too low. Real-time CGM is also known as *personal CGM* because you use it mostly independent of your health care professionals. Ideally, if you are using real-time CGM, you would use it all the time.

- ✔ **Professional CGM:** This type continuously measures your glucose level, but rather than displaying your readings, it stores them on the CGM device for your health care provider to download and view later. Because professional CGM does not display the readings it is also known as *blinded CGM*. (It is called "professional" CGM because the equipment is typically used under the direct guidance of a health care professional.) Professional CGM is typically used just occasionally, for about a week at a time.

Understanding continuous glucose monitoring

Real-time continuous glucose monitoring systems have three components: a sensor, a transmitter, and a receiver (or display).

Two real-time systems are available in Canada:

- **Medtronic** (www.medtronic.ca) has two types of CGMS. The main difference is that in one system the display unit is a stand-alone device and, as illustrated in Figure 9-7, in the other system the display unit is integrated into an insulin pump.

- **Dexcom** (www.dexcom.com) makes a CGMS. This is shown in Figure 9-8.

Transmitter   Sensor   Display

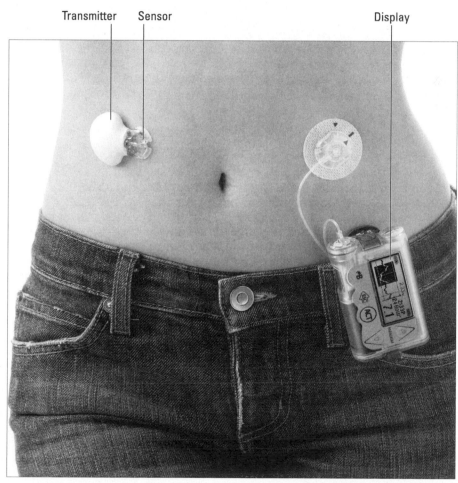

Figure 9-7:
A Medtronic continuous glucose monitoring system.

Photo printed with permission of Medtronic, Inc..

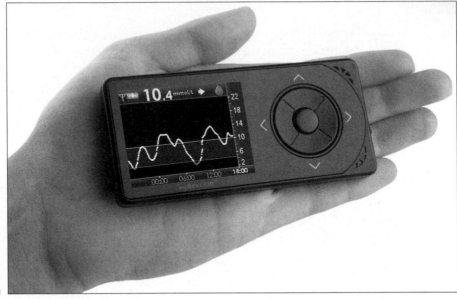

Figure 9-8:
Dexcom's
continuous
glucose
monitoring
system.

Figure 9-9 shows a close-up view of the Medtronic sensor and transmitter.

Sensor   Transmitter

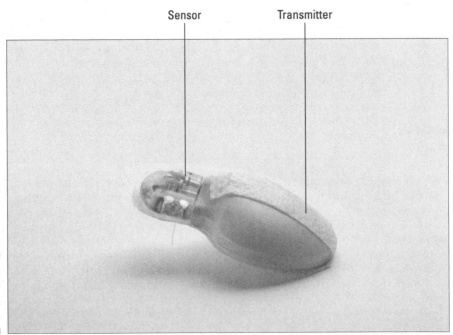

Figure 9-9:
Medtronic
sensor and
transmitter.

Here's how the different components of a real-time CGMS work:

- ✔ **Sensor:** A sensor is a disposable device with an electrode-containing tiny tail that's inserted under the skin — typically on the abdomen or buttock, but you can also put it on your arm or leg. Like your blood glucose test strips, the sensor measures your glucose level; however, unlike your blood glucose test strips, it measures your glucose level in your *interstitial* fluid (just under the skin surface), not your blood. The sensor then passes this information along to the transmitter.

- ✔ **Transmitter:** The sensor is directly connected to the transmitter. The transmitter receives your glucose level reading from the sensor and, using wireless technology, sends this data to the display (receiver).

- ✔ **Receiver (display):** The display, well, displays. It shows your current glucose level, your glucose levels over the past number of hours, and whether your glucose level is going up or down (this is indicated both by a continuous line and by arrows pointing — as you might imagine — up or down). It also has an alarm that will alert you if your glucose level is too low or too high. (The alarm thresholds are adjustable.)

  The display updates every five minutes; that means you will have a total of 288 measurements displayed per 24 hours. (Imagine doing 288 finger-prick samples per day!)

  Because the display is wireless, you can keep it anywhere up to several feet from the transmitter. This means that at night, for instance, you can put it on your bedside table and it'll still work. You can also upload the data to a website where both you and your health care team can review it.

Medtronic makes the only professional CGMS. Like real-time continuous glucose monitoring systems, professional CGMS has a sensor and a "transmitter" but, as we note earlier, the professional CGMS transmitter does not transmit data; rather, it stores data on a memory chip in the transmitter so your health care professional can download it later. As such, professional CGM has no receiver/display unit.

Checking out the benefits of continuous glucose monitoring

No matter how often you do a finger prick blood glucose test, you won't know what your glucose levels are for much of the day. Indeed, even if you test your blood a whopping ten times per day (and not many people are going to do that, thank you very much), you still only know your glucose level for a tiny fraction of the time. Sorting out your overall blood glucose control with this limited information is like trying to figure out the plot of a 300-page novel by reading only one word per page. With such limited information, at the very best you get only a vague sense of the plot and need to liberally "fill in the blanks" to guess what the story is all about. This holds true for managing your diabetes as well. You test your blood a certain number of times per day and you then need to "fill in the blanks" and guesstimate what your blood glucose level is for all those times between tests.

Despite these limitations, checking one's blood glucose a limited number of times per day (or even less often) in conjunction with periodic A1C testing (see earlier in this chapter) works surprisingly well and for the great majority of people with type 2 diabetes, this strategy provides enough information about one's blood glucose control. It works far less well, however, for many people with type 1 diabetes. It also works far less well for certain people with type 2 diabetes who are giving multiple daily injections of insulin.

Looking at the benefits of real-time continuous glucose monitoring

Here are some of the ways that *real-time* continuous glucose monitoring can help you:

✔ By providing you with a continuous display of your glucose levels (see Figure 9-10), real-time CGM gives you immediate feedback to tell you the impact on your glucose of the food you just ate, the exercise you just did (or are doing), and your insulin doses. This will then allow you to modify your diet, your exercise, or your insulin dosing if necessary.

✔ Up and down trending arrows alert you to an impending high or low blood glucose level so you can take corrective action *before* your glucose level gets too far out of whack. If your glucose level is heading up you can take extra insulin before your glucose level is too high; if you're glucose level is heading down you can take some sugar before you develop hypoglycemia.

Ian's friend, Jeremy, a physician with diabetes, has a nice way of explaining the importance of trending arrows. He says relying on isolated blood glucose readings to gauge your glucose control is like being a pilot whose altimeter says you're flying at 10,000 feet. Well, if the plane just took off and is climbing, that's well and good. But what if the plane is unexpectedly descending and you need to do something to avoid a crash landing? Either way you're at 10,000 feet, but what you do about it is as different as night and day. In other words, *the direction* that things are going provides essential information to tell you what to do — be it the up or down direction of a plane or the up or down direction of your glucose level. (Charlie Kimball, one of the best car racers in the world, lives with type 1 diabetes and relies on real-time CGM and these trending arrows to help keep his glucose levels in check as he whizzes around the racetrack at over 320 kilometres per hour! His website is www.charliekimball.com.)

✔ You can set (sound and vibration) alarms to go off if your glucose level is heading (or is) too low. These alarms alert you to an impending (or actual) episode of hypoglycemia so you can quickly take corrective action. These protective alarms are especially helpful if you experience hypoglycemia during your sleep or have hypoglycemia unawareness (refer to Chapter 5). *Low glucose suspend* is a feature available on Medtronic pumps when used along with a Medtronic CGMS. If you experience low blood glucose and do not take corrective action the pump automatically stops delivering insulin for a few hours. Without insulin being delivered, your blood glucose starts to rise, helping correct your hypoglycemia and reducing your risk of a catastrophic, prolonged episode of low blood glucose.

✔ You can set (sound and vibrations) alarms to go off if your glucose level is too high. This allows you to take corrective action such as giving yourself additional rapid-acting insulin.

Glucose levels for the past 24 hours   Current glucose level

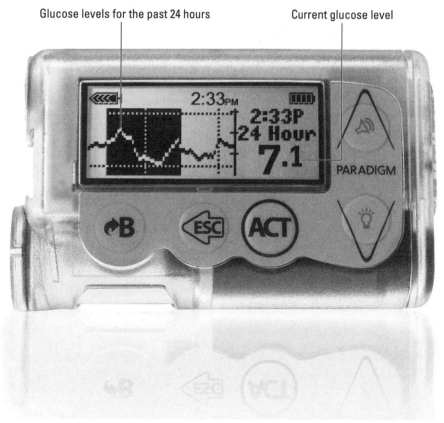

Figure 9-10:
Examples
of the
information
displayed on
a real-time
continuous
glucose
monitoring
system.

Real-time CGM can be so invaluable, so life-enhancing (even *lifesaving*), it's not surprising that more and more people living with diabetes (particularly type 1 diabetes) are using and benefiting from this technology. It does, however, have limitations and drawbacks as we discuss later in this section.

Looking at the benefits of professional continuous glucose monitoring

As we mention earlier, professional CGM does not provide information to you in real time; rather, the information is made available to you (and your health care provider) when you download the information from your device onto a computer. As such, it does not give you immediate feedback about your nutrition or exercise program, nor does it have alarms or a low glucose suspend feature. It does, however, provide invaluable *retrospective* information regarding:

- **The influence of your diet and exercise on your glucose level:** Thus, keeping a careful diary of what you've eaten and what activity you've done while you wore the CGM is very important.

- **An explanation for an A1C level that doesn't fit with your blood glucose readings:** For example, say your A1C was 9.2 percent despite your blood glucose readings being consistently less than 7.0 mmol/L. Professional CGM may reveal that your glucose level is well above target at times (such as after meals and overnight) that you are not routinely testing your blood. This helpful information may help guide changes to your therapy (such as, for example, needing to introduce — or increase the dose of — mealtime rapid-acting insulin or bedtime long-acting insulin).

- **Episodes of asymptomatic hypoglycemia:** Ian and his patients with type 1 diabetes are routinely shocked when they review professional CGM data and observe just how often prolonged and totally asymptomatic hypoglycemia happens during sleep. These patients had no inkling that anything was amiss. As they often say to Ian, "Sure, I noticed that my blood glucose was kind of low when I checked it in the morning, so I treated it and then I was fine. I had no idea that what I was seeing was the tail end of hours of hypoglycemia."

Being a fairly new and evolving technology, professional continuous glucose monitoring is not routinely available at many diabetes education centres or diabetes specialists' offices. If you and your health care providers feel you would benefit from professional CGM, have them contact Medtronic to find out the nearest facility where it is available.

A professional CGM study helped Martha, a patient of Ian's, who was testing her blood frequently using a blood glucose meter. (Her test results are marked as *x*'s in Figure 9-11. Note that for the sake of clarity we show only one day's CGM results; a typical professional CGM study provides several days' results superimposed on one another.)

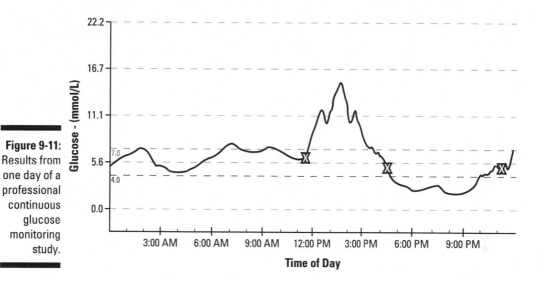

Martha's blood glucose levels, measured using her blood glucose meter, were excellent and, indeed, consistently within target. Her A1C was also excellent (6.5). However, the continuous line in the graph — which represents the data obtained from her CGMS — reveals that she had elevated glucose from about 1 p.m. until 3 p.m., and low blood glucose from 6 p.m. to 10 p.m. If Martha and Ian relied exclusively on her blood glucose meter results, they would have mistakenly thought everything was fine, whereas, in fact, her levels were often high and often low. Using the information from the CGMS, Ian, Martha, and her diabetes educators were able to adjust her insulin doses and diet, and her glucose levels were much more consistent thereafter.

Looking at the drawbacks of continuous glucose monitoring

Like all technology — especially new technology — CGM has some short-comings. These include the following:

✔ **Cost:** CGM uses disposable sensors. Each of these sensors costs about $50. Most people using real-time CGM replace these sensors about once a week. Needless to say, this cost quickly adds up. Also factor in the cost of the transmitter (about $700) and the receiver/display unit (this cost depends on whether you are using your pump as the receiver/display or a standalone unit). If you are using professional CGM your cost will be limited to a single sensor, because the other components will be lent to you free of charge for the duration of your CGM study. Also of note, whereas more and more provincial jurisdictions are funding pump therapy (at least for people with type 1 diabetes), such funding is not available for CGM, and private payers typically don't provide funding either.

- ✓ **Discomfort:** Some people find that inserting the sensor is uncomfortable or even somewhat painful. This is typically fleeting.

- ✓ **Inaccuracy:** Sensors are very accurate, but not perfect. Indeed, on occasion a value can be way off. For this reason, if you are using real-time CGM and get a value that's low enough or high enough to require corrective action, you must first do a blood glucose meter test to verify that the CGM result is accurate. (Just imagine if the sensor told you your glucose level was 14.0 — and you gave extra insulin — but in reality your glucose level was only 4.0. This would be very dangerous.)

- ✓ **Time lag:** Sensors measure the glucose level in your interstitial fluid, not in your blood. Most of the time the source is not important because interstitial fluid and blood have similar glucose levels. However, when your blood glucose level is quickly rising (such as immediately after eating) or quickly falling, your interstitial glucose level is different from your blood level. (It takes about 15 minutes for the interstitial fluid glucose level to catch up to the blood glucose level.) For this reason, you may notice symptoms of hypoglycemia, for example, even though the number you see on a real-time display is not low because the interstitial fluid glucose has yet to catch up. When you suspect your glucose level differs from what you see on the display, you need to test your blood to be certain what your level truly is.

- ✓ **Alarm fatigue:** A few years ago, when car theft alarms first became popular, it seemed like not a minute went by without some car horn blaring a false alert. The result? Most people stopped paying attention. Real-time CGM has a variety of alarms and alerts, all designed to help ensure the device is working properly and helping to keep you safe. The problem is, these warnings aren't always important and aren't always valid and, moreover, sometimes the CGM produces many alarms over the course of the day. Just like in the car alarm story, users can get tired from all this and start ignoring the CGM alarms or shutting them off altogether (which, of course, markedly reduces the CGM's value).

- ✓ **Calibration:** The sensors need to be taught how to interpret interstitial glucose readings. The way you teach them is by periodically doing a blood glucose test and entering the result into the CGMS. For this and for the other reasons in this list, having a CGMS does not mean you can throw away your blood glucose meter.

CGM is far from perfect, but every year the technology improves. Ultimately this will lead to the development of a feedback loop (essentially, an artificial pancreas) allowing your glucose sensor to continually and reliably measure your glucose level and automatically instruct your insulin pump to give just the right amount of insulin to match your needs. As one of Ian's patients said, "I'll simply wear my pancreas on my belt instead of having it inside my body."

You can learn more about continuous glucose monitoring systems by visiting the manufacturers' websites (www.medtronic.ca and www.dexcom.com), or by speaking to your diabetes educator or diabetes specialist. Note, however, that many health care providers, unless very involved with managing patients with type 1 diabetes, may not be all that familiar with CGM technologies.

Chapter 10

You Are What You Eat: Staying Healthy with Good Nutrition

*I*an has always believed that his power to help someone with diabetes gain control of their blood glucose (indeed, their health in general) pales in comparison to the unbridled power and influence of another source — *you* (the person living with diabetes)! Time after time, patient after patient, when someone who has not customarily looked after their health begins to take charge of the way they live, what they eat, what they drink, what exercise they do, what weight they shed, Ian smiles in awe. He not only gets to put away his prescription pad, but, often, is able to advise someone that their new lifestyle is working so well that they can withdraw some of their medications.

In this chapter we look at the key nutrition (diet) strategies you can follow to achieve and maintain good diabetes health. We also look at effective ways that people who are overweight (as most people with type 2 diabetes are; indeed, as most Canadians with or without diabetes are) can safely and effectively lose weight. (In Chapter 11 we explore the important ways that exercise can help you manage your diabetes.)

If diabetes is brand new to you, you may be reading this chapter before having the opportunity to meet with a dietitian. If so, in addition to reading this chapter, we recommend you have a look at the Canadian Diabetes Association (CDA) "Just the Basics" resource (www.diabetes.ca/basics). This short document is a summary of the essential CDA dietary recommendations you can follow until you meet with the dietitian. (If your doctor hasn't yet referred you to a dietitian, ask your doctor to do this as soon as possible.)

The Key Ingredients

Our diets are made up primarily of carbohydrates, proteins, and fats. These basic groups are rounded out by the other things we need to consume to survive, including minerals, vitamins, and, of course, water. And, for most of us, our diets also include some amount of alcohol and, often, non-nutritive sweeteners.

The CDA recommends that people with diabetes follow *Eating Well with Canada's Food Guide* (you can find it online at www.hc-sc.gc.ca/fn-an/food-guide-aliment/index-eng.php). This helpful guide recommends that you do the following:

✔ Enjoy a variety of foods.

✔ Emphasize cereals, breads and other whole grain products, fruits, and vegetables.

✔ Choose lower-fat dairy products, leaner meats, and food prepared with little or no fat.

✔ Select foods that are "low in energy density" (meaning that they aren't jam packed with lots of calories in a small volume of food) and are "high in volume." (This helps you feel full faster and avoid overeating.)

✔ Achieve and maintain a healthy body weight by enjoying regular physical activity and healthy eating.

✔ Limit salt, alcohol, and caffeine.

The CDA also recommends that you divide your diet (based on energy, or calories) as follows:

✔ **Carbohydrate:** 45 to 60 percent

✔ **Protein:** 15 to 20 percent

✔ **Fat:** 20 to 35 percent

Carbohydrates and proteins provide a different amount of energy (measured in calories) than fats. The number of calories in 1 gram of each group is as follows:

> ✔ **Carbohydrate:** 4 calories
>
> ✔ **Protein:** 4 calories
>
> ✔ **Fat:** 9 calories

Of course, you and your dietitian have to determine the best diet for you based on your particular needs. Your diet will include not only the best food choices for you, but also the appropriate number of calories you should consume. With unrestricted calories, you could limit your carbohydrates to 45 percent of your diet and still have enough energy to power a Boeing 777.

Technically speaking, there is a *calorie* and there is a *Calorie* and there is a *kilocalorie* (1,000 calories equals 1 Calorie equals 1 *kilo*calorie). However, almost no one speaks of kilocalories in normal, day-to-day discourse — and capitalizing the *c* every time is a chore — so we use the conventional term *calorie* whenever we talk about nutrition issues. Sure, doing so is not perfectly scientific, but we won't tell if you won't. (Also, you may come across the term *kilojoules*. One Calorie is equal to about 4.2 kilojoules. Again, few people use this unit of measure, so we don't either.)

Carbohydrates

Carbohydrates do much more than just fuel our bodies. They also fuel debate. Indeed, probably no other area of diabetes management offers quite the same degree of controversy. In this section we look at the important issues for you to be aware of, including the pros and cons of low versus higher carbohydrate diets.

Although *glucose* gets most of the attention, within our bodies we also have other forms of carbohydrate, including glycogen (which is stored in the liver and muscles). Dietary carbohydrates include starches, cellulose, and gums (not the chewing type).

Food sources of carbohydrate are found primarily in things grown in the ground and in dairy foods. Some of the common dietary sources of carbohydrate are bread, potatoes, grains, cereals, rice, dairy products such as milk and yogurt (cheese has very small amounts of carbohydrate), fruits, and some sweet, usually fleshy vegetables (such as parsnips and squash).

These are some important roles that carbohydrates play in the body:

- ✔ Carbohydrates are the main source of energy for muscles.
- ✔ Glucose is the carbohydrate that causes the pancreas to release insulin.
- ✔ When your body doesn't have enough insulin or your insulin doesn't work sufficiently well, ingesting carbohydrates raises the blood glucose above normal.
- ✔ Sugars (in sweet items such as candy) are not directly harmful (except, perhaps to your teeth if you don't look after them very well) as long as the total number of calories you ingest is not excessive.

Consuming sugar does *not* cause diabetes. Furthermore, don't let any well-meaning friend or relative tell you that because you have diabetes you cannot eat sugar. You can tell them Ian said so. (We'll leave it up to you if you also want to tell them that you recognize that you have to eat appropriate amounts and types of sugar.)

A few years back an elderly man was referred to Ian after having had type 2 diabetes diagnosed a few months earlier. He was a charming gentleman and clearly was working diligently to maintain his traditionally good health. As they spoke, Ian couldn't help but get the impression that something was bothering his new patient. Finally, because the gentleman was not volunteering anything in this way, Ian asked him if something was on his mind. "Well, Doctor," he said, "I guess I'm just feeling kind of sad that I had my 80th birthday yesterday and everyone got to eat my birthday cake except for me. And it was my favourite, too. Chocolate. I couldn't have any because I have diabetes." Whatever reply this gentleman was expecting, it was clearly not the one that Ian supplied. "Well, sir," Ian said, "I have a prescription I want you to fill. Right after you leave this office I want you to go *not* to the drugstore, but to the *bakery.* Buy the biggest chocolate cake they sell and cut yourself as big a slice as you want. And if anyone tells you that you 'can't eat it because you have diabetes,' you tell them that your diabetes specialist *ordered* you to." The patient left the room literally singing.

Cake is not a four-letter word! (Well, not *that* kind of four-letter word.) If you have diabetes, you can eat not only cake, but other sweets too. The point is, nothing is forbidden, sweets (in the form of products that contain added sucrose or fructose) just have to be consumed in moderation (not exceeding ten percent of your total daily calories) and, most importantly, not at the expense of other, healthier foods that you need. So long as your total number of carbohydrates and calories is appropriate, nothing is wrong with having occasional treats. Happy birthday!

Because carbohydrate is the food that raises the blood glucose — and high glucose is responsible for many of the complications of diabetes — consuming the proper amount of carbohydrates is important.

If you are on a 2,000-calorie diet and are consuming 50 percent of your calories as carbohydrate, that would work out to 1,000 calories of carbohydrate per day. Because a gram of carbohydrate is 4 calories, you could eat 250 grams of carbohydrate in a day. Most people with diabetes do very well on this amount of carbohydrate, but for others a lower percentage works best. In Appendix A we look at the number of grams of carbohydrate contained in a variety of foods and how this information can be used to help you come up with a healthy menu.

The CDA recommends a minimum intake of 130 grams of carbohydrates per day. Many of our patients ask us if they should follow a much lower carbohydrate intake (a "low-carb diet"). Often they've experimented with this and observed their blood glucose readings to have improved. Indeed, research studies do show that *short-term* use of a low-carbohydrate diet does indeed improve blood glucose control. However, low-carb diets present a few problems: They are difficult to follow for a long period of time; the long-term safety of low-carb diets is not established; and these diets may not provide sufficient vitamins, minerals, or fibre. For all these reasons, we advise against following a low-carb diet.

Glycemic index

All carbohydrates aren't alike in the degree to which they raise blood glucose. This fact was recognized some years ago, and a measurement called the *glycemic index* was created to quantify the amount that each food raises blood glucose. The glycemic index (GI) uses oral glucose as the standard (or indicator) food and assigns it a value of 100. Another food containing an equal amount of carbohydrate is rated according to its ability to raise blood glucose and is assigned a value in comparison to oral glucose. A food that raises glucose one quarter as much as oral glucose has a GI of 25, while a food that raises glucose three quarters as much has a GI of 75. A glycemic index of 70 or more is considered high; 56 to 69 is medium; and 55 or less is low. The point of the index is to select carbohydrates with low GI levels to try to keep the glucose response as low as possible.

Choosing carbohydrates with a low glycemic index can help to improve blood glucose control (and lipids). You might think, therefore, that you should make a concerted effort to choose low-GI foods. Alas, the story is much more complicated:

✔ The GI of a carbohydrate-containing food may be different when it is eaten alone than when it is part of a mixed meal.

✔ The GI of a food may differ depending on how it's processed and prepared.

✔ Some low-GI foods contain a lot of fat.

✔ Figuring out the GI can be difficult and can lead to confusion.

We can think of no better illustration of the fact that a low GI food is not automatically a good food choice than this: A Snickers candy bar rates better on the GI than a bowl of cornflakes. (We are not making this up!) Does the fact that a Snickers bar has a better GI than cornflakes make it a better food choice? Of course not! The glycemic index, in and of itself, doesn't make a food choice healthy or good. The GI is just one component among many (as we discuss in this chapter) that determines if a particular food is a good choice.

Because following a low glycemic index diet can help control blood glucose and lipids the Canadian Diabetes Association recommends following a low GI diet, however the CDA notes that this "should be based on the individual's interest and ability."

We recommend you start your nutrition therapy with the standard Canadian Diabetes Association recommendations, as you will learn from your dietitian. If you have been working with this meal plan and not succeeding the way you should, speak to your dietitian about possibly following a low-GI diet.

Should you elect to proceed with a low-glycemic-index diet, you can easily make some simple substitutions in your diet, as Table 10-1 shows.

Table 10-1	Simple Diet Substitutions
High-GI Food	*Low-GI Food*
Whole-meal or white bread	Whole-grain, multigrain, pumpernickel, or rye bread
Processed breakfast cereal such as corn flakes, puffed rice, puffed oats, and puffed wheat	Unrefined cereals like steel-cut oats, large-flake rolled oats, or processed low-GI cereals like muesli
Plain cookies and crackers, puffed rice cakes	Cookies made with dried fruits or whole grains like oats
Cupcakes and doughnuts	Cakes and muffins made with fruit, oats, and whole grains
Potatoes	Pasta (cooked al dente) or legumes
White rice	Basmati, brown, wild, or parboiled rice
Tropical fruit such as pine-apple, mango, papaya, can-taloupe, and watermelon	Temperate fruit such as apples, pears, oranges, peaches, plums, apricots, cherries, and berries

Because bread and breakfast cereals are major daily sources of carbohydrates, these simple changes can make a major difference in lowering your glycemic index. Foods that are excellent sources of carbohydrate but have a low GI include legumes such as peas or beans, pasta, grains like barley, par-boiled rice, and whole grain breads.

You can discover more about the glycemic index online at `www.diabetes.ca/for-professionals/resources/nutrition/glycemic-index` (or, easier, type "CDA glycemic index" into your search engine of choice and it will be the first hit).

Carbohydrate counting

Glucose levels rise after you eat mainly because of the carbohydrates in your meal (or snack). Also, in general, the greater the number of grams of carbohydrate, the more your blood glucose level will rise. People who are on an insulin program that includes frequent administration of rapid-acting insulin can gauge the amount of insulin to give themselves based on the number of grams of carbohydrate they are about to ingest. This is especially helpful if you have type 1 diabetes. (We discuss carb counting further in Chapter 13.)

Fibre

Fibre is the part of the carbohydrate that is not digestible and, therefore, adds no calories. It is found in most fruits, grains, and vegetables. Fibre comes in two forms:

- **Soluble fibre:** This form of fibre can dissolve in water and has a lowering effect on blood glucose and lipids, particularly cholesterol. Soluble fibre gets gooey and sticky when mixed with water. Examples of soluble fibre are oatmeal, eggplant, okra, oat products, beans, psyllium, and barley.

- **Insoluble fibre:** This form of fibre cannot dissolve in water and remains in the intestine. It absorbs water and stimulates movement in the intestine. Insoluble fibre also helps prevent constipation and possibly colon cancer. This is the fibre called *bulk* or *roughage*. Insoluble fibre doesn't change much when mixed with water. An example is the skin of an apple.

Consuming soluble fibre can help improve your after-meal blood glucose levels. Also, diets rich in fibre — especially cereal fibre — are associated with a reduced risk of cardiovascular disease.

The Canadian Diabetes Association recommends you ingest 25 to 50 grams of fibre daily.

Because too much fibre causes diarrhea and gas, increase the fibre level in your diet fairly slowly.

Proteins

Protein in your diet is usually in the form of muscle of other animals, such as chicken, turkey, beef, or lamb. Vegetable sources of protein include soybeans, legumes, nuts, and seeds. The main role that protein has in your diet is to maintain the health of tissues such as your muscles. For these reasons, people used to believe that you could build your own muscle by eating lots of other animals' muscle. The truth, however, is that you can build up your muscle only by exercising or weightlifting. You need little protein to maintain your current level of muscle, or increase it for that matter. Unlike carbohydrates, proteins do not raise blood glucose levels significantly.

Your choice of protein sources is very important because some contain very high quantities of fat while others are relatively fat-free. The following lists give you an idea of the fat content of various sources of protein.

About 30 grams (1 ounce) of **very lean** meat, fish, or substitute has 7 grams of protein and 1 gram of fat. Examples are

- Skinless, white-meat chicken or turkey
- Flounder, halibut, or tuna canned in water
- Lobster, shrimp, or clams
- Fat-free cheese

If you're looking for a source of protein with no fat, try Greek yogurt. Two ounces (about 60 grams or one quarter cup) of Greek yogurt contains 6 grams of protein and 0 grams of fat.

About 30 grams (1 ounce) of **lean** meat, fish, or substitute has 7 grams of protein and 3 grams of fat. Examples are

- Lean beef, lean pork, lamb, or veal
- Dark-meat chicken without skin or white-meat chicken with skin
- Sardines, salmon, or tuna canned in oil
- Other meats or cheeses with 3 grams of fat per 30 grams (1 ounce)

About 30 grams (1 ounce) of **medium-fat** meat, fish, or substitute has 7 grams of protein and 5 grams of fat. Examples are

- Most beef products
- Regular fat pork, lamb, or veal

- ✔ Dark-meat chicken with skin or fried chicken
- ✔ Fried fish
- ✔ Cheeses with 5 grams of fat per 30 grams (1 ounce) such as feta and mozzarella

About 30 grams (1 ounce) of **high-fat** meat, fish, or substitute contains 7 grams of protein and 8 grams of fat. Examples are

- ✔ Pork spareribs or pork sausage
- ✔ Bacon
- ✔ Regular cheeses such as cheddar and Monterey Jack
- ✔ Processed sandwich meats

You'll find a huge difference in the number of calories depending on whether you choose a high- or low-fat protein source. For instance, 30 grams (1 ounce) of skinless white-meat chicken contains about 40 calories, whereas 30 grams (1 ounce) of pork spareribs has 100 calories. Because most people eat a minimum of about 120 grams (about 4 ounces) of meat at a meal, they're eating from 160 to 400 calories depending upon the source. That's why looking carefully at the food you are about to eat is so important: The company your protein source keeps can make the difference between you successfully losing weight or not.

If you're on a 2,000-calorie diet of which 20 percent is protein, 400 calories would come from protein sources. Because a gram of protein is 4 calories, you could eat 100 grams of protein in a day.

Fats

When we think of fat, we tend to think of the fat we see on a steak or in hamburger meat. But you can find quite a variety of fats and fat-like substances. Although many of these are unhealthy and to be avoided, some, in fact, help to protect our health. This section looks at these different issues.

Cholesterol

Cholesterol is the fat-like substance everyone knows. It has been shown to be a major contributor leading to atherosclerosis (such as coronary artery disease, as we discuss in Chapter 6). It is recommended that no more than 300 milligrams a day of fat come from cholesterol. (One large egg has about 210 mg of cholesterol.) Other sources of cholesterol include organ meat such as liver or kidney, whole milk, and hard cheeses such as Monterey Jack and cheddar.

Most people do not realize the extent to which our bodies (our liver in particular) contribute to our cholesterol levels. In fact, our liver makes the majority of our body's cholesterol. And many people have a genetic predisposition for their liver to make too much cholesterol. That's why so many people with diabetes, even if faithfully following a low-fat diet, still require medication to achieve optimal blood cholesterol levels.

Other types of fat

In addition to cholesterol are several other types of fat:

- **Saturated fat** is the kind of fat that comes from animal sources. The streaks of fat in a steak are saturated fat. Butter, bacon, cream, and cream cheese are other examples of foods rich in saturated fat. Eating a lot of saturated fat can make your bad (LDL) cholesterol level go up. And that's not a good thing. The Canadian Diabetes Association recommends that saturated fat be no more than 7 percent of your total calorie intake.

- **Unsaturated fat** comes from vegetable sources such as olive oil, canola oil, and margarine. It comes in several forms:

  - **Monounsaturated fat** raises HDL (this is the good cholesterol) and does not affect LDL (bad cholesterol). Avocado, olive oil, and canola oil are examples. The oil in nuts, such as almonds and peanuts, is also monounsaturated.

  - **Polyunsaturated fat** lowers LDL but, depending on how much you consume, may also lower HDL. Examples of polyunsaturated fats are soft fats and oils such as corn oil, mayonnaise, and margarine. Polyunsaturated fats should be less than 10 percent of your total calorie intake.

One particularly healthy polyunsaturated fat is *omega-3 fatty acids*. Omega-3 fatty acids can help protect you from atherosclerosis, help improve your lipids, reduce blood pressure, and can also protect against the formation of blood clots in the coronary arteries (reducing your chances of having a heart attack). Omega-3 fatty acids are found in certain fish (such as salmon, tuna, mackerel, and trout) and plant sources (such as flax, soy, chia seeds, walnuts, and sea weed). You can also find certain brands of milk, eggs, and other foods that have added ("fortified") omega-3 fatty acids. It's recommended that you eat fish rich in omega-3 fatty acids at least once (better still, two or three times) per week.

Despite their widespread use, no convincing scientific evidence shows that taking omega-3 supplements (such as capsules) provides the same proven health benefits as getting your omega-3 fatty acids in the foods you eat. Therefore, we recommend you try to get this nutrient the way nature intended: in the foods you eat, not in the form of supplements.

Trans fatty acids (also called *trans fats*) raise LDL levels and are particularly unhealthy. You should minimize the amount you consume. Trans fatty acids are formed when liquid oil goes through a process of hydrogenation, turning it into a semi-solid form, like shortening and many margarines. These fats are used widely in the food industry in many commercially baked goods such as cookies, cakes, potato chips, doughnuts, pastries, French fries, and breaded foods. However, partly because of legislation, partly because of good business smarts, and partly because it's simply the right thing to do, more and more food manufacturers are reducing or eliminating trans fats from their products. You can significantly reduce your intake of these fats by avoiding commercially fried foods and high-fat bakery products. Looking at the nutrition facts table on a food label will tell you how much trans fat a given product contains.

If we go back to your hypothetical 2,000-calorie diet — lest you slowly starve while waiting for us to figure out how much fat to feed you so that you get your final 600 calories — fat has 9 calories per gram, so you can eat about 67 grams of fat daily. Seeing as you may have consumed much of this with your protein source, you may not have much fat left to add.

Getting Enough Vitamins, Minerals, and Water

Your nutrition plan must contain sufficient vitamins and minerals. If you eat a balanced diet that comes from the various food groups, you'll generally get enough vitamins for your daily needs. Indeed, the Canadian Diabetes Association guidelines advise that "routine vitamin and mineral supplementation is generally not recommended." Table 10-2 lists the vitamins and their food sources.

Table 10-2	Vitamins You Need	
Vitamin	*Function*	*Food Source*
Vitamin A	Needed for healthy skin, bones, and eyes	Milk, and green and orange vegetables
Vitamin B1 (thiamine)	Converts carbohydrates into energy	Meat and whole grain cereals
Vitamin B2 (riboflavin)	Needed to use food properly	Milk, cheese, fish, and green vegetables
Vitamin B6 (pyridoxine)	Needed for growth	Liver, yeast, and many other foods
Vitamin B12	Keeps the red blood cells and the nervous system healthy	Animal foods (for example, meat) and eggs
Folic acid (also called folate)	Keeps the red blood cells healthy	Green vegetables

(continued)

Table 10-2 *(continued)*

Vitamin	Function	Food Source
Niacin	Helps maintain healthy metabolism	Lean meat, fish, nuts, and legumes
Vitamin C	Helps maintain supportive tissues	Fruit and vegetables
Vitamin D	Helps with absorption of calcium	Dairy products, and is made in the skin when exposed to sunlight
Vitamin E	Helps maintain cells	Vegetable oils and whole grain cereals
Vitamin K	Needed for proper clotting of the blood	Green, leafy vegetables

As you look through the vitamins in Table 10-2, you can see that most of them are readily available in the foods you eat every day.

In certain situations, such as if you are pregnant or breastfeeding, elderly, a strict vegetarian, or on a very low-calorie diet, you should take a multivitamin daily. (If you could become or are pregnant you should also take a folic acid supplement. We discuss vitamin therapy and pregnancy in Chapter 7.) The CDA recommends taking 400 IU (international units) of vitamin D daily if you are older than 50. Apart from these special circumstances, taking vitamin supplements is seldom helpful (except for the people selling them!).

Minerals are also key ingredients of a healthy diet. Living with diabetes your mineral needs are essentially the same as if you didn't have diabetes. You only need most of your minerals in tiny amounts and can easily get them from a balanced diet. Take special note of two minerals:

- **Calcium:** Be sure to consume between 1,000 and 1,500 milligrams of calcium per day to maintain strong bones and help avoid osteoporosis. (If you aren't consuming enough calcium in your diet, you should take calcium supplements.)

- **Sodium:** Avoid adding sodium (salt) to your food, and if you have high blood pressure, make a point of buying foods that are low in salt. Try to restrict your sodium intake to less than 1,500 mg per day if you are under 50 years of age (less than 1,300 mg per day if you are between 50 and 70 years of age; and less than 1,200 mg per day if you are over 70 years of age).

Don't waste your money taking chromium supplements. Taking chromium supplements isn't proven to help control your diabetes.

Although we've saved our discussion about water to last, it is by no means the least important. Water makes up 60 percent or more of your body. All the nutrients in the body are dissolved in water. You can live without food for some time, but you won't last long without water. Water can help to give a feeling of fullness that reduces appetite. Make a point of drinking at least 1½ litres (50 ounces) of water per day.

Counting Alcohol as Part of Your Diet

Alcohol is a substance that has calories but no particular nutritional value. It has, however, been shown that a moderate amount (a drink or two per day) may reduce your risk of a heart attack.

If you like to have a drink, it's fine so long as you limit yourself to the following:

✔ No more than two drinks per day and less than ten drinks per week if you're a woman. (Of course, if you're pregnant you should not drink any alcohol at all.)

✔ No more than 3 drinks per day and less than 15 drinks per week if you're a man.

Having two drinks per day is *not* the same as having no alcohol all week and then quaffing 14 cold ones on a Saturday evening while you watch *Hockey Night in Canada.* Even if the game goes into overtime.

Because alcohol has calories, you must account for the alcohol you drink in your diet. Depending on the strength of the individual product, 350 millilitres (12 ounces) of beer, 150 millilitres (5 ounces) of wine, and 45 millilitres (1½ ounces) of hard liquor all have similar quantities of alcohol.

Despite what many people think, drinking beer or wine is not better for you than drinking hard liquor. To your liver they all taste the same.

Apart from the consequences of the calories it provides, keep in mind several other important points about alcohol:

✔ Alcohol — especially if taken without food — can cause low blood glucose if you are on insulin or some other types of antihyperglycemic medication (see Chapter 12). It does so by reducing your liver's ability to produce glucose. You can lessen this risk by making sure you eat some food when you drink alcohol.

- Alcohol reduces your awareness of symptoms of low blood glucose (refer to Chapter 5) and, as a result, makes you less likely to take appropriate corrective action.

- Alcohol can interact with sulfonylurea medications (see Chapter 12), which causes a variety of unpleasant symptoms, including nausea and flushing (even if you are not inebriated). This was more of a problem with older, now seldom-used sulfonylurea medications and rarely occurs with modern sulfonylurea drugs.

- If you're taking insulin or certain medicines that stimulate insulin production, drinking alcohol two or three hours after your supper can result in hypoglycemia occurring as late as the next evening.

Non-nutritive Sweeteners

Unrestricted consumption of sugars doesn't fit with good diabetes management (or, of course, with good health in general). And because how much sugar we should consume is limited, non-nutritive sweeteners have a role to play. *Non-nutritive sweeteners* (or sugar substitutes) are products which provide few calories and are added to other foods or drinks to provide sweetness.

The CDA guidelines note that these non-nutritive sweeteners have been approved by Health Canada for use "as either table-top sweeteners, food additives, or for use in chewing gum:"

- Acesulfame
- Aspartame
- Cyclamate
- Neotame
- Saccharin
- Sucralose
- Tagatose
- Thaumatin

Some of the non-nutritive sweeteners in the list have (many) other names. You will need to carefully read food labels to determine if these products are in the food you are buying.

Stevia is another non-nutritive sweetener. It is, however, not approved by Health Canada for use in foods, but is sold in some natural health products.

Of the non-nutritive sweeteners in common use, aspartame is especially well known. In the amounts commonly used, aspartame provides virtually no calories, yet provides abundant sweetness. In fact, aspartame is 200 times sweeter than sucrose (table sugar). Aspartame has been the subject of many Internet rumours detailing its dangers. These are false. The truth of the matter is that aspartame is completely safe unless you have a rare genetic disease called PKU. The equal truth is that despite common use of aspartame in our society, we as a population are getting larger and larger, not smaller and smaller.

Little data exists on the use of neotame and thaumatin in people living with diabetes. The other non-nutritive sweeteners in the preceding list are safe to use if you have diabetes — unless you're pregnant or breastfeeding, in which case you shouldn't consume saccharin or cyclamate.

Sugar alcohols (erythritol, isomalt, lactitol, maltitol, mannitol, sorbitol, and xylitol) are another type of non-nutritive sweetener. They do provide calories, but typically have very little effect on blood glucose levels. Examples of products that may contain sugar alcohols are chewing gum, hard candies, some jams, and syrups. Consuming more than 10 grams per day of sugar alcohols can cause abdominal cramping and diarrhea.

A helpful website to learn more about non-nutritive sweeteners, including their various names, is www.sweetenerbook.com.

Looking at Other Dietary Strategies

In addition to general healthy eating principles as discussed in this chapter, you can undertake several other CDA-approved strategies to enhance your health.

- ✔ **The Mediterranean diet** can improve blood glucose control and lower the risk for cardiovascular disease. The Mediterranean diet emphasizes consuming olive oil, legumes, unrefined cereals, fruits, vegetables, nuts, seeds, dairy products, and fish. Meat is consumed in only small amounts.

- ✔ **A vegan or vegetarian diet** can improve blood glucose control and lipid levels. (Though definitions vary, generally speaking a vegan diet excludes all animal products including dairy products, and a vegetarian diet excludes meat, fish and poultry, but includes dairy products such as cheese, eggs, yogurt, or milk.)

- ✔ **A DASH ("Dietary Approaches to Stop Hypertension") diet** can lower blood pressure, improve blood glucose control, and lower the risk for cardiovascular disease. The DASH diet emphasizes fruits, vegetables, fat-free or low-fat dairy products, whole grains, fish, poultry, fibre, and nuts, and avoids saturated fats, cholesterol, and red meats.

The CDA also notes that diets high in "dietary pulses" (examples of dietary pulses are beans, peas, chickpeas, and lentils) can be consumed to improve blood glucose and lipid levels.

Eating Out

Canadians are eating more and more of their meals in restaurants. This is not necessarily a bad thing (especially if you happen to own a restaurant!), but it complicates managing your diabetes. At home you know what ingredients you're using, you can measure quantities, you can follow certain steps to avoid weight gain (see the section "Weighty Issues," later in this chapter, for behaviour-changing tips), and, if you're carbohydrate counting, you can fairly accurately measure the carbs in your food. In a restaurant, you mostly don't have control over many of these factors. Also, restaurants (including fast-food establishments) tend to serve food that is richer in fat, higher in salt, and bigger in volume than you might normally eat at home (see the section "Weighty Issues" for more about proper portion size). We may not consider *cake* to be a bad four-letter word, but *supersize* sure is!

Here are helpful tips you can follow to make eating out a healthful, not harmful, experience:

- **Make sure you eat foods from the major food groups.** Even fast-food restaurants have healthy food selections if you look hard enough.

- **If a portion size is big (ask the wait staff; they'll know), order one serving and split it with your dinner-mate.** (That's what Ian and his wife routinely do; and the wait staff don't even blink.)

- **Avoid buffets.** Few people can go to an all-you-can-eat place and leave the restaurant feeling less than stuffed. Also, buffets often serve carbohydrate-rich foods, which will make your blood glucose level go up.

- **Order foods that are baked, steamed, or broiled rather than deep fried.** Fried foods are typically less healthy than are these other choices.

- **Ask for salad dressings, toppings, and sauces on the side, not on top of your food.** This way, you can be in control of determining how much or how little of these items you have.

- **Avoid foods that are heavily battered or breaded or that are served with rich, creamy, or cheesy sauces.** Heavy battering and breading and these types of sauces are typically less healthy choices.

- **Make sure the wait staff are paying attention when you order a diet soft drink.** Wait staff sometimes bring a non-diet soft drink to the table by mistake.

✔ **If you take rapid-acting insulin before your meals, don't take your dose until you're certain your food is on its way.** Better still, wait until it's in front of you. More than one person has had an insulin reaction because they took their dose only to then find their food was delayed in arriving. (This is a concern especially if you're on a plane. The food cart is on its way, you give your insulin, when, oops, turbulence hits and the cart disappears. But your dose has already been administered, putting you at risk of hypoglycemia. Better to not give your rapid-acting insulin until your yummy — or not — airline food is right in front of you.)

Making sense of nutrition food labels

Prepackaged foods for sale in Canada have nutrition food labels. Understanding these sometimes confusing labels will help you make healthy food selections when you're at the grocery store. In this sidebar we look specifically at those aspects of nutrition food labels that are especially important for people with diabetes.

These are the most important things about nutrition food labels for you to be aware of:

✔ **The serving size:** In theory, this is the amount of the item that one person would be expected to eat during one meal (or snack, and so on). This amount is set by the manufacturer. It is, however, very easy to buy a package and, based on its size, assume it to be one serving size whereas, in fact, it may contain two or more servings. (You may be astonished to find out how tiny one serving of a favourite snack actually is.) Remember that you may or may not want to eat one serving size. If you eat two servings, for example, you'll be consuming twice as many calories and twice as much fat as what the label lists the product to contain for just one serving size.

✔ **% daily value:** This indicates the percent of your daily nutrition requirements you will meet by eating one serving size of the food.

✔ **The amounts, in one serving, of calories, total fat, saturated fat, trans fat, total** cholesterol, sodium, total carbohydrates, fibre, sugars, protein, vitamin A, vitamin C, calcium, and iron.** This is a detailed list indeed, but provides key information regarding these essential nutrients.

These are other important things for you to know about food labels:

✔ Prepackaged foods are often rich in sodium, so keep an especially close eye on this part of the label.

✔ If you're carbohydrate counting, note that although fibre is listed on the label, because it doesn't raise blood glucose, you should subtract it from the total amount of carbohydrate listed when you perform your calculations.

If you have questions about a specific product's nutrition food label, remove it from the package (ah, that would be *after* you've bought the product) and take it with you to your next appointment with your dietitian. (Alternatively, take a picture of the label — whether or not you've bought the product — and bring the picture with you when you next see the dietitian.) You can learn more about food labels at the Dietitians of Canada website: www.dietitians.ca. You can find out more about "nutrient content claims" at www.hc-sc.gc.ca/fn-an/label-etiquet/nutrition/cons/claims-reclam/table1-eng.php.

Weighty Issues

If you're overweight and have diabetes (refer to Chapter 4 if you're not sure how much you should weigh), these are some of the benefits you may experience from even small weight loss:

- Improved blood glucose control. (If you have type 2 diabetes, you may even find that your antihyperglycemic medications — which may not have been working sufficiently well for you — work much more effectively to the point that, in consultation with your physician, some — or possibly all — of them can be reduced in dose or even discontinued altogether.)
- Improved blood pressure
- Improved lipids (cholesterol and triglycerides)
- Enhanced self-esteem
- Better sex life
- More energy and more incentive to exercise
- Reduced risk of some types of cancer
- Increased life expectancy

Weight-loss challenges

Losing weight is difficult for many reasons, but perhaps foremost among them is the immense challenge of trying to change lifestyle patterns and habits that you may have lived with for decades. No one should ever tell you that the changes you're being asked to make are easy. They are *not* easy. In fact, for most people they are downright difficult. But *you can do it.*

Another obstacle to losing weight is expecting too much too soon. If you need to lose 23 kilograms (about 50 pounds) and after a month you have lost only 2 kilograms (about 4 pounds), you may start to feel frustrated, as if you're never going to get there. But don't think for a second that you haven't had success. You've had great success! So pat yourself on the back (something, by the way, that many people living with diabetes do not do often enough).

Diabetes is a long-term disease. Achieving your target weight doesn't have to occur overnight, or even over weeks or months. Slow and steady surely does win the weight-loss race. In fact, if you lose weight too quickly you'll be more likely to regain it.

Nothing is as likely to frustrate your efforts to follow proper nutrition therapy as trying to figure it out without professional help. We strongly recommend that in addition to reading this chapter, you see a registered dietitian who has expertise in helping people with diabetes. If your doctor hasn't referred you to one, as soon as you finish reading this chapter, pick up the phone, call your doctor's office, and ask them to book you an appointment. You'll be glad you did.

If **you have** loved ones who are overweight, be sure to share with them how weight loss can markedly reduce their likelihood of developing diabetes. Indeed, you and your loved ones can embark together on a journey of healthy eating, weight loss, and good health.

The best strategy for losing weight

The best strategy for losing weight is to combine reduced calorie intake with increased calorie expenditure. Indeed, to lose weight successfully you typically need a willingness to make exercise a part of your daily life. If, for some reason, you cannot move your legs to exercise, you can get a satisfactory workout using your upper body alone. We look in depth at exercise and diabetes in Chapter 11.

If you need to lose weight, you should aim to shed 1 to 2 kilograms (about 2 to 4 pounds) per month, losing 5 to 10 percent of your initial body weight over 6 to 12 months. Try to burn off 500 calories more per day than you ingest. (See Chapter 11 to find out what type and duration of exercise allows you to accomplish this.)

Half a kilogram (about a pound) of fat contains 3,500 calories. Therefore, in order to lose this much fat, you must eat 3,500 calories less than you need or you must burn off these calories by exercising.

As we discuss in the section "The Key Ingredients," earlier in this chapter, we advocate healthy eating following the recommendations of the Canadian Diabetes Association and Health Canada. We do *not* recommend following any of the numerous fad diets. Although these diets often provide success, it is almost always short-lived, with all (or more) of the weight that was lost being regained later. Many of these diets are so restrictive, they can make you feel unwell with constipation, fatigue, muscle aches, hair loss, and so on. (Hmm, a diet that doesn't provide long-term weight loss, can make you feel unwell, and often costs lots of money to boot; not exactly a recipe for success — except for the people selling the books and running the fad clinics.)

Portion control for weight loss

Although many factors help to explain why Canadians (and most others in the world, for that matter) have become heavier and heavier, one unavoidable fact is that supersized food portions — whether consumed in or outside of the home — have been a major factor leading to our supersized waists. You can find very helpful information on the CDA website to help you estimate the best portion sizes (go to www.diabetes.ca then, in the search box on the upper right of the page, type in "portion guide").

Medication therapy for losing weight

We're not big fans of medication therapy for weight loss. Almost every drug ever created for this purpose has, because of safety concerns, been stopped in development or withdrawn from the market. Not a good track record, to say the least.

Xenical (orlistat) has been — and continues to be — available, but is of limited benefit for most people. Xenical is taken three times daily (with your meals). It works by blocking your small intestine from absorbing ingested fat into your blood stream. Unfortunately, most people lose only small amounts of weight while taking this medicine, and, significantly, many people run into problems with oily deposits escaping from their rectum and soiling their underclothes. Ugh! Having said all that, some people tolerate the drug well and lose some weight. Also, Xenical can help reduce blood glucose levels.

Recently two new drugs (Qsymia and Belviq. . . gee, we would have loved to have been a fly on the wall during the meetings where these names were decided upon!) have been approved for use in the United States. Qsymia is actually a combination medication containing two already available drugs (phentermine and topiramate). The long-term safety and effectiveness of these drugs is not known. Whether or not these new drugs (or ones that will follow) prove to be helpful medicines to assist with weight loss, they do not and will not replace ongoing healthy eating strategies (coupled with exercise).

Surgery for weight loss (bariatric surgery)

Bariatric surgery is increasingly used to help people lose weight if they've been unable to succeed with calorie restriction (and exercise) and if they're very overweight.

As you might imagine, surgery — *any* surgery — is not to be undertaken lightly. (An old expression says that minor surgery is surgery that someone else has.) Nonetheless, for select individuals it can be a very effective form of therapy, with multiple health benefits including improved glucose control, improved blood pressure control, reduced need for medications, and more.

Several different surgical treatments are available including *Roux-en-Y gastric bypass* and *laparoscopic gastric banding (lap banding)*. Gastric bypass (and other related procedures) involves rerouting a portion of the gut to reduce the amount of intestinal surface area available to absorb nutrients into your body. Laparoscopic banding is a far simpler procedure and involves placing a removable constricting band around the upper end of the stomach; as a result you feel full faster when you eat and you eat less.

Each of the available surgical options has its pros and cons. Gastric bypass, for example, is a much larger surgical procedure compared with lap banding, but, on the other hand, being a much older procedure it has a longer track record of success.

If you are considering bariatric surgery, you will need to do your homework, including meeting with surgeons who perform these procedures to find out what risks (both short- and long-term) the procedures would pose, the expected benefits, and the costs (health care plans may pay for the Roux-en-Y procedure, but typically don't cover the approximately $15,000 cost of laparoscopic banding). If you are looking online for information about the various procedures, one particularly helpful website is the Ontario Bariatric Network. (The site, though geared in some respects toward Ontarians, contains very helpful information for anyone wanting to learn about bariatric surgery.) To learn more about the different types of bariatric surgery go to www. ontariobariatricnetwork.ca then click on "Resources" then "Bariatric Surgery" then "Surgery Types."

Behaviour modification

In addition to the lifestyle changes we discuss earlier in this section, a number of other strategies are available to help you lose weight. You needn't adopt all of the following tips (though you are welcome to); adopting even a few of them can have a terrific impact.

Here (in no particular order) are some behaviour modification tips you may find helpful in your quest to lose weight:

- Eat at set times.
- Don't skip meals.

- Keep a food diary.

- Pack a healthy lunch rather than eating out at a restaurant.

- Slow down your eating.

- Put your cutlery down between mouthfuls.

- Don't put more food in your mouth before you have finished your last bite.

- Concentrate on the taste of each mouthful before you swallow.

- Every few minutes, pause and ask yourself if you're still hungry.

- Don't finish every morsel on your plate. There's nothing wrong with leaving some behind.

- After the food has been served, remove the serving dishes and bread-basket from the table.

- Don't keep high-calorie snacks visible in the kitchen or elsewhere in the house. Better yet, don't keep them in the house at all.

- Remember that seemingly innocent things like salad dressings can be very rich in calories.

- Add (low calorie) bulk to your food (by adding a vegetable to pasta for example). You can often satisfy your hunger by increasing the volume of food even if you reduce the number of calories.

- Avoid impulse buying when doing your grocery shopping. Bring a shopping list and walk the aisles specifically looking for the items you have written down rather than just wandering from aisle to aisle.

- Get a 5-kilogram (11-pound) weight and carry it around for a while to appreciate how even a small loss is important.

- Incorporate regular exercise into your weight-loss strategy.

- Most important of all, remember that there's no rush. As we say earlier, trying to lose weight too rapidly will make you more likely to regain the weight later.

A recent study suggested that the combination of keeping a food diary, avoiding eating lunch in a restaurant, and not skipping meals was a particularly effective strategy.

As you go about the difficult task of losing weight and keeping it off, remember to seek the help of those around you. A loving partner provides great help through the roughest days.

Coping with Eating Disorders

You might remember the expression "You can't be too rich or too thin." How much damage has this statement — or at least the sentiment (especially the "thin" part) — done to society? Young people, particularly girls, are often preoccupied with their body weight. When this preoccupation becomes too great, it can result in an eating disorder.

Young girls with eating disorders (and young boys about a tenth as often) either starve themselves and exercise excessively or eat a great deal and then induce vomiting and/or take laxatives and water pills (*diuretics*). Someone who starves herself has *anorexia nervosa,* while someone who binges and purges has *bulimia nervosa.* These conditions can result in severe illness and, when carried to extremes, even death.

Anorexia is usually found in girls who have a distorted body image and are fearful of weight gain. The girls may appear unusually thin and may not menstruate. Their malnutrition may be very severe.

Bulimia involves eating large quantities of food and then purging it by vomiting and taking laxatives or water pills. These people are usually not as severely thin as people with anorexia. Because their weight is closer to normal, they usually menstruate normally.

Managing diabetes requires a certain amount of routine from day to day, so if you have an eating disorder — and thus, inconsistent food intake — it complicates matters and makes achieving consistently good blood glucose levels virtually impossible.

It is imperative that a person with an eating disorder receive proper treatment. Eating disorders clinics specialize in providing this necessary care. If you have an eating disorder or if you care for someone who does, we recommend you see your family physician to let them know of the issue. Your doctor will want to assess your health and refer you to the appropriate specialist clinic as necessary.

Chapter 11

Exercising Your Way to Good Health

*I*t may well be that you look back at your high school grad photos and point out to your children or grandchildren how slim and trim you were way back when exercise was not a chore, but a routine. Perhaps it was not long thereafter that family and work commitments appeared, followed by some excess weight around your middle. And after your lifestyle had changed, maybe you were like millions of your fellow Canadians and simply could never find the time or enthusiasm to get on track with exercise and shedding the extra kilograms you had acquired.

But the wonderful thing is, you're not too late. You're *never* too late. Whether you're 25 or 85, you can still make changes in your lifestyle to enhance your health. And you don't have to feel intimidated by this. The changes don't have to occur overnight. And the changes don't have to be *all* or *none,* because any change is a change for the better.

And we can promise you that the changes you have to make are not quite so intimidating as those recommended by Hippocrates, the renowned physician of ancient times, who said, "Overweight people should perform hard work, eat only once a day, take no baths, and walk naked as much as possible."

Simply put, exercise is one of the most powerful weapons you have to stay healthy. In this chapter we look at how exercise can help you and how you can incorporate exercise into your diabetes treatment plan.

ANECDOTE

A prescription for exercise

Ian well remembers John, a middle-aged bus driver who had been living with type 2 diabetes for 13 years when they first met. John's family physician referred John to Ian because John's blood glucose levels were too high. The doctor had recommended — and John had declined — insulin therapy. John didn't exercise and he was considerably overweight. He had high blood pressure and high cholesterol. "Dr. Blumer," John said, "I'm already on seven different types of medicines. I take 25 pills a day. Geesh, I feel like I've become my father. Heck, I'm a walking drug store. Don't ask me to take insulin, too."

To John's surprise, Ian didn't. "John, it's your call. You don't have to be your father. You can make changes that will help to keep you healthy and, quite possibly, that could get your blood glucose levels down without requiring insulin."

John looked keenly at Ian. "You think so?" he asked.

"You bet," Ian replied. "And this is how to do it." Ian reviewed many of the key points contained in this book, including the importance of diabetes education, healthy eating, exercise, and so forth. John took this to heart, figuratively and literally. He improved his diet, he began and progressively increased his exercising, he lost weight, and, over the next 12 months his blood glucose, blood pressure, and cholesterol all improved without additional medicine. Indeed, things improved so dramatically that not only did he not need additional medicine, in fact he was able — under close medical supervision — to come off over half the pills he had been taking.

At the time of John's last visit to Ian he was beaming: "Dr. Blumer, I saw it like this. Either I made the time to exercise now or I made the time to look after my diabetes complications later. I think you can figure out which I chose."

How Exercise Can Improve Your Diabetes Health

Exercise is helpful for everyone, but is especially helpful if you have diabetes. Exercise can

- ✔ Lower your blood glucose.
- ✔ Lower your blood pressure.
- ✔ Improve your lipids (cholesterol and triglycerides).
- ✔ Help you both to lose weight and to keep off weight you've lost.
- ✔ Reduce your risk of a heart attack (and improve your prognosis if you've already had one).

✔ Increase your energy level.

✔ Reduce your stress level (and improve your ability to handle stress).

✔ Improve your general sense of well-being.

✔ Improve your sex life (more energy, more stamina . . . more merrymaking).

✔ Provide social interaction.

If we haven't convinced you yet, how about this: If you have diabetes and you exercise regularly, you can reduce your risk of dying in the next ten years or so by over 50 percent! So, do you need to exercise? Well, only as much as you need to breathe. Literally.

 As we discuss in Chapter 4, exercise, healthy eating, and weight control markedly reduce one's risk for developing type 2 diabetes. If you have diabetes, let your loved ones know of this benefit and encourage them to exercise with you to reduce their risk of developing type 2 diabetes.

Finding the Right Type of Exercise

People routinely ask Ian what the best exercise is. Whenever Ian is asked this, he recalls the time many years ago when he asked the bicycle store owner what the best helmet was for his very young son. Her wise answer: "The one he will actually wear." So, too, with exercise. The type of exercise you do is far less important than simply finding one that you enjoy and will stick with.

 Exercise can be defined and categorized in different ways. The Canadian Diabetes Association (CDA) clinical practice guidelines look at exercise in three broad types:

✔ **Aerobic exercise** (also called *cardiovascular exercise* or simply "*cardio*") is "physical activity, such as walking, bicycling, or jogging that involves continuous, rhythmic movements of large muscle groups lasting for at least 10 minutes at a time."

✔ **Resistance exercise** is "physical activity involving brief repetitive exercises with weights, weight machines, resistance bands, or one's own body weight (e.g., pushups) to increase muscle strength and/or endurance."

✔ **Flexibility exercise** is "a form of activity, such as lower back or hamstring stretching, that enhances the ability of joints to move through their full ranges of motion."

(The CDA points out that "some types of exercise, such as yoga, can incorporate elements of both resistance and flexibility exercise.")

Because the benefits of the different types of exercise are complementary, you should do all three types.

Cardiovascular exercise and you

The most important thing in choosing an exercise is that you like it enough to carry on with it. Another factor that may influence your decision is the number of calories an exercise burns. Table 11-1 supplies this information.

Table 11-1	Exercise and the Amount of Calories You Burn in 20 Minutes at Different Body Weights	
Activity	*Calories Burned (57 kg/125 lb.)*	*Calories Burned (80 kg/175 lb.)*
Running, 11 kph/7 mph	236	328
Skiing, cross-country	196	276
Skiing, downhill	160	224
Football	138	192
Tennis	112	160
Walking, 6.5 kph/4 mph	104	144
Swimming	80	112
Baseball	78	108
Dancing	70	96
Golfing	66	96
Carpentry	64	88
Gardening	60	84
House painting	58	80
Typing	38	54
Writing	30	42
Standing	24	32

Everything you do burns calories. Even sleeping uses 20 calories in 20 minutes if you weigh 57 kilograms (125 pounds).

When Rajeev, a 35-year-old dentist, found out that he had diabetes, he decided to start exercising. Since his best friend golfed, he thought he would try that too. A couple of months later, despite playing golf several times a week, his glucose control and his weight hadn't shown much improvement. As it turned out, he had joined one of the few golf courses in Canada that require you to use a cart. He switched clubs (so to speak) and was soon walking up and down the fairways, burning calories with each and every step. Only a small minority of golf courses in Canada have rules making cart use mandatory. That leaves you with lots and lots of walkable courses in Canada to choose from. So the next time you are on the links, make sure the only driving you're doing is with your clubs. Fore!

Virtually everyone can do cardiovascular exercise. If you have a limitation that makes it difficult to do some types of exercise such as walking, try a different one, such as swimming.

You do *not* have to go out and spend a whole bunch of money on exercise machines, fitness clubs, and the like (though of course you're welcome to). We wish we had a dollar for every treadmill that now functions as a full-time clotheshorse or dust collector. Some comfortable clothes and shoes are all you need to begin your exercise program.

The Canadian Diabetes Association has some excellent "how-to" videos on exercise. You can find these "Physical Activity Exercise Videos" on the CDA website (www.diabetes.ca/for-professionals/workshops/physical-activity-and-exercise-workshops).

Starting cardiovascular exercise

Perhaps you have heard the famous Chinese proverb, "A journey of a thousand miles begins with a single step." Proverbs are proverbs for a reason.

In our experience, people face two main obstacles to taking up exercise:

- Feeling overwhelmed by the task
- Inertia

Well, neither of these obstacles is insurmountable. We can assure you — in fact, we can guarantee you — it doesn't have to be too big a task. Set your sights low. Very low. Very, very, low. Get the point? If you never exercise, start your new program by simply walking daily to the end of your block and back. Do that for a few days, then try circling the block daily. A few days later, walk several blocks. Every week try to cover a slightly greater distance, and when you have succeeded with that, increase your pace. When you have gotten into a routine, you will find that your inertia is a thing of the past.

A good rule of thumb is to increase your daily exercise by five minutes every week. Using this approach, you will be up to half an hour of daily exercise within a month and a half. Not too shabby.

If you think you may want to start getting out for a regular walk but need something else to motivate you, consider getting a dog. Dogs love going for walks. And, just like you, they also need to exercise. Not sure you want the responsibility? Offer to take the neighbour's dog for a daily walk. Both your neighbours and their dog will be thrilled.

Determining the right amount of cardiovascular exercise

The Canadian Diabetes Association recommends that people with diabetes perform at least 150 minutes of moderate-to-vigorous-intensity cardiovascular exercise each week, spread out over at least three days of the week (with no more than two consecutive days without exercise). That's not to say that you have to rest on your well-deserved laurels if you've accomplished this. Indeed, try to build up to at least four hours of weekly exercise.

These are examples of moderate exercise:

- Brisk walking on a level surface. (Think of the pace of a brisk walk as being similar to the pace you would use if you were late for the bus. It is walking "with a purpose" unlike sauntering around the mall.)
- Biking
- Swimming at a moderate pace
- Dancing at a moderate pace
- Raking leaves
- Water aerobics

These are examples of vigorous exercise:

- Brisk walking up an incline
- Jogging
- Aerobics
- Hockey
- Basketball
- Swimming at a fast pace
- Dancing at a fast pace

Do you eat your entire week's calories in one meal? Do you do your entire week's breathing with one deep breath? No? Then remember, you shouldn't try to do your entire week's exercise in one session either. It's simply not as effective if you do it that way. Rather, you need to exercise at least several days per week.

If on the days you are exercising, you are unable to set aside 30 or more consecutive minutes for this task, feel free to divide up your daily exercise into several ten-minute sessions; it will work just as effectively.

The following are several ways to determine if you are pushing yourself to the right extent:

- ✔ **The talk test:** You should be able to talk while exercising.
- ✔ **The breath sound check:** When you hear yourself breathing (not panting), you are going at the right pace.
- ✔ **Perceived exertion:** Work at a level that feels moderate to somewhat hard, but not beyond that.

These three techniques are particularly helpful because they allow you to adjust your exercise according to your own needs.

Do not continue exercising if you have chest discomfort or severe shortness of breath. These can be symptoms of heart problems.

Resistance exercise and you

Weightlifting is a form of resistance exercise. It involves moving heavy weights, which can be moved only for brief periods of time. It strengthens muscles significantly, improves bone density (and therefore helps both prevent and treat osteoporosis), and increases endurance. And, as a nice bonus, pioneering studies by a Canadian researcher, Dr. Ron Sigal, have shown that resistance training also helps improve blood glucose control and lipid levels in people living with type 2 diabetes. (And, though not nearly as important as these other benefits, you may find it a nice plus to discover your more toned appearance as you look in the bathroom mirror.)

Weight training, which uses lighter weights, can be a form of cardiovascular exercise. Because the weights are light, you can move them for prolonged periods of time. The result is improved cardiovascular fitness along with strengthening of muscles and bones.

The Canadian Diabetes Association recommends performing resistance exercise at least twice weekly (and, preferably, at least three times weekly) *in addition to performing aerobic exercise.*

The CDA recommends, when performing resistance exercise, that you progress in the following way:

1. **Start with one set using a weight with which you can perform 15 to 20 repetitions while maintaining proper form.**

2. **Progress to two sets and decrease the number of repetitions to 10 to 15 while increasing the weight slightly. If you cannot complete the required repetitions while maintaining proper form, reduce the weight.**

3. **Progress to three sets of eight repetitions performed using an increased weight and maintaining proper form.**

If you choose to do resistance exercise, first meet with a qualified exercise specialist and then keep in touch with him or her periodically.

Taking Precautions Before You Start Exercising

Although exercise is typically very safe to do, before you embark on a new exercise program, talk to your family doctor. He will need to consider certain factors including:

- **Whether or not you may have heart disease:** Before you start exercising, your doctor may choose to send you for an *exercise stress test* (this is a test where your heart is monitored while you walk on a treadmill) to look for evidence of coronary artery disease (see Chapter 6) — even if you have no heart symptoms.

- **Whether or not you have high blood pressure:** Although exercise is good treatment for hypertension, it can be dangerous if you have severely elevated blood pressure.

- **The state of your blood glucose control:** Exercise is terrific therapy for elevated glucose levels, but it can be dangerous if you have severe hyperglycemia, in which case your blood glucose levels will have to be reduced to a safer level — generally under 15.0 mmol/L or so — before you start an exercise program. This is especially important if you have type 1 diabetes and you have ketones present. (We discuss high blood glucose emergencies in chapter 5.)

✔ **The state of your eyes:** Some forms of exercise can aggravate retinopathy (see Chapter 6). If you have not been to your eye doctor within the past year, have your eyes checked before you undertake any form of vigorous exercise; especially heavy weightlifting.

✔ **Whether or not you have peripheral neuropathy:** You can still exercise if you have peripheral neuropathy, but we suggest you read the section (in Chapter 6) on foot care and footwear first. (Whether or not you have foot problems, be sure to obtain proper socks and shoes for you to wear when exercising. And remember that in order to avoid getting blisters, you need to gradually wear in your new shoes.)

✔ **Physical limitations:** Things such as obesity, arthritis, peripheral arterial disease (refer to Chapter 6), and amputations may influence the nature of the exercise you undertake.

✔ **The medications you are on:** Your doctor may need to adjust your anti-hyperglycemic medications (in particular, your insulin doses) if you're going to be exercising. We look at this subject in more detail in the following section.

Exercising if You Are Taking Antihyperglycemic Medication

Exercise helps improve *overall* blood glucose control, but, depending on the intensity of the exercise you're doing and the medications you're taking, can cause blood glucose levels to *temporarily* go up or down. To see how your blood glucose levels are responding to your exercise, for the first few days after you begin (or increase) your exercise program, check your blood glucose more often than usual including:

✔ Before you exercise

✔ An hour or two after you've completed your exercise

✔ In the middle of the night (if you're taking insulin).

If your numbers are higher or lower than you expect, contact your physician to see what changes to your medications need to be made. (If you're taking insulin also contact your diabetes educator.)

To the surprise of most people with diabetes, *vigorous* exercise often makes blood glucose level go up, not down, during, and briefly after exercising. The reason is this: if you perform vigorous exercise certain hormones in your body — such as adrenaline (epinephrine) — go up, which makes your insulin (from your pancreas or from an injection) work less well and your muscles will temporarily not be able to properly use the glucose in your blood, causing your glucose level to rise. Within a few hours your blood glucose levels will return to normal (or may even fall below that).

If you are experiencing hypoglycemia when you exercise (or later that day or evening), your health care provider may need to adjust your blood glucose-lowering medications:

- ✔ *If you are on oral antihyperglycemic medications*, your dose may need to be reduced or you may need to change to a different medication.

- ✔ *If you are on insulin therapy,* options include eating a carbohydrate-containing snack before you exercise or reducing the amount of insulin you give yourself before you exercise or, in some circumstances, reducing the dose of the next scheduled insulin injection you give *after* you exercise.

Also, if you are on blood glucose-lowering medications that have the potential to cause hypoglycemia, whenever you exercise:

- ✔ Carry treatment for hypoglycemia. (We discuss treatment for hypoglycemia in Chapter 5.)

- ✔ Wear a medical alert necklace or bracelet that states you have diabetes.

- ✔ If you use rapid-acting insulin, do not inject it into a limb that you are about to exercise. (Injecting rapid-acting insulin into a limb that you then exercise increases the absorption rate of the insulin, which increases the risk of hypoglycemia.) Therefore, for example, do not inject rapid-acting insulin into your leg if you are about to go for a run or into your dominant arm if you're about to play tennis.

If you are on insulin therapy and you exercise in the evening you may experience hypoglycemia overnight. If you begin to exercise in the evening, for the few days set your alarm to wake you up in the middle of the night to test your blood glucose.

When it comes to diabetes and exercise, in almost all circumstances you should have your medications and diet adjusted to accommodate your exercise. You should rarely, if ever, have to change your exercise to accommodate your treatment!

Finding a Supervised Exercise Program

Although pretty well any way you choose to exercise is better than not exercising at all, exercise is particularly likely to help you control your diabetes and enhance your fitness if you perform *structured* exercise *supervised by a qualified trainer.*

You can find the appropriate program by contacting these sources:

- Your physician

- Your diabetes educator

- Your regional CDA office (You can find your nearest CDA office by going to www.diabetes.ca/about-us/where/regional)

- Your local YMCA/YWCA (Your YMCA/YWCA will likely offer exercise programs run by excellent fitness leaders who will be sensitive to your needs and can fit you into a class that's suitable for you. These facilities are often far less threatening — and far less expensive — than large, commercial fitness establishments.)

- Your local fitness facility

- The Canadian Society for Exercise Physiology (www.csep.ca)

- The Canadian Association of Cardiac Rehab (www.cacr.ca)

- The Canadian Kinesiology Alliance (www.cka.ca)

Chapter 12

Controlling Your Blood Glucose with Non-insulin Antihyperglycemic Medications and Alternative Therapies

*I*f you have read earlier chapters of this book before arriving here you likely noticed a recurring theme: Taking charge of your diabetes is paramount, and doing so with appropriate healthy eating strategies, exercise, and weight control are incredibly powerful tools. The great majority of people living with type 2 diabetes achieve additional benefits by coupling these lifestyle measures with blood glucose-lowering medication.

In this chapter we look at non-insulin medications that can help you control your (type 2) diabetes. (In Chapter 13 we discuss insulin therapy — which is helpful for many people with type 2 diabetes and is mandatory for all people with type 1 diabetes.)

The traditional terms to describe non-insulin blood glucose-lowering medications are *oral hypoglycemic agents* and *oral antidiabetic agents*. These terms are used less often nowadays and have been largely replaced by the more contemporary (and more accurate) term *antihyperglycemic agents* (or its equivalent terms: *antihyperglycemic drugs* and *antihyperglycemic medications*). In this book we use the term *antihyperglycemic medications* when referring to non-insulin blood glucose-lowering medications.

To Take or Not to Take: That Is the Antihyperglycemic Medication Question

If you're like most people, you'd rather not take medication, and who could blame you? Table 12-1 lists some of the possible reasons you may have for *not* wanting to take antihyperglycemic medicines. We take the liberty of quoting some things you might say (even though we probably haven't even met you — how presumptuous!), and we even indicate if we agree with your concern or not.

Table 12-1   Reasons Not to Take Antihyperglycemic Medications

I Don't Want to Take Antihyperglycemic Medications Because They . . .	Our Opinion
Are not "natural."	We agree.
Can have side effects.	We agree.
Are not as good a treatment as proper nutrition therapy, exercise, and weight control.	We agree.
Occasionally (depending on the type) cause hypoglycemia.	We agree.
Can (depending on the type) sometimes interact adversely with other medicines.	We agree.
Can be hard to remember to take.	We agree.
Are a sign that I'm unable to control my blood glucose levels without them.	We agree.

Surprised that you're right (or at least that you're in agreement with us and so must be right!) on each point? But of course you're right. Who wants to take medicines if you can avoid them? No one.

But consider the other side of the coin. Table 12-2 lists of some of the possible reasons you may have for *wanting* to take antihyperglycemic medications.

Table 12-2	Reasons to Take Antihyperglycemic Medication	
I'm Willing to Take Antihyperglycemic Medications Because . . .		*Our Opinion*
They'll help me reduce my blood glucose levels if lifestyle efforts alone can't do the trick.		We agree.
By improving my glucose control, they'll help protect my eyes, nerves, and kidneys.		We agree.
They seldom have serious side effects.		We agree.
Minor side effects can usually be corrected easily by adjusting the dose or changing to a different antihyperglycemic medication.		We agree.
With the appropriate drug and dose, I can usually avoid hypoglycemia.		We agree.
Serious drug interactions seldom occur.		We agree.
I know diabetes is a progressive disease and that's not my fault. Taking an antihyperglycemic medication doesn't mean that *I* have failed; it simply means that *my pancreas* has.		We agree.
Remembering to take medicines is a pain in the butt, but it's a heck of a lot better than remembering to go for eye surgery and dialysis appointments.		We agree.
Enough already. I give up!		'Nuff said.

Choosing the right medication for you

In recent years, tremendous strides have been made in developing new and innovative medications to help control blood glucose. As a result, your doctor can choose from many different drugs. And over the next few years more and more types of blood glucose-lowering medications will become available. This is wonderful; having additional weapons in the medical arsenal to help you stay healthy is great. But — there's always a *but* — with so many new drugs becoming available, each with their own unique properties (both good and bad), your doctor is going to have an increasingly difficult time knowing which one to choose for you.

That's where you come in. By becoming aware of the different medicines we discuss in this chapter and, in particular, by discovering their pros and cons, you can work with your doctor to find the best medicine for you and your specific situation. (In Chapter 8 we discuss other ways you can be a key member of your health care team.)

Antihyperglycemic medication therapy (or insulin for that matter) should *never* be considered a substitute for lifestyle treatment. Relying exclusively on drugs to keep you healthy, and ignoring proper nutrition, exercise, and weight control, is a sure-fire way to fail with your diabetes management. Medications are *complementary* to what *you* do for you, and how you live your life.

Understanding how antihyperglycemic medications work

As we discuss in detail in Chapter 4, people develop type 2 diabetes due to two main factors: *insulin resistance* (a condition where your tissues do not respond to insulin properly) and *insulin deficiency* (wherein your pancreas is unable to manufacture sufficient insulin to keep up with your body's needs). Many of the drugs doctors use target these specific issues. Some newer drugs also target other areas — such as reducing appetite — to help control blood glucose. Figure 12-1 illustrates how the different antihyperglycemic medications work.

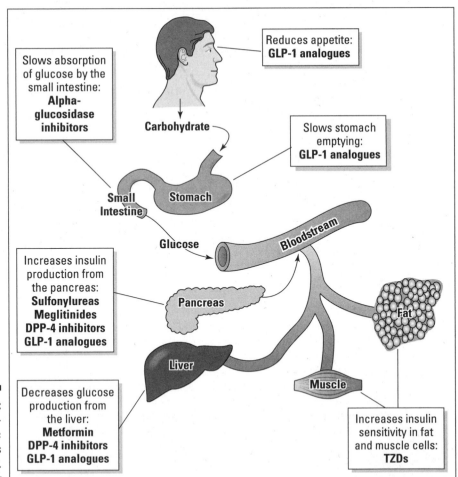

Figure 12-1: How antihyperglycemic medications work.

Reduces appetite: **GLP-1 analogues**

Slows absorption of glucose by the small intestine: **Alpha-glucosidase inhibitors**

Slows stomach emptying: **GLP-1 analogues**

Carbohydrate

Small Intestine

Stomach

Glucose

Bloodstream

Increases insulin production from the pancreas: **Sulfonylureas Meglitinides DPP-4 inhibitors GLP-1 analogues**

Pancreas

Fat

Liver

Muscle

Decreases glucose production from the liver: **Metformin DPP-4 inhibitors GLP-1 analogues**

Increases insulin sensitivity in fat and muscle cells: **TZDs**

Investigating the Types of Antihyperglycemic Medications

All classes of antihyperglycemic medication have at least two things in common:

✔ They help to reduce blood glucose.

✔ They have unpronounceable names.

In this section we look at the different types of antihyperglycemic medication that are available to assist you. (We also discuss several types of medication that are *un*available to assist you — at least so far — but will likely become available within the next few years.)

The label on your prescription drug bottle will have both the trade name *and* the generic name of your medicine; just like Shakespeare's rose, any way you say it, it's the same medicine. In this section we use generic names.

Although most people with type 2 diabetes are treated with antihyperglycemic medication long before they are treated with insulin, be aware that insulin is a perfectly suitable treatment for type 2 diabetes — at *any* stage of the disease, even as early as the day it's diagnosed. (We discuss insulin therapy in Chapter 13.)

Metformin

The Canadian Diabetes Association — and pretty well every other diabetes organization on the planet — recommends (for reasons we include in the following list) metformin as the preferred antihyperglycemic medicine for most people with type 2 diabetes. Therefore, if you have type 2 diabetes and you aren't taking metformin, we suggest you discuss with your doctor whether or not metformin would be a good choice for you.

Metformin is available as a single medication and is also available in combination with certain other types of blood glucose-lowering medication (including TZD and DPP-4 inhibitor drugs; we discuss these drugs later in this chapter).

 Metformin is taken twice (or, sometimes, three times) per day. If you would prefer to have to take it only once daily, speak to your doctor about taking the long-acting form of metformin, called Glumetza, as this only needs to be taken once daily.

Metformin is part of the family of drugs called *biguanides*. But it's a small family indeed, seeing as metformin is the only member.

These are important things for you to know about metformin:

- ✔ Lowers blood glucose mainly by reducing the production of glucose from the liver.

- ✔ Does not cause hypoglycemia.

- ✔ Does not cause weight gain.

- ✔ Reduces your risk of having a heart attack or stroke (if you have diabetes).

- ✔ Can improve your lipids.

- ✔ May improve your fertility if you're a woman with infertility due to polycystic ovary syndrome (PCOS).

- ✔ Reduces your risk of developing type 2 diabetes if you have prediabetes. (We discuss prediabetes in Chapter 4.)

- ✔ Tends to cause nausea, abdominal cramping, and diarrhea. These symptoms can be lessened (or avoided altogether) if you take your metformin with food and if you begin taking it in a low dose and slowly increase the dose over a few weeks.

- ✔ Can make it harder for your intestine to properly absorb vitamin B12 from food. For that reason you should have your vitamin B12 level checked from time to time; if your level is low, taking an oral B12 supplement typically corrects the problem.

Many physicians are unaware that taking metformin can cause low vitamin B12, so be sure to ask your doctor if they are monitoring your B12 level and, if they aren't, ask them to do so.

Metformin can cause — rarely — a serious adverse effect called *lactic acidosis*. (Symptoms of lactic acidosis include nausea, vomiting, abdominal pain, poor appetite, and malaise.) For this reason, you should not use metformin if you have significant liver disease, *active* heart failure, or kidney failure. *Mild* kidney malfunction does *not* prevent you from taking metformin. Your doctor should check your kidney function with a blood test that measures creatinine and GFR (we discuss these tests in Chapter 6) before prescribing this medication.

If you're having certain types of X-rays where you'll be given intravenous dye, your doctor will likely advise you not to take your metformin for a few days before and after the test. This precaution ensures that if the dye causes kidney problems, you won't have excess metformin accumulating in your body.

Sulfonylureas

All sulfonylurea drugs have, with a few exceptions (which we discuss later in this section), quite similar properties. These are the different types of sulfonylurea medication:

- Glyburide
- Gliclazide (This drug is also available in a long-acting form — gliclazide MR — taken once daily.)
- Glimepiride

(In theory, other sulfonylurea medications are still technically available; however, they are virtually never used nowadays.)

Of the three sulfonylurea medications, glyburide is *least* preferred as it is the most likely of the drugs in this group to cause low blood glucose. If you take glyburide and are experiencing hypoglycemia, ask your physician to change you to gliclazide or glimepiride.

These are important things for you to know about sulfonylureas:

- Lower blood glucose by stimulating your pancreas to produce more insulin.
- Can cause hypoglycemia.
- Can cause weight gain.
- Can occasionally cause a photosensitive skin rash (a rash that occurs upon sun exposure).
- Can cause allergic reactions in people who have sulfa-drug allergies. (This does not happen often.)
- Can interact with alcohol in some cases, causing unpleasant symptoms such as nausea and flushing (even if you aren't inebriated). This was more of a problem with older, now seldom-used sulfonylurea medications and rarely occurs with modern sulfonylurea drugs.

Meglitinides

We admit to taking liberties here, but practicality trumps fussing over nomenclature. So we're going to do what the whole medical world does and group together two very similar (but not identical) classes of drugs — meglitinides and D-phenylalanine derivatives — and simply refer to them collectively as meglitinides. Do you care? We didn't think so. (Incidentally, meglitinides are also sometimes referred to as *glinides* for short.)

These are the different types of meglitinide medication:

✔ Repaglinide (also called GlucoNorm)

✔ Nateglinide (also called Starlix)

Because repaglinide is more potent than nateglinide, nateglinide is seldom used.

These are important things for you to know about meglitinides:

✔ Lower blood glucose by stimulating your pancreas to produce more insulin.

✔ Are particularly effective at reducing after-meal blood glucose levels, compared with other antihyperglycemic medications.

✔ Can cause hypoglycemia (but are less likely to do so than are sulfonylureas).

✔ Can cause weight gain.

Thiazolidinediones

There are two thiazolidinediones (more easily referred to as TZDs, and sometimes referred to as *glitazones*):

✔ Pioglitazone (which goes by several other names, including Actos)

✔ Rosiglitazone (also called Avandia)

TZDs were commonly used drugs until a few years ago when controversies and concerns arose. Because of concerns that rosiglitazone may increase the risk of heart problems, this drug has fallen from favour and is now rarely used. Pioglitazone is still used in Canada and many other countries, however in certain nations — including several in Europe — it has been taken off the market because of concerns it *may* (this is unproven) increase the risk of bladder cancer.

These are important things for you to know about TZDs:

✔ Lower blood glucose mainly by helping glucose move from the blood into fat and muscle. They do this by reducing insulin resistance (refer to Chapter 4).

✔ Do not cause hypoglycemia.

✔ Can cause fluid retention leading to swollen ankles. This can be a nuisance but is not serious.

✔ Typically cause some weight gain. This is partially related to fluid retention.

✔ May cause mild anemia. (This is important in only one way: If your doctor is not aware that TZDs can cause mild anemia, you could end up having unnecessary tests done.)

✔ Increase your risk of having a fracture of a forearm, hand, or foot if you're a woman. The reason for this is not yet known. (It may turn out that it's related to loss of calcium from the bones.)

✔ May improve your fertility if you're a woman with infertility due to PCOS.

✔ Can affect your lipids. (Whether this is a meaningful difference is controversial.)

✔ Reduce your risk of developing type 2 diabetes if you have prediabetes. (We discuss prediabetes in Chapter 4.)

✔ Increase your risk of heart failure. This is more likely if you have previously had a heart attack or if you're taking insulin. The great majority of people taking TZD therapy do *not* develop heart failure; nonetheless, the risk remains real.

If you develop breathing difficulty while you're on a TZD, you may have heart failure and you should seek immediate medical attention. Also, if you have significant heart damage, you should not take a TZD.

It can take a few weeks of treatment before blood glucose levels start to improve. (Patience is a virtue with these drugs.)

Alpha-glucosidase inhibitors

Because of a limited ability to reduce blood glucose levels, alpha-glucosidase inhibitor medication is not often used. On the other hand, it's very safe therapy with virtually no serious side effects. The only member of this class of medicine available in Canada is acarbose, which goes by the trade name Glucobay — as in keeping your *glucose* at *bay* (although we must admit it does bring to mind images of, ahem, a sweet Caribbean beach destination).

These are important things for you to know about acarbose:

✔ Lowers blood glucose by slowing the rate of absorption of glucose from the small intestine into the blood. (It does this by blocking the action of an enzyme — alpha-glucosidase — that breaks down larger carbohydrates into smaller ones such as glucose.)

✔ Is less effective than other antihyperglycemic medicines at reducing blood glucose levels.

✔ Has a greater effect on reducing after-meal blood glucose levels than on fasting blood glucose levels.

✔ Does not cause hypoglycemia.

✔ Does not cause weight gain.

✔ Reduces your risk of developing type 2 diabetes if you have prediabetes. (We discuss prediabetes in Chapter 4.)

✔ Virtually never causes severe side effects and is, therefore, a very safe medicine. But acarbose frequently causes *non*-severe, unpleasant gastro-intestinal side effects (including gas, bloating, and flatulence). A helpful way to avoid these side effects is to start with a very low dose and then slowly increase it.

Given acarbose's side-effect profile, you could say that the best candidates for this drug are those people who are "loud and proud."

If you develop hypoglycemia when you're on this medication, you must treat yourself with glucose or dextrose (such as Dextrosol), not sucrose. That is, do not treat yourself with table sugar, fruit juice, or colas.

DPP-4 inhibitors

In the short period of time that DPP-4 inhibitors have been available, they have quickly become very popular. They're now widely used in Canada and elsewhere.

In your Internet travels, you'll come across two terms for this class of drug: DPP-4 inhibitors and DPP-IV inhibitors. Both are correct, and both refer to the same thing (the IV is simply the Roman numeral equivalent of the number 4). DPP-4 inhibitors block the action of the *di*peptidyl *p*eptidase type 4 enzyme. By doing so they increase the level in the blood of hormones called *incretins*. The higher level of incretins is responsible for the blood glucose-lowering effect of these drugs.

There are currently three different DPP-4 inhibitors available in Canada, but more will likely come onto the market over the next few years. DPP-4 inhibitors are very similar to one another in terms of their blood glucose-lowering effectiveness. These are the available DPP-4 inhibitors:

✔ **Sitagliptin:** The trade name for this drug is Januvia. It is also available in combination with metformin (called Janumet).

✔ **Saxagliptin:** The trade name is Onglyza. It is also available in combination with metformin (called Kombiglyze).

✔ **Linagliptin:** The trade name for this drug is Trajenta.

These are important things for you to know about DPP-4 inhibitors:

✔ Lower blood glucose by

- Stimulating the pancreas to produce more insulin production, and

- Decreasing glucagon production by the pancreas. (As we discuss in Chapter 3, because glucagon causes the liver to release glucose into the blood, reducing glucagon levels reduces blood glucose.)

✔ Reduce blood glucose levels only modestly (that is, better than some drugs; not as well as some others).

✔ Don't cause hypoglycemia.

✔ Don't cause weight gain.

✔ *May* cause inflammation of the pancreas (pancreatitis). This is not proven. If you are taking a DPP-4 inhibitor and you develop severe upper abdominal pain this may be a symptom of pancreatitis, and you should notify your physician straight away.

✔ Don't cause side effects for the majority of patients. (Indeed, these drugs tend to be remarkably well tolerated, which is a strong point.)

GLP-1 analogues

GLP-1 analogues have been a member of the diabetes arsenal for a few years now. There are currently two GLP-1 analogues available in Canada:

✔ **Exenatide:** Its trade name is Byetta. You take this medication by injection twice daily. Not yet available in Canada is a once-weekly form called Bydureon.

✔ **Liraglutide:** Its trade name is Victoza. It is taken by injection once daily.

Many other GLP-1 analogues will likely come onto the market over the next few years.

GLP-1 stands for glucagon-*l*ike *p*eptide type 1. Despite the name, apart from some biochemical similarity to glucagon, GLP-1 analogues share nothing in common with glucagon. The term *analogue* derives from GLP-1 analogues acting analogous (that is; similar) to the body's naturally occurring GLP-1. GLP-1 analogue therapy is said to be *incretin-based*, meaning that, like DPP-4 inhibitors (which we discuss earlier) the drug works by acting on the body's incretin hormone system. Want another term? Of course you do. Okay, here it is: Because GLP-1 analogues act like, or mimic, the way the body's naturally occurring GLP-1 incretin hormone works, GLP-1 analogues are also called *incretin mimetics*.

These are important things for you to know about GLP-1 analogues:

✔ Lower blood glucose by these four means:

- Stimulating the pancreas to produce more insulin

- Decreasing glucagon production by the pancreas (As we discuss in Chapter 3, because glucagon causes the liver to release glucose into the blood, reducing glucagon levels reduces blood glucose.)

- Reducing appetite (and, therefore, food intake)

- Slowing how quickly the stomach empties food (which makes you feel full faster)

✔ Rarely cause hypoglycemia.

✔ Often cause weight loss. As the great majority of people with type 2 diabetes are overweight — and as most other antihyperglycemic therapies cause weight *gain* — (or at best, are weight neutral) the ability of GLP-1 analogues to help you lose weight is clearly a very nice benefit indeed. Although most people lose weight on these medications, the amount of weight that is lost can vary considerably; some people lose just a few pounds, some considerably more. Also, some people do not lose any weight at all and on occasion someone even gains weight. For these reasons, these drugs should not be considered "weight loss drugs;" rather, they are *diabetes* drugs that just happen to usually cause weight loss.

✔ Frequently cause nausea.

Nausea is most likely to develop during the first few days of therapy and typically goes away after a week or so. To prevent nausea — and help minimize it if it does develop — you start these drugs in a small dose then, if you are free of adverse effects, the dose is increased. *Do not* increase the dose if you are still having nausea on the lower dose. Doing so will make your nausea worse!

✔ Reduce your risk of developing type 2 diabetes if you have prediabetes. (This has been proven for liraglutide, but is likely also true of other members of this family of drugs.) (We discuss prediabetes in Chapter 4.)

✔ *May* cause inflammation of the pancreas (pancreatitis). This is not proven. If you are taking a GLP-1 analogue and you develop severe upper abdominal pain this may be a symptom of pancreatitis, and you should notify your physician straight away.

__ **Chapter 12: Controlling Your Blood Glucose with Non-insulin**
Antihyperglycemic Medications and Alternative Therapies

249

> ✔ Should not be taken if you or a family member has had *medullary* thyroid cancer. This is a very rare form of thyroid cancer. A theoretical concern is that GLP-1 analogues may increase the risk of developing this cancer. They should also not be taken if you have another rare disease called *multiple endocrine neoplasia syndrome type 2* (MEN2).

Other antihyperglycemic medications

Several antihyperglycemic medications are either not currently available for use in Canada or are available for use, but are seldom used. We discuss these drugs here as, regarding the former, they may become available in Canada over the next few years and, regarding the latter, those drugs that are available may be prescribed for you.

Pramlintide

Pramlintide (trade name Symlin) is a drug that mimics the action of a pancreatic hormone called *amylin*. Pramlintide is an injectable drug that, though entirely different in chemical structure from GLP-1 analogues, has many similar actions in terms of how it helps control blood glucose. Pramlintide reduces appetite, slows down stomach emptying, increases insulin production, and reduces glucagon production. Pramlintide is not currently available for use in Canada.

Orlistat

Orlistat (trade name Xenical) is a drug developed and used to help people lose weight. Some evidence suggests that orlistat helps lower blood glucose levels independent of its weight-losing properties (which we discuss in Chapter 10). If so, this effect is weak. Orlistat is rarely prescribed primarily for blood glucose control.

Bromocriptine

Bromocriptine is a drug that has been available for many years to treat diseases unrelated to diabetes. In recent years it has been discovered that a rapid-acting form of bromocriptine (called Cycloset) can help reduce blood glucose to a modest extent. Cycloset is not available for use in Canada.

Colesevelam

Colesevelam (brand name Welchol) is a drug developed to reduce LDL cholesterol. It does so by trapping bile acids in the intestine and enhancing their excretion from the body. (For this reason drugs in this class are called *bile acid sequestrants*.) Incidentally, and by an unknown mechanism, it has been observed that people with type 2 diabetes taking colesevelam may have a modest improvement in their blood glucose control. Colesevelam is not currently being marketed in Canada.

Why a drug may be available elsewhere but not in Canada

You might wonder why certain drugs are available in other countries, such as the United States, but not in Canada. (The converse seldom occurs.)

Many reasons are possible. One reason is that pharmaceutical companies need to seek approval for their drug from each respective government (Health Canada in, yup, Canada; the FDA in the United States; and so forth). Each regulatory body has its own policies, procedures, and criteria, so a drug may be approved for use in one country, but not another. The most common reason, however, is simple economics. For example, a drug manufacturer may look at the 300 million plus population of the United States and the comparatively tiny 30 million or so Canadian population, and decide that the economics favour the larger population. Thus they either don't seek approval for their drug in Canada or they do seek and get approval, but defer launching the drug here until it has been launched in larger jurisdictions. This isn't always a bad thing by the way, as sometimes a drug is found to be unsafe before ever coming to Canada and never gets used here. On the other hand, certain drugs that are proven both safe and effective get to be used by people in other countries often years before Canadians are able to benefit from these medicines. Having seen this occur with a number of helpful diabetes medications and technologies, Ian can tell you it is immensely frustrating.

SGLT-2 inhibitors

SGLT-2 inhibitors are new drugs not yet available in Canada or most other countries. (At least, they weren't available at the time of this writing; depending on when you're reading this they may now be available.) These drugs have a very novel way of reducing blood glucose. Unlike most antihyperglycemic medications, which work primarily by helping glucose move from the blood into the body's tissues, SGLT-2 inhibitors work by helping the body excrete glucose (by facilitating the passage of glucose from the blood across the kidneys into the urine). Because glucose contains calories, eliminating glucose from the body also helps people lose weight. Regulatory bodies are currently studying whether or not these drugs are proven safe enough to use. Data so far available suggests they are, indeed, very safe, however they do fairly often cause one particular side-effect which, though not serious and though easily treated, can be a nuisance: yeast infections of the vulva and vagina in women (vulvovaginitis) and the penis in men (balanitis).

Using Antihyperglycemic Medication Effectively: The CDA-Recommended Approach to Treating Type 2 Diabetes

Every few years the Canadian Diabetes Association (CDA) assembles a group of experts who volunteer to review all the available medical evidence on diabetes management, and come up with recommendations on how best to manage this condition. (Ian is one such volunteer.) This whole book is based on these recommendations. In this section we look at the CDA's recommended drug strategy to get your blood glucose control in order.

The overarching goal is to get rid of symptoms of hyperglycemia as quickly as possible and to achieve a target A1C (less than or equal to 7.0 percent) within three to six months. (Refer to Chapter 9 for more on A1C.)

These are the CDA recommendations (based on what should be done from the day of diagnosis) for managing type 2 diabetes:

✔ As soon as your diabetes is diagnosed you should

- Be referred to diabetes educators to receive appropriate diabetes education.

- Start lifestyle therapy. All the other recommendations noted in this list are *in addition to* (not instead of) lifestyle treatment.

- If your A1C is 8.5 percent or higher, immediately begin taking metformin either alone or along with a second blood glucose-lowering medication, one of which *may* be insulin. If your blood glucose levels are particularly elevated and you are unwell as a result, you *should* be immediately started on insulin.

✔ After two to three months, if your A1C remains above target (that is, it remains above 7.0) and you are not yet taking metformin, it should now be prescribed. If you're already taking metformin, a second antihyperglycemic medication or insulin should be added (this is especially important if your A1C is above 9.0).

In choosing which antihyperglycemic medication to add to metformin, your doctor needs to consider the pros and cons of the different drug classes and select the most suitable drug from the most suitable class for you. Your doctor should take into account both how the medication may help you, and also, what kinds of side effects might occur.

Wilson's excellent blood glucose adventure

Wilson, a 49-year-old small-business owner with no known health problems apart from being overweight (BMI 31), had recently seen his family physician for a routine physical. Blood tests were performed and it was found that he had diabetes. He was not having symptoms of hyperglycemia and his A1C was 8.3. His family physician referred him to Ian. This was how Ian and Wilson decided to proceed:

✔ **Day one:** Wilson was referred to a diabetes education centre, where he met with a diabetes educator and dietitian (refer to Chapter 8). Lifestyle therapy (refer to Chapters 10 and 11) was started immediately.

✔ **After two months:** Wilson was working with his diet and had lost 2 pounds (1 kilogram), but after showing some initial improvement, his fasting blood glucose levels had plateaued at about 9 to 10 mmol/L. Ian prescribed metformin because it would improve Wilson's blood glucose levels without causing weight gain or hypoglycemia, and because it could help protect against heart disease. Wilson was started on a low dose of metformin and over the span of 4 weeks progressively increased his dose until the dose was optimized.

✔ **After four months:** Wilson had been doing some regular exercise, though not as diligently as he had hoped and had not lost any more weight. His fasting blood glucose levels were now about 8 mmol/L and his A1C was 7.6. Wilson was instructed to continue his metformin and, in addition, was started on a GLP-1 analogue to help bring down his blood glucose levels and potentially help him lose weight.

✔ **After five months:** Since starting the GLP-1 analogue Wilson had lost 4 pounds (2 kilograms), he was exercising more regularly, and his fasting blood glucose levels were now running within goal (4 to 7 mmol/L). No change was made to his therapy.

✔ **After six months:** Ian tested Wilson's A1C and it was within target at 6.8 (target 7.0 or less). Success!

Ian's choice of a GLP-1 analogue was a somewhat arbitrary decision; he could just as appropriately have chosen another class of antihyperglycemic medication such as a DPP-4 inhibitor. Each class has its advantages and disadvantages, and there is seldom a right or wrong way to do things — with the exception of doing nothing and letting blood glucose readings remain too high on an ongoing basis, which is never right.

Here are important messages to take from these CDA recommendations:

✔ From the day you are diagnosed with type 2 diabetes, consider yourself racing against the calendar. Your goal is to achieve a target A1C (7.0 percent or less) within three to six months. (Refer to Chapter 9 for more on A1C.)

✔ As you race against the calendar, you may well find yourself requiring more and more medication to achieve your target A1C. This doesn't mean you're sicker than someone who requires fewer medicines. It may well mean that you're wiser than the person who declines taking necessary medicines, runs blood glucose levels that are too high, and develops (what would have been avoidable) diabetes complications as a consequence.

✔ Insulin therapy is never a bad choice. As we discuss in Chapter 13, taking insulin — in addition to or instead of other forms of antihyperglycemic medication — doesn't mean you are less healthy than the person who doesn't require insulin therapy.

✔ Achieving target blood glucose control is more important than which drug (or drugs) you use to achieve this goal.

✔ Lifestyle therapy is *always* a key component of therapy.

Write a note with the date six months from when your diabetes was diagnosed. Stick the note on your fridge and look at it periodically; that's your due date (even if you're not pregnant!), the date by which you and your health care team are striving to deliver a healthy blood glucose level. And this is one delivery that is quite fine if it comes early.

As Time Goes By: Antihyperglycemic Medications, Type 2 Diabetes and You

The good news about controlling your blood glucose is that, shortly after your type 2 diabetes is diagnosed, an excellent chance exists that you can achieve target blood glucose readings (refer to Chapter 9) with intensive lifestyle therapy and often just one type of antihyperglycemic medication. The bad news is that, as Figure 12-2 illustrates, with each passing year your pancreas's ability to produce insulin goes down, so the therapy that worked so well initially works less well with time. This information was first published in the journal *Diabetes* in 1995. When you were diagnosed with type 2 diabetes your pancreas was making only one half the insulin it should. And with each passing year it makes less and less of what you need. That's *not* your fault. But it does mean you and your doctor should continually review your glucose control and reassess your treatment.

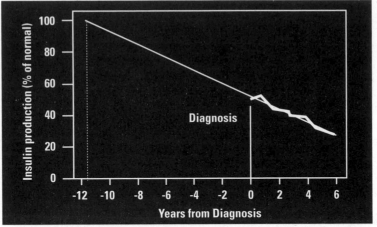

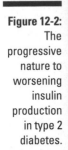

Figure 12-2:
The
progressive
nature to
worsening
insulin
production
in type 2
diabetes.

As doctors have learned more and more about the importance of excellent blood glucose control, they are introducing antihyperglycemic medications sooner to help patients manage their diabetes and protect them from diabetes complications. And, equally importantly, they are increasingly recommending *multiple* antihyperglycemic medications early on, sometimes from the day diabetes is diagnosed (particularly if your blood glucose levels are especially high). Doctors are also using insulin more often and earlier in the course of therapy.

If your blood glucose control is not sufficient on a moderate dose of a single antihyperglycemic medication, adding a second drug is generally better than increasing the dose of your existing medication. This approach will improve your blood glucose control more rapidly and cause fewer drug side effects than using a higher dose of a single medication.

Though you may hate the idea of taking a whole bunch of medications, consider the alternative. Do you really want toxic levels of glucose poisoning your system day after day after day? Now, we recognize that some people would say that they don't want medications poisoning them either. True enough. All we can say to that is that the medicines doctors use have proven themselves safe for the overwhelming majority of the millions of people who use them, but high glucose levels are dangerous to everyone. And that includes you.

Complementary and Alternative Therapies

Many people with diabetes use complementary or alternative therapies (also known as *natural health products* or *complementary or alternative medicines — CAMs* for short). Alternative and complementary therapy refers to non-traditional treatment, typically offered or recommended by people outside of the mainstream medical community. Suffice it to say, a fair bit of controversy surrounds these treatment options. Some CAMs have been around for many years, while others are fairly recent. Importantly, although CAMs are commonly used to lower blood glucose, none have been definitively proven to have a significant effect. (Perhaps this will change in the future.) The Canadian Diabetes Association advises against taking CAMs for blood glucose control due to the lack of proven effectiveness and safety.

Cautions concerning CAMs

The media frequently mention how this or that nutrient/herb/mineral may help you if you have diabetes. Disappointingly, what we invariably discover is that the evidence of improvement comes not from a research study involving real people or, for that matter, even laboratory animals. Rather, the new "discovery" is typically that a substance, which *theoretically* should help diabetes, has been found to be present in a berry or leaf or root or some such place. Ah, if only theory and reality were the same (or, often, even close facsimiles).

 Carefully evaluate non-traditional therapy in the same way that we hope you would consider prescription medication: Know what it's supposed to do, what it's *not* supposed to do (that is, side effects), and, most important, whether certain health problems or other medicines you're taking would make it dangerous to take at all. In other words, you need to be an informed consumer. Never assume that because something is natural it must be safe. After all, arsenic is natural, too.

 Because some non-traditional therapies can interact with your prescription drugs, let your physician know if you are taking non-traditional therapies. Bring them (in their original bottles) to your doctors' appointments. You can also go online to www.drugdigest.org to check for potential adverse interactions between your CAM and your prescription medicine.

Determining the value of complementary and alternative therapies in managing diabetes is very difficult for several reasons:

- ✔ Very few scientific studies have investigated these treatments.

- ✔ Potential side effects have not been adequately assessed.

- ✔ The strength of non-traditional agents can vary enormously from bottle to bottle, even if the label on the bottle says the same thing.

- ✔ The purity of non-traditional agents can vary enormously and may even contain toxins and contaminants.

- ✔ Alternative and complementary therapies have not been required to pass much in the way of government scrutiny, so long as they are marketed as foods, not drugs. This is a surprise to most people, who think — quite understandably — that a company could not say its product performs in such and such a way without evidence to back the claim. (The federal government introduced the Natural Health Products Regulations in 2004 in an attempt to improve this situation. You can learn more about these regulations at www.hc-sc.gc.ca/dhp-mps/prodnatur/index-eng.php.)

If CAMs are helpful for diabetes (and, as we discover in this chapter, very little evidence supports this), most likely they would be of benefit only if you have type 2 diabetes. If you have type 1 diabetes, your problem is lack of insulin, and no CAM is going to change that. If you have type 2 diabetes, a main problem is insulin resistance and CAMs may possibly exist that could reduce this.

Limited scientific information is available to guide decision-making regarding CAMs. So if you are considering taking an alternative or complementary therapy, you're making your decision based as much (or more) on hope as on science. That's fine if medical science knows the product has no potential for harm. But in the same way that science doesn't know about all the benefits that some remedies may hold, science doesn't know about all the potential downsides they may have. So please use caution.

Looking at some types of CAMS

Here's the lowdown on some of the more frequently used complementary and alternative therapies:

- ✔ **Chromium** deficiency is associated with an increased risk of developing type 2 diabetes. However, in North America chromium deficiency is rare, whether or not you have diabetes. Also, if you already have type 2 diabetes, taking chromium supplements is not of proven value.

✔ **Cinnamon** taken for medicinal purposes became very popular a few years ago. Although early evidence suggested a theoretical benefit in controlling blood glucose levels, later studies cast doubt on this. Cinnamon does, however, continue to be of proven benefit on French toast and cappuccinos!

✔ **Fenugreek** is a legume grown in India, the Mediterranean, and North Africa. Its use in treating diabetes goes back many centuries, and some evidence suggests that it may be effective in slightly improving blood glucose levels. This is not proven.

✔ **Garlic** is used for many purposes. Sometimes, it is even used for cooking! Some suggestions exist that garlic could help lower glucose levels, though the evidence for this is contradictory.

✔ **Ginkgo** is one of the oldest living tree species. Innumerable people take ginkgo to treat dozens of different ailments. Some very preliminary evidence suggests ginkgo may offer some benefit in the treatment of diabetic retinopathy. On the other hand, experimental evidence suggests it could make your blood glucose levels go *up*.

✔ **Ginseng** is a plant that exists in a variety of species. *American* ginseng has been found to improve glucose control to a small degree in some studies. These observations are preliminary.

✔ **Gymnema sylvestre** is a tropical plant found in central and southern India. In Hindi, it goes by the name "destroyer of sugar," based on folklore that chewing the leaves results in the inability to taste sweet things. Some *preliminary* evidence suggests that, apart from suppressing appetite, it has the ability to reduce blood glucose levels, possibly by improving the function of the pancreas's beta cells (these are the cells that make insulin).

Chapter 13

Using Insulin Effectively

*T*he discovery of insulin over 90 years ago was a miraculous event. Indeed, since Banting, Best, Macleod, and Collip's famous breakthrough in 1921 (refer to Chapter 3 for the inside scoop), the lives of untold millions of people have been enhanced or, often, saved by insulin therapy. However, as the years have passed, along with insulin's justified reputation as a wondrous medicine, so, too, has insulin gained the reputation, for many individuals, of being something intimidating or even something to be feared. In this chapter we look at the many benefits insulin therapy has to offer and we clear up misconceptions surrounding one of Canada's most famous contributions to the world.

What Is Insulin?

If you have type 1 diabetes, insulin is your saviour. Simply put, without insulin you could not survive. And if you have type 2 diabetes, though insulin may not very often be the difference between life and death (not in the short term, anyhow), it frequently is the difference between good health and bad health. As we explain in Chapter 3, insulin is a hormone that's produced in the pancreas and released into the bloodstream, where it travels to different parts of your body. Insulin acts on certain cells (such as fat cells and muscle cells) to allow glucose to enter so that these cells can carry out their normal functions. If you don't have insulin in your body to allow glucose to enter into the tissues, the glucose hangs around in the blood, damages your organs, and starts to spill out into your urine.

Looking at the Types of Insulin

A healthy pancreas functions on autopilot. When one eats, the blood glucose level goes up and the pancreas immediately responds by releasing insulin into the bloodstream, which promptly brings the glucose level back to normal. If your pancreas is malfunctioning and you require insulin injections, the goal is to try to reproduce what a healthy pancreas would normally do. You can consider this "thinking like a pancreas." We're aided by having a variety of different insulins to choose from, each with its own set of properties. When you're prescribed insulin, your doctor should try to match your body's needs with the most appropriate insulin. Because each person is different, the type of insulin you first start on may be changed to a different one, depending on how your body responds.

When you switch from one insulin to another, you may have unused doses of the first insulin. If it hasn't expired and the package is unopened, consider donating the insulin to Insulin for Life (www.insulinforlifecanada.org). This charity will send your insulin to individuals in developing nations who don't have access to insulin and may get sick or even die without it.

Table 13-1 lists insulins (and their properties) available in Canada. Note that the times we give are approximations and can vary significantly — even for the same person.

Table 13-1   **Types of Insulin Available in Canada and Their Properties**

Classification	Generic Name	Trade Name(s)	Manufacturer	Onset of Action	Peak Action	Duration of Action
Rapid-acting	aspart	Novorapid	Novo Nordisk	10 to 15 minutes	1 to 2 hours	3 to 5 hours
	glulisine	Apidra	Sanofi Aventis			
	lispro	Humalog	Eli Lilly			
Short-acting	regular	Humulin-R	Eli Lilly	30 minutes	2 to 3 hours	5 to 8 hours
		Novolin ge Toronto	Novo Nordisk			
Intermediate-acting	NPH	Humulin-N	Eli Lilly	1 to 3 hours	5 to 8 hours	14 to 18 hours
		Novolin ge NPH	Novo Nordisk			
Long-acting	detemir	Levemir	Novo Nordisk	90 minutes	Virtually none	16 to 24 hours
	glargine	Lantus	Sanofi-Aventis	90 minutes	None	24 hours
Premixed (the numbers after the names refer to the ratio of rapid- or short-acting insulin to intermediate-acting insulin)		Humalog Mix25	Eli Lilly	Depends on specific type	Depends on specific type	Depends on specific type
		Humalog Mix50	Eli Lilly			
		Humulin 30/70	Novo Nordisk			
		Novolin ge 30/70	Novo Norcisk			
		NovoMix 30				

ANECDOTE

Moving away misperceptions: How Dorothy overcame her fears about insulin

Dorothy was 50 years old when she was diagnosed with type 2 diabetes. Her initial treatment was lifestyle therapy, and she was thrilled when a change in her diet, modest weight loss, and a daily walk brought her glucose levels down to normal. A couple of years later, however, her glucose levels started to climb and she began taking non-insulin antihyperglycemic medications. That helped, but only temporarily, and her blood glucose readings had now risen to an average of 11 mmol/L and she was feeling fatigued. Her family doctor referred her to Ian to see if she should be on insulin. When Dorothy came to Ian's office, she was sad, angry, and frightened all at once. She felt like a failure. She told Ian she was "terrified of the needle" and added, "I would hate jabbing myself. I simply couldn't do it. You can't convince me otherwise." As she spoke to Ian she was on the verge of tears.

"Dorothy," Ian said, "we will do whatever you want. I can't force you to do anything. And I wouldn't want to even if I could. *You* are the boss and *you* will decide what you want to do. But I think you would be unfair to yourself if, whatever you decide, it wasn't an informed decision. So let's make sure you know the most important information to help you make your decision." Dorothy was certainly agreeable to that.

Ian said a few things to Dorothy that day. He remembers telling her, "It is crucial that you know that *you* are not a failure, your *pancreas* is, and that's not your fault. It happens to most people with diabetes. And as for hating jabbing yourself, why would you like it? Who would? But you are *already* jabbing yourself each time you test your blood glucose. And doing a finger stick jab is more uncomfortable than giving insulin. With the tiny needles we use nowadays, giving insulin is virtually pain free. And as for not being able to do it, look at the other obstacles that you have overcome; you've changed your diet, you've lost some weight, you're exercising regularly, you're taking a whole bunch of pills that I'm sure you'd rather not have to, and you're testing your blood every day. You've managed all those things. And if you can handle all those things, I'm sure you could manage giving insulin also."

Dorothy became more at ease but was still apprehensive. "But, Doctor, when you start insulin, you're on it forever."

"That's usually true, Dorothy," Ian replied, "but not because insulin creates dependency. It's because your pancreas is failing and it's not going to be rejuvenated. It can no longer make enough insulin, so we have to supplement it. We're simply giving your body back the hormone it's lacking. One other thing: Medical science is always progressing. Other ways of giving insulin are being developed. And better pills are always coming along. I don't know if you'll be on insulin injections forever. Maybe in a few years you won't have to be."

Well, Dorothy still wasn't thrilled with the prospect of giving insulin. And of course she had no reason to be thrilled. But she met with the diabetes educator and was pleasantly surprised to find that giving insulin wasn't nearly as bad as she had thought. And as her glucose levels returned to normal and her energy improved, she was very glad she had decided to take insulin after all.

One common misunderstanding is equating Humulin with Humulin-N. Humulin is a trade name and refers to a *variety* of types of insulin marketed by one particular company (Eli Lilly in this case). Humulin-N refers to Eli Lilly's brand of NPH insulin.

New insulins are under development. One is called degludec (trade name Tresiba), which is a very long-acting insulin; indeed it lasts considerably longer than any currently used insulin. Insulin degludec will likely be available for use in Canada in the near future (or, depending when you're reading this, already is!).

Understanding Insulin Terminology

Medicine, like many other fields, is chock-a-block full of jargon and hard-to-understand terminology. That's not a big deal when one physician is speaking to another. It's more of an issue, however, if you're a person living with diabetes and you're trying to understand what the heck a doctor is trying to tell you.

Here are some definitions regarding the classification of insulin to help you out:

- **Rapid-acting insulins:** Insulins with the quickest *onset of action* after they've been injected.

- **Short-acting insulin:** Insulin with a short *duration of action*. (Regular insulin is the only member of this group.)

- **Intermediate-acting insulin:** This type has a duration of action in-between (that is, intermediate between) rapid-acting insulin (or short-acting insulin) and long-acting insulins.

- **Long-acting insulins:** These have, well, a long duration of action.

- **Premixed insulins:** These are, as you may surmise, a mixture of two different types of insulin

Basal-bolus insulin therapy is the state-of-the-art insulin strategy used to manage type 1 diabetes (and is also the optimal insulin strategy for many people living with type 2 diabetes). Basal-bolus insulin has, as you might guess, two components:

- **Basal insulin** (Levemir, Lantus, NPH): Insulin you give once or, in some cases, twice a day to prevent your blood glucose levels from climbing between meals and overnight. (NPH when taken at breakfast time will, to a small extent, also help control after-lunch blood glucose levels, but not nearly as effectively as bolus insulin taken before lunch; see the following bullet.)

✔ **Bolus insulin** (Apidra, Humalog, NovoRapid, regular insulin): Insulin you give before each meal to prevent your blood glucose levels from climbing after a meal. It is also called mealtime insulin. (Although regular insulin is considered a bolus insulin, because it less closely replicates normal insulin release from the pancreas, it is typically not as good a choice as Apidra, Humalog, or NovoRapid.)

The other way of using basal-bolus insulin therapy is with an insulin pump (see "How to Give Insulin" later in this chapter).

Basal-bolus insulin therapy is also commonly called *intensified insulin therapy.* Although we do use this term, we admit to not being overly fond of it. That's because *all* people with diabetes need to be treated intensively regardless of whether with diet and exercise, non-insulin antihyperglycemic medication, or one, two, three, or more doses of insulin.

Rapid-acting insulin

Three types of rapid-acting insulin are available: Apidra (glulisine), Humalog (lispro), and NovoRapid (aspart). All the rapid-acting insulins have similar actions and thus one is not preferred over the other.

Rapid-acting insulin

✔ Is taken with meals to prevent your blood glucose levels from rising too high after your meal.

✔ Is taken in-between meals to bring down ("correct") high blood glucose.

✔ Is a bolus component of basal-bolus insulin therapy.

✔ Is the only insulin used with insulin pump therapy

✔ Usually works most effectively when taken about 15 minutes before eating. (As this timing can be a hassle, many people give it immediately before eating; the insulin will still work but not as effectively.)

✔ Wears off within a short period of time (three to five hours).

✔ Compared to regular insulin, is less likely to cause hypoglycemia and provides better after-meal blood glucose control. (For these reasons rapid-acting insulin is preferred over regular insulin.)

If you have gastroparesis (a condition in which your stomach becomes less efficient at propelling food into your small intestine; refer to Chapter 6) *and* erratic blood glucose control, you may benefit from taking rapid-acting insulin an hour or so *after* your meal. Your diabetes specialist can help you determine if this would be a good option for you.

Regular insulin

Regular insulin is, confusingly, sometimes referred to as a short-acting insulin and is sometimes referred to as a fast-acting insulin. We don't think either of these terms is all that accurate; we think simply calling regular insulin, well, *regular insulin*, is best.

Regular insulin is also called Toronto insulin, but it is seldom called that anymore. (Too bad; it reminded people around the world of insulin's Canadian roots.)

Regular insulin

✔ Is a mealtime insulin, given to prevent your blood glucose levels from rising too high after your meal.

✔ Is a bolus component of basal-bolus insulin therapy. (Although both regular insulin and rapid-acting insulin are bolus insulins, the latter is preferred, as we discuss in the preceding section.)

✔ Works most effectively when taken about 30 minutes before eating. (As this timing can be a hassle, many people give it shortly prior to meals; the insulin will still work but not as effectively.)

✔ Has a longer duration of action than rapid-acting insulin.

✔ Compared with rapid-acting insulin, is more likely to cause hypoglycemia (including overnight if regular insulin is taken at suppertime), provides less effective after-meal blood glucose control, and is less convenient to use (as it needs to be given 30 minutes before a meal). For these reasons, rapid-acting is preferred over regular insulin.

Intermediate-acting insulin

NPH (often simply called *N*) is the only available intermediate-acting insulin. Intermediate-acting insulin

✔ Is given to prevent your blood glucose levels from going up too high between meals.

✔ Is a basal component of basal-bolus insulin therapy.

✔ Is often given at bedtime to prevent blood glucose level from going up too high overnight. (We discuss this *dawn phenomenon* later in this chapter.)

✔ Does not have much effect until a few hours after it's injected, so it doesn't help to reduce your blood glucose levels immediately after you inject it.

✔ Is more likely than long-acting insulin to cause hypoglycemia (including overnight). For this reason, NPH is being prescribed less and less, and long-acting insulin more and more.

If you take NPH insulin in the evening or at bedtime, having a bedtime snack will reduce your risk of having an episode of hypoglycemia overnight. Having a snack is particularly important if you know from experience that NPH causes you to have lows overnight and if your blood glucose at bedtime is less than 7.0 mmol/L. (Having said this, it is Ian's *strong* preference, for people on NPH who are experiencing overnight hypoglycemia, to not take NPH, but rather to take a long-acting insulin instead; see the next section.)

Long-acting insulin

Two types of long-acting insulin are available: Levemir and Lantus. Tresiba, a new, very long-acting insulin, will likely become available in Canada in the near future. Long-acting insulins

✔ Are given to prevent blood glucose levels from going up too high between meals and overnight.

✔ Are the basal component of basal-bolus insulin therapy.

✔ Are typically given at bedtime, but for most people work equally well when taken at other times.

✔ Don't have a quick action, so they don't help to reduce your blood glucose levels immediately after you inject it. For this reason, long-acting insulins are usually supplemented with rapid-acting (or regular) insulin given with meals or, in the case of type 2 diabetes, often with other anti-hyperglycemic medications.

✔ Have a very consistent action — they have pretty well the same effect on blood glucose levels two hours after the injection as they do eight or more hours after the injection. (Lantus has no peak action and Levemir has only a slight peak.)

✔ Last up to 24 hours, so they are typically taken just once per day. (This pattern does have many exceptions. Many people — particularly if taking Levemir, but also with Lantus — find they require it twice daily.)

✔ Result in more consistent blood glucose values (meaning that your blood glucose readings will be less variable) than with intermediate-acting insulin.

✔ Compared with intermediate-acting insulin, typically cause less weight gain for those people newly starting insulin therapy. (This may be particularly true of Levemir insulin.)

✔ Are less likely to cause hypoglycemia (including overnight) than intermediate-acting insulin. For this reason, long-acting insulins are prescribed increasingly often and intermediate-acting insulins less and less often.

✔ Should not be mixed in the same syringe with any other insulin.

✔ Cost much more than intermediate-acting insulin

✔ Cause discomfort in a small percentage of people upon injection. With Levemir insulin, an even smaller percentage may develop a sore, red rash at the injection site.

If you experience more than minimal discomfort when injecting these insulins or if you develop a rash at the injection site, inform your physician right away because you may need to change the insulin to a different type.

Because insulin cartridges all look similar, if you are taking two or more types of insulin it is essential that you read the label on the cartridge before you give yourself an injection; otherwise you may give yourself the wrong one.

Premixed insulin

Premixed insulin combines, in a single cartridge (or vial), both a mealtime insulin (either Humalog, NovoRapid, or regular insulin) and an intermediate-acting insulin (either NPH or another insulin that acts similar to it). The percentage of mealtime insulin and intermediate-acting insulin differs depending on the specific type of premixed insulin. Determining which of the various available premixed insulins provides the best blood glucose control for a given individual is largely a matter of trial and error. The various types of premixed insulin are listed in Table 13-1, earlier in this chapter.

If you ever need to buy premixed insulin in the United States, be aware that what we call 30/70 insulin in Canada is called 70/30 insulin there.

The advantage of a premixed insulin is that you have to take it only twice per day (before breakfast and before supper). If you were to separately take bolus insulin (three injections per day) and basal insulin (one or two injections per day), you would need more frequent injections.

The huge disadvantage to premixed insulin is that, because it is premixed, you can't independently adjust each of its two insulin ingredients to match your body's specific requirements. Although some diabetes specialists use it often, we find premixed insulin seldom provides sufficient flexibility and blood glucose control. We don't routinely recommend it for people with type 2 diabetes and we never recommend it to people with type 1 diabetes.

Inhaled insulin

Many companies have cumulatively spent many billions of dollars developing insulin you can inhale (similar to the way that asthma inhalers are used). Alas, for myriad reasons (including reimbursement issues, dosing difficulties, safety concerns, and other challenges), all these efforts have fallen by the wayside and no inhaled insulin therapy is currently available anywhere in the world. One company (MannKind at www.mannkindcorp.com), however, has continued its efforts and hopes to eventually bring their version (Afrezza) of inhaled insulin to the market.

Not to be confused with inhaled insulin is *Oral-lyn*, an aerosol form of insulin you spray on the inside of the cheek. It's available for use in a few countries, but not in Canada (or the United States). Whether it will prove to be a safe, effective, and useful product remains to be seen.

Animal insulins

In very rare circumstances, people with diabetes are treated with animal insulins. The two available products are Hypurin Regular and Hypurin NPH, made by Wockhardt UK. You can find further information on this topic at http://hc-sc.gc.ca/dhp-mps/brgtherap/activit/fs-fi/qa_qr_insulin-eng.php. (Daunting task indeed to type this web address into your browser; instead, just type the terms "Hypurin health Canada" into your search engine and this link to Health Canada's information on animal-sourced insulins will show up.)

Type 1 Diabetes and Insulin Therapy

The best insulin treatment strategy if you have type 1 diabetes is *basal-bolus* therapy, meaning that you either use an insulin pump or you take basal insulin (Lantus, Levemir, or NPH) once or twice a day and bolus insulin (Apidra, Humalog, or NovoRapid) prior to meals. Of these two methods, pump therapy is the best treatment available for type 1 diabetes because it most closely mimics what a normal pancreas does.

If you have type 1 diabetes and aren't being treated with basal-bolus therapy (with or without an insulin pump), contact your doctor to discuss changing to basal-bolus therapy.

Because Levemir and Lantus insulins, compared with NPH insulin, cause less hypoglycemia (including nocturnal hypoglycemia) and less blood glucose variability, they are the preferred basal insulin for people with type 1 diabetes. (On the other hand, long-acting insulins cost considerably more than NPH insulin. So if cost considerations are a factor in your choice of insulin therapy *and* if using NPH insulin gives you excellent blood glucose control and only infrequent hypoglycemia, you don't *have to* change to Levemir or Lantus insulin.)

Type 2 Diabetes and Insulin Therapy

Unfortunately, insulin therapy for people with type 2 diabetes has typically been looked at as a sign of failure, a last resort greeted with equal parts doom and gloom. What a shame! Insulin is simply one more treatment option — one that's terribly underused. Goodness knows how many people might have been spared complications if only insulin had been used sooner in the course of their therapy.

The right time for you to start insulin if you have type 2 diabetes is when you cannot achieve appropriate blood glucose control without insulin or when very quick blood glucose lowering is required (for example, if your blood glucose readings are very high and you are having symptoms from this; refer to Chapter 2). For some people that means starting insulin at the time of diagnosis; for others, after years of combined use of two or more non-insulin antihyperglycemic medications (we discuss these in Chapter 12).

The key point is that you and your health care team must always be looking at ways to optimize your glucose control. If lifestyle change does the trick, great. If oral medications or non-insulin injectable medications (GLP-1 analogues; refer to Chapter 12) bring your readings into target, terrific. What you want to avoid is the all-too-common scenario where you and your physicians spend month after month, year after year (all the while risking — or actually incurring — damage to your body), awaiting a magical improvement in glucose control that simply isn't going to happen without insulin therapy.

No insulin is "best" if you have type 2 diabetes; however, these strategies are particularly effective:

✔ Basal insulin (Levemir, Lantus, or NPH) at bedtime and one or more non-insulin antihyperglycemic medicines (particularly metformin) during the daytime. This is Ian's preferred way to begin insulin therapy for most type 2 diabetes patients who require insulin. The insulin (if given in sufficient dose) prevents blood glucose levels from rising unduly overnight, and the other antihyperglycemic medications keep blood glucose levels under control during the day.

✔ Basal-bolus insulin therapy (see "Looking at the Types of Insulin" earlier in this chapter).

✔ Premixed insulin twice daily. (Because of the limited flexibility of this strategy, we seldom use this.)

✔ Insulin pump therapy. (This is underused and is an excellent option for people with type 2 diabetes who are active, lean, have not had a sufficient response to basal-bolus insulin therapy, and whose insulin dose requirements are not inordinate.)

Because metformin therapy complements the action of insulin for people with type 2 diabetes, it's typically used regardless of which of the aforementioned insulin strategies you follow.

An excellent and increasingly popular strategy is to add GLP-1 analogue therapy to insulin and metformin when the latter two medications alone aren't achieving sufficient blood glucose control. This strategy helps control blood glucose and, for many people, results in some weight loss.

Your diabetes educator, family physician, and diabetes specialist can help you decide which treatment program is best for you.

Never minimize the importance of following a program of proper nutrition and exercise. Doctors often see people who, despite being on huge doses of insulin and numerous other antihyperglycemic medications, are still having problems with glucose control — problems that improve virtually overnight when those people have made appropriate dietary changes and renewed efforts with exercise.

Debunking Insulin Myths

The longer Ian has been in practice, the greater is his sadness when he meets patients with diabetes complications that could have been avoided if only they had known that their beliefs about insulin therapy (and which led them to avoid it) were based on incorrect information. Well, in case you, too, have any misperceptions regarding insulin therapy, here we list a few of the most common insulin myths:

✔ **Giving insulin is difficult.** In fact, giving insulin is very, very simple and straightforward. And as a bonus, taking insulin often means you can discontinue a whole bunch of pills you might be presently (unsuccessfully) taking for blood glucose control.

✔ **Insulin needles hurt.** Nowadays needles have incredibly fine points, are *really* short (as short as 4 millimetres or 0.15 inches), and are specially coated to make inserting them under your skin virtually pain-free.

✔ **Injecting insulin in front of people is embarrassing.** With current techniques, such as using insulin pen devices, giving insulin is typically very discrete; indeed, the odds are good that you've sat near — or even right beside — someone in a restaurant who injected insulin and you never noticed. Not only that, but insulin use is so commonplace that most people seeing someone giving themselves an injection wouldn't bat an eye anyhow.

✔ **Insulin will make you feel like you're a prisoner to your diabetes therapy.** Many people find taking insulin liberating as they discover how it allows for flexibility with meal timing, when they exercise, and so forth.

✔ **Insulin will make you feel unwell.** In fact, on insulin therapy you will likely feel *better* as your blood glucose levels improve — typically after many months (or even years) of suboptimal therapy on other medications that are no longer working well for you.

✔ **Taking insulin means you've failed.** Taking insulin means your *pancreas* has failed, not you. Indeed, taking insulin means you've *succeeded* in adopting an excellent form of therapy.

✔ **Taking insulin creates a dependency for it.** Insulin is used when your own pancreas can no longer do its job. And because medical science doesn't have a way of making your pancreas rejuvenate itself, most people who start insulin need to stay on it. But this *isn't* because insulin is addictive or creates dependency; it's because your underlying diabetes isn't going to go away. (A good example of this is the fact that some people with type 2 diabetes are able to discontinue insulin therapy if they've succeeded with sufficient lifestyle change.)

✔ **Insulin leads to complications.** Perhaps your Aunt Sally went blind after she started insulin. If so, the insulin didn't cause it; in fact, the delay in starting insulin may have led to this.

✔ **Insulin will make you pass out.** Although taking insulin can lead to low blood glucose, which has the potential to cloud your thinking and even cause you to lose consciousness, this seldom happens to people with type 2 diabetes. And if you have type 1 diabetes, taking appropriate precautions minimizes this risk.

Insulin therapy has been improving and saving lives for over 90 years, yet it remains very underused, and as a result, many people get unnecessarily sick. We think that's a tragedy — and that's no myth.

How to Give Insulin

The best way to learn how to give yourself insulin is by sitting down with a diabetes educator and having her or him teach you. Therefore, if your doctor has prescribed insulin for you, unless your doctor is both very knowledgeable about how to give insulin *and* is a good teacher, you should be referred — at the time you get your prescription — to a diabetes educator so you receive their expert teaching *and* their ongoing guidance.

You can't be expected to have a single teaching session regarding insulin therapy and then to be expected to "know it all" and manage your insulin dosing and adjustment on your own. When your educator teaches you how to give insulin, arrange for *ongoing* follow-up, be it in person, by phone, e-mail, or some other means.

Using an insulin pen

Have you ever seen a movie where the actor says, "We can do this the easy way or we can do this the hard way. You decide." Well, the same applies to giving insulin.

Though insulin syringes are still available and some Canadians still use them, the overwhelming majority of people in Canada who take insulin do so with an insulin pen device. Compared with syringes, insulin pens are much easier to use, are more accurate, easier to carry, and the list goes on. (Of the thousands of patients in Ian's practice, he can count the number of syringe users on the fingers of one hand). Unless you have been using syringes from day one, are perfectly happy with them, and really, *really* don't want to change, speak to your diabetes educator about switching to a pen.

Pen devices come in two broad categories:

✔ **Refillable pens** use insulin-filled cartridges. You insert the cartridge into the pen and, when the cartridge is used up, you replace it with a new cartridge. Each insulin manufacturer (Eli Lilly, Novo Nordisk, Sanofi Aventis) makes a refillable pen designed for use specifically with their company's insulin.

✔ **Disposable pens** come prefilled with insulin. When the insulin in the pen is used up you dispose of the pen. Each insulin manufacturer makes a disposable pen, however not all insulins are available in a disposable pen format. Two of these are illustrated in Figure 13-1.

Eli Lilly and Novo Nordisk also make insulin pens that can give insulin in 1⁄2 unit increments. These pens can be helpful for small children (and the occasional adult) where very small doses of insulin are being given and even a 1⁄2 unit dose change can make a big difference. Also, pens are available that have a memory of the amount and time administered for the previous dozen or so doses. These can be helpful for people who may be prone to forgetfulness and would benefit from being able to see when they gave their last dose.

Here are some other things to know about insulin pen devices:

- In the event that you change from one type of pen to another you needn't waste your needles; the same type of needle can attach to any of the various pen devices.

- Refillable pen devices are available, free of charge, from diabetes education centres and pharmacies.

- When you first start insulin, your diabetes educator will likely provide you with an initial, small, free supply of insulin for your pen device.

- Insulin pens have a display that tells you how much insulin you are about to inject. If your dose exceeds the maximum amount that can be delivered with one injection, you don't need to remove the needle and inject yourself again. Instead, you can re-dial the pen while the needle is still inserted under your skin.

- To help people who may have a hard time reading a pen's display, pens make a clicking sound as you dial your dose; this helps you ensure you dial up the correct dose. Also, for some devices you can obtain a miniature magnifying glass that fits over the display to make reading the numbers easier.

Figure 13-1:
Example of disposable pens: Humalog KwikPen (13-1a) and NovoRapid FlexTouch (13-1b).

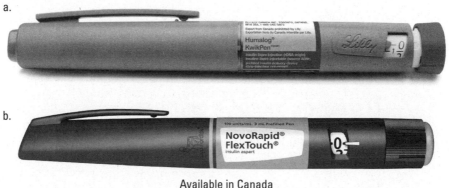

Available in Canada

Printed with permission from Eli Lilly Canada Inc (13-1a) and Novo Nordisk (13-1b).

Insulin jet injectors

If neither pen devices nor syringes nor a catheter such as the Insuflon suit your fancy, and if you don't mind spending a whole bunch of money (many hundreds of dollars), you can obtain a jet injection device (such as the AdvantaJet injector — www.advantajet. com — distributed in Canada by Activa Brand Products; 800-991-4464). The idea behind these is that because they don't have needles, using them to give insulin won't hurt as much. Although that's true for some people, it's not for others, and in any event, giving insulin with a pen device is virtually pain-free anyhow. Jet injectors are rarely used in Canada.

Whether you've been taking insulin for 20 days or 20 years, a time may well come when you accidentally give yourself either the wrong insulin or the wrong dose, or even forget to give a dose altogether. Fortunately, such a slip-up seldom leads to anything serious. Don't feel guilty or stupid if you make a mistake with your insulin; it happens to everyone. The way to deal with this type of oversight will depend on many factors, including the type of insulin you are taking (or, ahem, not taking), the dose, your blood glucose control, and the type of diabetes you have. Because so many factors must be taken into account, speak to your diabetes educator to formulate a plan of action if you make an error with your insulin.

Giving insulin is both easy and essentially pain-free. There are, however, certain people who have a tremendous aversion (*needle phobia*) to giving *any* form of injection to themselves. If you have a needle phobia to the point that you are unable to give yourself insulin, you may benefit from using a replaceable, disposable, catheter that you insert under your skin every few days and through which you can give your insulin without actually piercing your skin each time. This doesn't completely eliminate giving yourself a needle, but does make it necessary far less often. One example is the Insuflon catheter. You can learn about this product at www.autocontrol.com/ACM/ portfolio/insuflon-catheter.

Using an insulin pump

Ian loves insulin pumps. Why? Well, as Ian likes to say, medical research convinced him of its scientific rationale and merit, but it was Ian's *patients* who made him a believer. When patient after patient (after patient after patient after. . .) who has gone on a pump comes in with the biggest of smiles and says, "Wow, I love this pump! I should have gone on this years ago," it would take a pretty hardened soul indeed to not be persuaded. But insulin pumps aren't for everyone with diabetes; indeed, they are of value only for certain individuals. In this section we look at this and other issues regarding insulin pump therapy.

What is an insulin pump?

Simply put, *insulin pumps* are pumps that pump insulin. But calling an insulin pump "just a pump" is like calling Usain Bolt "just a runner." Insulin pumps are highly intricate, finely honed, precision instruments.

Insulin pumps continuously deliver (or infuse) insulin into the subcutaneous tissue (that is, the tissue just under the skin surface); as such the medical term for insulin pump therapy is *continuous subcutaneous insulin infusion* therapy or CSII. CSII is one form of *basal-bolus insulin therapy,* which we discuss earlier in this chapter. It is also a type of *intensified insulin therapy.*

Insulin pumps come in two main types (see Figure 13-2 for an illustration of some of the pumps available in Canada):

✔ **Pumps that use tubing:** Three main types of such pumps are available in Canada (each manufacturer may make several different models):

  • **MiniMed Paradigm Veo** (usually just called the Veo) is made by Medtronic (www.medtronic.ca)

  • **OneTouch Ping** (usually just called the Ping) is made by Animas (www.animas.ca)

  • **ACCU-CHEK Spirit Combo** (usually just called the Spirit) is made by Roche (www.accu-chekinsulinpumps-ca.com)

✔ **Pumps that don't use tubing:** These are typically referred to as *patch pumps.* Currently one such pump is available in Canada; the OmniPod (www.myomnipod.ca) which is made by Insulet and distributed in Canada by GlaxoSmithKline. (Many other companies are currently developing their own patch pumps.)

Figure 13-2: Insulin pumps: The Veo (13-2a), ACCU-Chek Spirit Combo (13-2b), and OmniPod (13-2c).

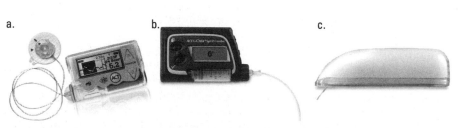

a.   b.   c.

Printed with permission from Medtronic (13-2a), Roche Diagnostics (13-2b), GlaxoSmithKline (13-2c)

Some features of insulin pump therapy are common to all insulin pumps and some are unique to a given device.

These are some key features common to *all* insulin pumps. They all

- Are small, computerized devices.

- Have an insulin reservoir that you fill with insulin.

- Use only rapid-acting insulin. If you use pump therapy, you no longer administer insulin by syringe or pen and you no longer give intermediate- or long-acting insulin. Rapid-acting insulin most closely mimics insulin from a healthy pancreas.

- Have a very small motor that controls a cylinder that pushes the insulin from the reservoir out of the pump.

- Deliver small amounts of (basal) insulin into your body 24 hours a day. You must program the pump to tell it how much basal insulin to give.

- Deliver extra (bolus) insulin into your body at mealtimes and, typically, with snacks. Extra insulin is also delivered in-between meals if your blood glucose level is elevated.

- Require you to carbohydrate count. You must tell the pump — based on the type and amount of food you are about to eat — how much bolus insulin to give (typically, within 15 minutes prior to beginning your meal). For this reason, carbohydrate counting is a crucial element of successful pump management. (We discuss carbohydrate counting later in this chapter.)

- Don't measure your blood glucose levels. If you use a pump, you must continue to do blood glucose meter tests.

- Are supported by excellent toll-free help lines and, in the event of a pump suddenly failing (which doesn't happen often), astonishingly quick couriered delivery of a replacement pump when necessary. (Ian is consistently impressed by the high quality of service and support that the pump manufacturers provide.)

- Have a 90-day grace period during which, should you decide that insulin pump therapy isn't the right choice for you, you can return your pump to the manufacturer for a full refund.

These are key features of *tube-requiring insulin pumps*:

- They require, as you would expect, tubing.

- The tubing connects to an *insertion set* which has a small plastic *catheter* that you insert under your skin (to about the same depth as an insulin needle) in any location that you would normally inject insulin (such as the back of the arm, the abdomen, the thigh, and so forth).

✔ The tubing and insertion sets are replaced every three days. The pump itself typically lasts three or four years before needing to be replaced.

✔ The pumps have buttons that you press to program the pump and also to have the pump give you a bolus of insulin when needed (such as when you're about to eat).

✔ Most of these pumps have a remote control which replicates the same functions as the buttons on the pump and also serves as a blood glucose meter.

✔ They can be disconnected for brief periods of time (typically not to exceed 30 or, at most, 60 minutes).

✔ Some tube-requiring pumps are waterproof and you can wear them while swimming or bathing. (Nonetheless, in general we feel you should avoid getting them wet in case the protective seal is compromised, which could allow water to get into the pump and interfere with its function. Briefly disconnecting your pump while you take a dip — or shower — is usually a better option than wearing it.)

These are key feature of *patch pumps*:

✔ They do not use tubing. Rather, their catheter goes directly from the pump into the skin. The catheter inserts itself automatically. The absence of tubing is the single most important difference between patch pumps and pumps that require tubing.

✔ They have an adhesive backing and you stick the pump directly on your skin wherever you would normally inject insulin. The pump does not come off until you remove it to replace it with a new one.

✔ They do not have buttons; rather they are controlled with a remote control (that also serves as a blood glucose meter).

✔ They are waterproof. (And, as they don't come off, you wear them when swimming or showering.)

✔ The pumps are single use only. That is, after wearing a patch pump for three days you take it off and put on a new one. (You package up the used ones about once a month or so and send them to a facility for recycling and proper disposal of certain of its materials.)

One advantage of having a remote control is that it allows you to give boluses of insulin particularly discretely. For example, if you are eating in a restaurant or in the middle of a business meeting when you need to give yourself a bolus of insulin, you don't need to even touch your pump; instead you can pull the remote out of your purse (or pocket), press the buttons on the remote, and you're done.

The pros and the cons of insulin pump therapy

Insulin pump therapy is considered the "gold standard" for managing type 1 diabetes. Indeed it is far and away the best way of administering insulin for most people living with type 1 diabetes and for some people living with type 2 diabetes. It is, however, definitely not for everyone.

These are some benefits from using an insulin pump (compared with other ways of giving insulin):

- ✔ **It provides better blood glucose control.** This is the single most important and compelling reason to use an insulin pump. It can help smooth out blood glucose levels — with fewer episodes of hypo-and hyperglycemia — because problems with inconsistent and erratic insulin absorption of longer-acting insulins are no longer an issue. (Pumps use only rapid-acting insulin.) For many pump users, pump therapy also results in improved A1C readings.

- ✔ **It's very convenient.** Whenever you need to give yourself a bolus of insulin, you just press a button on the pump or the remote. You don't have to get out an insulin pen (or syringe) and inject yourself. This makes giving your insulin boluses much more convenient, not only with meals, but with snacks. It also more conveniently allows you to bring down ("correct") high blood glucose between meals. (No more debating whether or not your blood glucose is high enough or your snack big enough to make getting out your pen device and injecting yourself worthwhile; with a pump it's so easy that you don't need to think twice.)

- ✔ **You require fewer injections.** When you use an insulin pump you change the catheter every three days. Which means that you go from giving yourself 12 or more needles over three days when using an insulin pen to one needle every three days when using a pump. Or, looked at differently, you go from giving yourself 120 (or more) needles per month to giving yourself 10 needles per month.

- ✔ **It's discrete.** If being discrete is important to you, you will like being able to give yourself a bolus of insulin without anyone knowing (not that this is an issue for most people).

- ✔ **It provides flexibility and improved quality of life.** Insulin pump therapy makes many aspects of living with diabetes much easier. It allows for greater flexibility regarding meal timing, exercise, shift work, sleeping in, travelling across time zones, and other routine day-to-day aspects of life. (One of the things that most people new to pump therapy quickly discover — and often to their surprise — is the feeling of freedom that insulin pump therapy provides.)

Simply put, going on an insulin pump makes life easier. Not *easy* (living with diabetes is seldom easy), but *easier*.

Here's one additional (and often under-recognized) benefit of insulin pump therapy. For some people who have had type 1 diabetes for many years and are "fed up" and have lost interest in managing their diabetes (with, perhaps unsurprisingly, not very good blood glucose control), going on an insulin pump can be re-energizing. "Finally, a different way to look after my diabetes," Ian often hears patients in this situation say. When using this new strategy, many of these patients develop renewed interest in their diabetes and develop the best blood glucose control they've had in years.

If you have type 1 diabetes and you find yourself in the situation where you have lost interest in your diabetes and your blood glucose control is poor, speak to your diabetes specialist about whether or not you might be a candidate for insulin pump therapy.

Insulin pump therapy is not, however, a panacea. These are some drawbacks to insulin pump therapy:

- **It is *very* expensive.** A tube-requiring pump will cost you about $7,000 and supplies will run you about $250 per month (and that doesn't even include the cost of insulin or blood glucose test strips). Each individual patch pump is relatively inexpensive and you don't need to buy insertion sets or tubing, however, as patch pumps need to be replaced every three days the total cost over time works out to be similar to tube-requiring insulin pump therapy. However, more and more provinces in Canada are covering nearly all the costs of insulin pumps and pump supplies (though not insulin or test strips) for people living with type 1 diabetes. Check with your provincial government or contact a pump manufacturer to find out if your province covers these costs.

- **You and your pump are virtually inseparable.** As the preceding lists mention, you wear patch pumps 24/7, and although you can disconnect tube-using pumps, you should do so for only minutes at a time. Indeed, just like a teenager and a phone, when it comes to you and your insulin pump, separations are kept to a minimum.

- **Pumps do not think for you.** As one of the diabetes educators with whom Ian works says, "Insulin pumps are smart, but they're not geniuses." You need to be taught (by a "pump trainer" diabetes educator) how to operate and adjust your pump based on your glucose levels, your exercise, your diet, and so on.

- **You have to do lots of blood glucose testing.** You must test your blood glucose 6 to 12 times per day (unless you are also using continuous glucose monitoring — which we discuss in Chapter 9 — in which case testing your blood glucose less often is possible).

> ✔ **Mastering the pump requires time, energy, and work.** Insulin pump therapy has a significant learning curve. Mastering it will entail lots and lots of time, energy, and work. Initial education is a *minimum* of 12 to 15 hours and education is ongoing and indefinite. You don't go on a pump on day one and have great blood glucose control on day two. Mastering the pump can take weeks or even months of teaching sessions (some in person, some by phone, some by e-mail) with the diabetes educators and repeated tweaking of your pump settings before your control is optimized. If you aren't up to this type of commitment, then that nearly $7,000 insulin pump you just got will become nothing more than one very, very expensive paperweight.

> ✔ **It can bring hassles and frustrations.** Learning how to use — and continuing to use — an insulin pump entails a certain degree of hassle and frustration. Pump alarms, insertion set issues, and so on all require attention and can aggravate you.

So should you switch to an insulin pump? Well, you'll base your decision on how you feel about all the pros and cons in this chapter. Taking all those things into account, Ian feels the people most likely to succeed with insulin pump therapy are those individuals with type 1 diabetes (or type 2 diabetes being managed on small to moderate doses of insulin four or more times daily) *who are committed to working very hard* at their diabetes management.

When Ian first suggests pump therapy to his patients, the usual response he hears is, "Doctor, I can't imagine having that thing attached to me all the time. It would make me feel like a prisoner." But as surprising as this may seem, what Ian almost always hears after a previously hesitant patient goes on a pump is, "This is *so* much better. I love the freedom!"

And as for the extra work involved with pump therapy, that's a trade-off that pump users are invariably happy to make.

If you want to discover more about insulin pump therapy start by reading the information on the pump companies' websites (we list these earlier) and by discussing this option with your diabetes educator and, if you have one, your diabetes specialist. Also, speak to people who already use a pump; they can share their own experiences with you. (If you don't know anyone who uses a pump, ask your diabetes educator or physician if they have a patient who would be willing to speak to you.)

Insulin pump therapy is sadly underused (both for people with type 1 and type 2 diabetes). Sometimes (fortunately, less and less often) this is because members of one's own health care team aren't all that familiar or comfortable with the technology. Thus they don't advocate using it even for people whom it might benefit. If your health care team members are uncomfortable with — or insufficiently familiar with — the technology, they can refer you to their colleagues who have greater expertise with insulin pumps.

Choosing the right pump

If and when you decide you want to use insulin pump therapy, your next decision will likely be which pump to use. All the pumps available in Canada work very well and all the pump companies provide excellent customer support. Therefore in making your decision you need to look at other considerations such as:

- ✔ **Do you want a patch pump or a tube-requiring pump?** This is the main question for many people. When making your decision take the following into account:

  - Patch pumps are convenient because they don't require tubing. On the other hand, some people find patch pumps — even though they're small — to feel bulky or appear obvious. (Tube-requiring pumps are bigger, but you can stow them discretely clipped to your bra or in your pocket.)

  - Patch pumps require you to always have your remote control with you because you can't give a bolus of insulin without it. On the other hand, the remote also acts as a blood glucose meter, and you need to carry around a meter regardless of which pump you use.

  - Patch pumps cannot be taken off (unless you are replacing it with a new one), whereas tube-requiring pumps can be disconnected for brief periods of time.

- ✔ **Is the pump's display easy enough to read?** Some displays are easier to read than others.

- ✔ **Are the navigation menus to your liking?** Some pumps' navigation menus are easier to sort through than others. (In Ian's opinion none of the currently available pumps have sufficiently easy navigation menus.)

- ✔ **Can the reservoir size accommodate the amount of insulin you use?** Different pumps have different size reservoirs.

- ✔ **Do you want to use a remote?** All pumps have remotes, but the remotes used with some pumps are much more sophisticated than others.

- ✔ **Will you want to use continuous glucose monitoring?** The Medtronic Veo is the only pump which can be coupled with continuous glucose monitoring (see Chapter 9) to display your glucose level continuously on the pump's screen. The Veo, when coupled with continuous glucose monitoring also has the ability to automatically stop delivering insulin if you have low glucose (a feature called *low glucose suspend*). This can be an important safety feature, particularly if you are prone to low blood glucose overnight.

Portrait of a pumper

Bill, a 34-year-old shift worker, was an active man who was very attentive to his diabetes management. He tested his blood glucose at least four times per day, sometimes even more. He was giving himself Humalog insulin with meals and Lantus insulin every evening. Bill's blood glucose readings and A1C were both good, though not optimal. "Bill," Ian said to him at the time of an appointment, "I think you should consider getting a pump." Bill was surprised and wondered why he should. "Because you are working hard at managing your diabetes, but your glucose control isn't as good as it should be for all the work you put in. Also, with you working shifts and playing hockey, I think you'd really enjoy the flexibility that insulin pump therapy would provide."

Bill was hesitant at first but then decided to try the pump. A few months later he was back in the office. "How's it going?" Ian asked. "Well," Bill said, "I must admit I was a bit skeptical

of your advice, but I decided to try the pump anyhow." Bill paused for a moment then continued; "And I have to tell you it was a *fantastic* decision. And like you said, life isn't now *easy*, but it is *easier*. When I need a bolus, presto, it's done. Now, no one even notices when I give my insulin, not that that would bother me anyhow. And guess what? I'm having fewer lows than I was." Ian asked Bill if he would ever go back to his insulin pen injections. "Not on your life. They'd have to shoot me to get this pump from me!"

Bill was a very good candidate for an insulin pump. He was testing and injecting many times per day. He was motivated and interested in putting in the considerable time and energy necessary to learn how to use a pump. Without this devotion, switching to a pump is no more likely to make your glucose control better than driving a Porsche rather than a Hyundai would make you a better driver.

Caring for Your Insulin

Although insulin is not particularly difficult to look after, you should be aware of some handling issues:

- ✔ Do not use insulin after the expiration date marked on the label.
- ✔ Before its first use, store an *unopened* vial or cartridge of insulin in the refrigerator. (Refrigeration helps to preserve the insulin's potency.)
- ✔ After you use it for the first time, you can keep your vial or cartridge of insulin either refrigerated or at room temperature.

You'll find that injecting insulin that is at room temperature is more comfortable than injecting insulin you have just taken out of the refrigerator.

✔ After its first use, your vial or cartridge of insulin has a limited time (usually about four weeks) before you will need to discard it. The package insert that came with your insulin will indicate the precise time recommended by the manufacturer of the particular insulin you are using.

✔ Insulin doesn't take well to excessive heat (such as being kept inside a car on a hot summer day) or, contrarily, to excessive cold (as Ian's patient found out when he returned to his car after his son's mid-winter hockey practice only to find his insulin resembled a Popsicle). You should not use insulin that has been frozen or subjected to extreme heat.

✔ If you will be travelling to a destination where you won't have access to refrigeration facilities for insulin storage, use an insulated travel pack to keep your insulin protected from the elements. Frio (www.frious.com) makes a particularly good and quite novel line of travel packs that, when dunked in water, automatically start to cool. After a few days the cooling effect diminishes and it's time for another dunk.

✔ Many a person has successfully injected insulin through clothing, but we don't recommend you do it routinely.

✔ Because with repeated use needles get dull very quickly (which can both increase the discomfort of an injection and lead to skin damage including *lipohypertrophy* — which we discuss in Chapter 6), we recommend you do not reuse your needles.

✔ Dispose of used needles in a puncture-proof "sharps" container that is sealed shut before being discarded. Most pharmacies will accept these containers and will dispose of them for you.

✔ If you're using cloudy insulin (some insulins are clear and some are cloudy), turn the vial upside down then right-side up 20 times to mix the contents before you inject it. If clumps are present, do not use the insulin.

Adjusting Your Insulin Dose

If you're taking insulin, you can pat yourself on the back; you have just been given the right to prescribe your own medicine. Well, not entirely, but to quite a significant extent.

Insulin is different from almost any other medicine your doctor will ever ask you to take. Unlike antibiotics, heart medicines, or, for that matter, other types of blood glucose–lowering medication, insulin is *not* designed to be taken in a set dose day to day. Quite the opposite, in fact. If your pancreas was working properly, it would constantly adjust how much insulin it was producing based on your body's needs at any given moment. When you give yourself insulin, you're trying to mimic what your pancreas would normally do, so that means you, too, should be constantly adjusting your insulin dose. In fact, when Ian ask patients how much insulin they are taking, it is music to his ears when they reply, "Oh, well that depends . . . ." Precisely right. It depends. It depends on many things including:

- What you are about to eat (This refers to both the *type* of food — particularly the carbohydrate content — and the *amount* of food you're about to enjoy. We discuss the importance of *carbohydrate counting* if you have type 1 diabetes later in this chapter. Some people with type 2 diabetes also benefit from carbohydrate counting.)
- Your current blood glucose level
- Your recent blood glucose levels
- Whether you will be exercising
- Which type of insulin you are using

The common denominator in this list is the need to make *proactive* insulin adjustments. The single greatest reason for failing to achieve good blood glucose control despite taking insulin is making *retroactive* insulin adjustments. To be proactive, you should be like a soothsayer, trying to predict what your reading is likely to be in a few hours and taking the amount of insulin *now* that will give you a good blood glucose level *later.* Far too often people simply say, "Oh, my reading is high, I need more insulin," or "My reading is low, I need less insulin." These statements are perfectly true, but they take into account far less information than is available and necessary.

Although insulin adjustment is essential for the great majority of people with insulin-treated diabetes, if you have type 2 diabetes and have excellent blood glucose control on the same daily dose of insulin, making routine changes wouldn't be necessary.

Many, many people have the mistaken impression that their insulin dose correlates to the severity of their diabetes. In case you're one of those people, we're glad you are reading this paragraph. Your insulin dose tells you (and your doctor) absolutely *nothing* about how good or bad your diabetes is. You can be on 10 units per day and have all sorts of complications and difficulties with your diabetes, or you can be on 300 units per day and sail along very nicely, thank you very much. Just like you should wear the shoe size that your feet require, so should you take the dose of insulin your body requires.

When you start insulin, you must consider it as just that, *a start.* You'll need to stay in regular touch with your diabetes educator for *ongoing* dosage adjustment guidance. Your educator knows you as an individual and can provide advice specific to you. For example, your educator will help you learn how to adjust your doses based on your blood glucose readings, your diet, your exercise, your travel schedule, and, for some women, your menstrual cycle. Without the educator's ongoing help, very few people ever master insulin adjustment and they typically end up feeling very frustrated.

As you might imagine, insulin doses need to be changed in *many* different situations. In the next few sections we look at a few select situations where insulin adjustment is warranted and discuss what kind of changes can improve things.

Adjusting your insulin dose to lower your fasting blood glucose

Bill was a 65-year-old man with type 2 diabetes. He was taking 10 units of Lantus insulin at bedtime. Although his readings were 5.0 to 7.0 mmol/L at bedtime, his before-breakfast blood glucose readings were running 10.0 to 12.0 mmol/L. Bill blamed the high readings on eating too big a bedtime snack, but when he reduced his snack, it didn't help. Ian suggested to Bill that he increase his bedtime insulin dose by one unit every night until his before-breakfast readings came down to target. Two weeks later, Bill was up to 24 units of insulin daily and his before-breakfast readings were down to 5.0 mmol/L.

Bill's problem is very common. Without sufficient quantities of insulin in your system, your blood glucose level tends to rise overnight as your liver releases glucose into the blood (starting at about 3 a.m.) in response to increasing levels of other hormones (such as cortisol, epinephrine, and growth hormone). This is called the *dawn phenomenon*. Intermediate- or long-acting insulin (the former routinely taken at bedtime; the latter usually but not always taken at bedtime) is the ideal way to combat this. The insulin provides a substantial effect overnight to combat the liver's tendency to release glucose at that time. To get this benefit from your insulin, however, the dose *has to be adjusted* to meet your body's demands, as Bill discovered.

Adjusting your insulin dose to avoid overnight hypoglycemia

Low blood glucose occurring overnight is dangerous because, compared with daytime hypoglycemia, you are less likely to notice it and you can go from being asleep to being unconscious without having awakened in-between.

Completely eliminating the risk of overnight hypoglycemia is not possible, but you can minimize the risk. The best solution will depend on what insulin you're taking. If you're having overnight hypoglycemia, we recommend, in consultation with your doctor and diabetes educator, the following options to help you avoid this problem:

- ✔ If you're taking NPH, replace it with Lantus or Levemir. (Lantus and Levemir cause far less hypoglycemia than does NPH). If cost considerations preclude you making this change then, if you're taking NPH at suppertime, switch the time you take it to bedtime and take a bedtime snack. If that still doesn't help then reduce the dose of your NPH.

- ✔ If you're taking regular insulin at suppertime, discontinue this and take a rapid-acting insulin at suppertime instead.

- ✔ If you're taking Levemir or Lantus at bedtime, reduce the dose. If that doesn't help, take it earlier in the day.

- ✔ Change to an insulin pump.

For generations, health care providers and people with diabetes have believed that high blood glucose readings first thing in the morning were often indicative of a "rebound" from having had (and slept through) a low blood glucose in the middle of the night. (This is called the *Somogyi phenomenon* or a *Somogyi reaction.*) With the introduction of continuous glucose monitoring (refer to Chapter 9), we now know that this type of rebounding rarely, if ever, occurs. So if you have a high blood glucose reading when you wake up in the morning, your glucose levels have likely been steadily creeping up overnight.

If you or your health care provider suspect you are having episodes of low blood glucose overnight, from time to time set your alarm for the middle of the night and get up and test your blood glucose at that time. Alternatively, wear a continuous glucose monitor for a week (an "iPro study"); refer to Chapter 9.

Adjusting your insulin dose to improve elevated after-meal blood glucose levels

Anita was a 52-year-old woman with type 2 diabetes. Her before-meal blood glucose readings were within target (4.0 to 7.0 mmol/L) yet her A1C level at 7.9 percent was above target of 7.0 percent or less. Anita was taking Levemir insulin 36 units at bedtime. Anita started testing her blood glucose two hours after the start of her meals and although her blood glucose after breakfast was good, after lunch and after dinner her readings were consistently in the 10.0 to 12.0 mmol/L range. Anita started taking NovoRapid (a form of rapid-acting insulin) in a dose of 4 units before her lunch and dinner and her after-meal readings slightly improved. She then increased these doses by 1 unit every day and in two weeks, now taking 18 units of NovoRapid before lunch and before dinner, her after-meal blood glucose levels were down to 5.0 to 8.0 mmol/L. Soon thereafter her A1C was also within target having come down to 6.8 percent.

As Anita discovered, if you have a good but not optimal A1C, the problem is often that your after-meal blood glucose is elevated. She corrected this by taking rapid-acting insulin before those meals that were followed by elevated blood glucose. She then progressively increased her doses until her readings came into target.

If your A1C is too high, you and your health care team need to figure out at what times your blood glucose is elevated. If your blood glucose is within target before meals but elevated after meals, then taking rapid-acting insulin before meals is helpful (in conjunction with ensuring you are eating healthfully). Taking rapid-acting insulin, however, is only going to help if you are taking the appropriate dose.

Carbohydrate Counting

As we discuss in Chapter 10, carbohydrates are *the* key nutrient in raising blood glucose readings after meals. You can take advantage of this by adjusting your insulin dose to fit with the likely effect on your blood glucose of the quantity of carbohydrates you are about to eat. This is called *carbohydrate counting* (*carb counting* for short) and is an essential part of type 1 diabetes management, especially if you're using an insulin pump. It can also be a helpful strategy for many people with type 2 diabetes if being treated with rapid-acting insulin.

The best way to learn how to perform carbohydrate counting is by meeting with a registered dietitian. They are expertly trained in this field and will likely spend at least an hour with you to go over the basics. Having a follow-up meeting (or meetings) with the dietitian to have the principles of carb counting reinforced is often a good idea.

Having a honeymoon — whether or not you're married

The *honeymoon period* is a brief period of time, typically lasting no more than a few weeks to a few months, that some individuals experience when, shortly after the onset of type 1 diabetes, some recovery of pancreatic function happens and less insulin is required. (Occasionally, an individual will even be able to temporarily discontinue their insulin.) All honeymoons are short, including — with rare exceptions — this one.

You're an award winner

Two companies that manufacture insulin in Canada give out awards to celebrate those individuals who have used insulin for many years. Novo Nordisk has the Novo Nordisk Half Century Award Program (recognizing, as you might surmise, 50 years of using insulin) and Eli Lilly has the Lilly Diabetes Journey Awards (one award is for 25 years of insulin use, one for 50 years of insulin use, and one for 75 years of insulin use). You can find out more about the Novo Nordisk award by calling 800-465-4334 and you can find out more about the Eli Lilly awards by calling 888-545-5972.

Mary was a 16-year-old girl with type 1 diabetes. She was taking Lantus insulin at bedtime to prevent her blood glucose from rising overnight and was taking Humalog insulin with each meal to prevent her blood glucose readings from climbing too high after she ate. Nonetheless, she found that sometimes her after-meal readings were excellent and other times they were poor, without rhyme or reason. Mary met with the registered dietitian and discovered a reason: Her consumption of carbohydrate was varying quite a bit from meal to meal, but she wasn't adjusting her insulin dose to match her carbohydrate intake. Mary learned how to adjust her insulin based on how much carbohydrate she was eating, and soon thereafter her after-meal readings were excellent.

The first step in carbohydrate counting is to calculate how many grams of carbohydrate you're about to consume and to then give a certain number of units of rapid-acting insulin based on that. (See the following tip.) Because each person responds differently, adults are typically arbitrarily started on a ratio of 1 unit of insulin for every 10 grams of carbohydrate, but it can range from 1 unit per 2 grams to 1 unit per 30 grams. (And even that's not written in stone.) Bear in mind that not all carbohydrates will raise your blood glucose to the same degree (refer to our discussion on the glycemic index in Chapter 10). Do not count the fibre you eat when totalling the number of carbs in your diet because, although it's a carbohydrate, it will not raise your blood glucose.

You can find out the carbohydrate (including fibre) content of foods by having a look at the nutrition facts label on the food you buy. (Refer to Chapter 10.) Also, some excellent books are available to help you learn and use carb counting. One particularly helpful book is *The Calorie King Calorie, Fat & Carbohydrate Counter* (Family Health). You can download various smart phone apps that will help you carb count. Also, most modern insulin pumps can perform the required calculations for you; all you have to do is tell the pump how many grams of carbs you're about to eat (and some of these devices make even that step easier by coming with a pre-loaded inventory of foods and their carbohydrate content). Bon appétit!

The Salter Nutri-Weigh Dietary Computer Scale (www.salterhousewares.com) can be a very helpful tool for determining the number of grams of carbohydrate that are present in foods you are about to eat.

If you're carbohydrate counting, you'll also benefit from using a *correction factor* (or *insulin sensitivity factor*). A correction factor tells you the amount of insulin you'll need to bring an elevated before-meal blood glucose level down to normal. In other words, your correction factor corrects your elevated blood glucose (and your carb counting-determined dose prevents your level from going up from the food you're about to eat).

Yolanda has type 1 diabetes treated with Humalog insulin with meals and Levemir insulin at bedtime. She's about to eat supper. Her before-supper blood glucose is 13.0 mmol/L. Her about-to-be-devoured scrumptious meal contains 40 grams of carbohydrate. She uses a carbohydrate counting ratio of 1 unit per 10 grams of carbohydrate (a 1:10 ratio) and a correction factor of 1 unit for each 2.0 mmol/L her blood glucose is above 7.0. To know how much insulin she needs to take, she does the following calculation:

1. **She uses her carbohydrate counting ratio:** 40 g of carbohydrate × 1 unit/10 g = 4 units.

2. **She uses her correction factor:** 13 mmol/L – 7 mmol/L = 6 mmol/L × 1 unit/2 mmol/L = 3 units.

3. **She adds these two amounts together and determines how much insulin she needs:** 4 units + 3 units = 7 units.

4. **She injects 7 units of insulin:** She then smiles to herself, thinking of how carb counting and using the correction factor quickly became second nature after spending an hour with the wonderful dietitian.

Carbohydrate counting may not be rocket science, but it isn't easy either, and it's certainly not for everyone. If you're doing very well without carbohydrate counting, don't feel you have to take on this additional task. If, however, things aren't going sufficiently well for you (and in particular if your glucose control is inconsistent and/or your A1C isn't as good as it should be), contact your dietitian to discuss whether carbohydrate counting would be good for you.

Donating blood

If you're on insulin therapy, Canadian Blood Services' current policy is that you are not a candidate to give blood. We are sure this policy is well intentioned, but we feel it's overly restrictive. If you are on non-insulin antihyperglycemic medications, you are eligible to donate blood unless some other health problem precludes this.

Travelling with Your Insulin

We live in a mobile society, and if you use insulin, where you go, your insulin goes too.

Breezing through the border

As you well know, airline security is now greater than ever. And this means you will need to take some additional measures when you are planning on travelling by plane.

Transport Canada has issued guidelines for when you are flying with diabetes supplies. The following information is from the Canadian Diabetes Association's reference to these guidelines:

- ✔ Advise the security personnel that you have diabetes and that you're carrying your supplies on board. Have a letter from your physician indicating that you have diabetes and that you need to carry your diabetes medication and supplies.

- ✔ Organize your medication and supplies into one separate container and take it with you in your *carry-on* (not your stowed) baggage.

- ✔ Ensure that your insulin needles have their guards (protective covers) in place and are accompanied by the insulin.

- ✔ Place your insulin and any other medications in a container with a professionally printed pharmaceutical label identifying the medication. If the pharmaceutical label is on the outside of the box containing the insulin, the insulin must be carried in that original packaging.

- ✔ Cap your lancets. Also, your lancets must be accompanied by a glucose meter imprinted with the manufacturer's name.

- ✔ If you have any difficulty throughout the screening process, request to speak to the screening supervisor.

- ✔ If you are travelling outside of Canada, consult with your airline for applicable international regulations.

If you use an insulin pump, you may wish to pre-emptively notify the screening officer that you are wearing the device. They will probably not bat an eye (insulin pumps are so commonplace they are likely seeing them routinely), but it may spare you some additional time and questions.

We know at least three important reasons to take your insulin and supplies (injection devices, blood glucose meter, lancets, and so on) with you as part of your carry-on (not your checked) luggage:

- ✔ If you are going to Sydney, Nova Scotia, for example, your *carry-on* luggage is not going to get mistakenly sent to Sydney, Australia.
- ✔ The baggage compartment temperatures may not be appropriate for your insulin.
- ✔ You will need it!

And although not technically an insulin supply, make sure you take extra snacks with you on board in case your meals are delayed.

And on the subject of insulin supplies, if you will be travelling for any sort of extended period, make sure you have lots of extra insulin, blood glucose test strips, and so on. Better to have too much than to try finding a pharmacy at midnight in an unfamiliar city.

The Canadian Diabetes Association has partnered with an insurance company to offer travel insurance to its members. We discuss this further in Chapter 16.

Because rapid-acting insulin works very quickly, even if you see the flight attendant moving the food cart down the aisle in your direction, do *not* take your insulin dose until your food has been set down in front of you. One patient of Ian's told him about the time when, anticipating imminent arrival of his meal, he took his rapid-acting insulin only to find the food cart quickly whisked away when turbulence interrupted food services. With his mealtime insulin having been given but no meal to go with it, he was at risk of having hypoglycemia. Fortunately, he had wisely taken some snacks with him in his carry-on luggage and substituted the snacks for the missed meal.

When flying, keep your low blood glucose treatment (such as your dextrose tablets) *on your person*, not in the overhead bin. In the event the seatbelt sign is illuminated and you need to treat a low, that overhead bin will be as out of reach as if it was on the other side of the ocean.

Adjusting your doses between time zones

Travelling between time zones seldom causes big problems with blood glucose control or insulin dosing, especially if you're on basal-bolus therapy (we define this earlier in this section), but following a few simple steps will help ensure things go smoothly:

✔ **Bolus insulin:** Take it at your new mealtimes, regardless of when they happen to be.

✔ **Basal insulin:**

- If you use Lantus or Levemir, take it at the same time in your new location as you did back home. For example, if you live in Vancouver and usually take, say, Lantus insulin at 8 p.m. *PST* and you then travel to Montreal — which has a three-hour time difference — you would take your Lantus insulin at 11 p.m. *EST* (which is still 8 p.m. PST).

- If you use NPH insulin at bedtime, take it at your new bedtime.

- If you use premixed insulin before breakfast and before dinner, take your insulin at your new before-breakfast and before-dinner times.

If on your travel day you anticipate a significant delay between meals, take a snack and a small amount of your rapid-acting or regular insulin halfway between those meals.

If your travels will take you beyond more than a few time zones, or if you will be staying in the new time zone for more than a few days, we recommend that you be in touch with your diabetes educator before you travel to get advice specific to your situation. Bon voyage!

Part IV
Particular Patients and Special Circumstances

The 5th Wave   By Rich Tennant

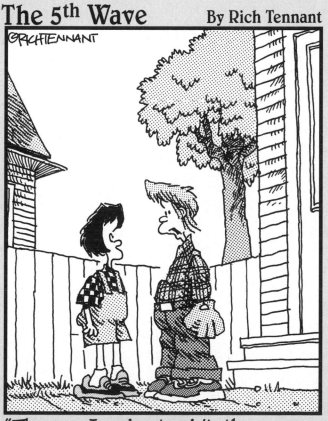

"The way I understand it, the reason I was getting cold and tired was because my body wasn't making enough insulation."

In this part . . .

We look at the unique challenges that diabetes poses to children, the elderly, and Canada's Aboriginal peoples. We also look at some very practical issues that confront people with diabetes, including employment, insurance, and driving. We also discuss taking precautions to ensure you are prepared to manage your diabetes as best you can in the event of a disaster.

Chapter 14

Your Child Has Diabetes

Children with diabetes present special issues that adults with diabetes don't have. Not only are they physically growing and developing, but they also are dealing with new social issues and trying to figure out their place in the world. Diabetes takes the challenges of growing up and makes them even more challenging.

When a child has diabetes, it's a concern. When *your* child has diabetes, you may see it as a disaster. If your child has diabetes, in a sense your whole family has diabetes; or at the very least your whole family has to deal with it. If something affects those with whom you share common interests (or, in your case, love), what affects them affects you, too.

In this chapter we look at how you can keep your child healthy and prevent diabetes from ruling his or her life, and yours. You find out how to manage diabetes in your child at each stage of growth and development, from infancy up to and including early adulthood. And as we look at these issues, remember that you're not to blame for your child's diabetes. You didn't cause it. And your child didn't cause it either. So neither of you should ever feel guilty about it.

Your Baby or Toddler Has Type 1 Diabetes

Having a young child with type 1 diabetes adds complexity and challenges to parenthood, but you can be assured that you won't have to make the journey alone. Indeed, you will have abundant support from a dedicated health care team working with you to help you and your child along the way.

Diagnosing type 1 diabetes in a baby or toddler

Although type 1 diabetes doesn't usually show up in babies, it can. The first evidence that your baby is developing diabetes will typically be repeatedly soaked diapers (as your baby will be passing urine in greater quantities and more often than usual), accompanied by — or shortly followed by — weight loss, vomiting, diarrhea, and lethargy. Because diseases unrelated to diabetes can also cause these symptoms, a doctor could initially diagnose your child with some other condition, such as gastroenteritis. By the time the diabetes is diagnosed, your child may be very ill.

Diagnosing diabetes in a toddler may be just as difficult as diagnosing it in a baby. The first signs are typically extreme thirst and frequent urination. Attempts at toilet training fail as bedwetting becomes an increasing problem. (Bedwetting happens because the child cannot control his constantly filling bladder.) Your child will also develop fatigue, irritability, and weight loss. Other symptoms can include vomiting and abdominal pain.

Blood glucose targets for your baby or toddler with type 1 diabetes

Blood glucose targets for a baby or toddler are higher than are the targets for older children and adults. Fortunately, keeping blood glucose readings within these higher targets in a very young child is highly *un*likely to lead to later diabetes complications.

For children 5 years of age and less, the Canadian Diabetes Association's recommended target before-meal readings are 6.0 to 10.0 mmol/L and the target A1C is up to 8.0 percent. (A target A1C of up to 8.5 percent is acceptable if this higher target is required in order to keep your child from experiencing hypoglycemia.)

Although blood glucose targets are higher in a very young child (compared to older children or adults), it is still very important to avoid blood glucose levels that are overly high. *Hyper*glycemia (high blood glucose) can lead to dehydration. A baby is fragile, and even losing small amounts of water can make your baby very sick, very quickly. It is also very important to avoid severe *hypo*glycemia (low blood glucose). Severe hypoglycemia — especially if happening repeatedly — can damage a young child's developing brain.

Managing your baby or toddler's type 1 diabetes

With the help and support of your child's physician and the diabetes educators, you will learn:

- ✔ **How to identify symptoms of hyperglycemia, hypoglycemia, and ketoacidosis** (Refer to Chapter 5.)

- ✔ **How to administer and adjust insulin doses** (Refer to Chapter 13; also see the tip later in this section.)

- ✔ **How to measure the blood glucose and ketones** (Refer to Chapter 9.)

- ✔ **How to treat hypoglycemia, and how and when to use glucagon** (In Chapter 5 we discuss the use of glucagon to treat *severe* hypoglycemia. In the tip that follows this list we discuss so-called "mini-dose" glucagon.)

- ✔ **How to nourish your child properly** (In Chapter 10 we talk about general nutrition principles, but of course with a child this young you'll need to get very detailed advice from a dietitian.)

- ✔ **What to do when your child is sick with another illness** (See "Sick Day Solutions for Your Child with Type 1 Diabetes," later in this chapter.)

Glucagon can be given in small amounts — *"mini-dose glucagon"* — to treat *mild* or *impending* hypoglycemia in a child who can't or won't ingest carbohydrates. The amount of the mini-dose depends on your child's body weight. Speak to your pediatrician or diabetes educator to find out the appropriate mini-dose for your child.

Because a child's eating habits may not be consistent, giving rapid-acting insulin (refer to Chapter 13) *after*, rather than *before*, meals may be helpful at times. First you can see how much of the meal your child ate and then give an amount of insulin based on that. Be sure to speak to your diabetes educators about this option.

Your responsibilities as the parent of a baby or toddler with diabetes are extensive and time-consuming, and the list above may seem (and is) rather daunting. But you can do it. Indeed, you must. Just remember that you don't have to do it alone. You will have your health care team working with you and, equally importantly, educate family members and friends who can help out, even for a short time. They will probably be happy to lend a hand. Without help, you may end up constantly emotionally and physically exhausted (as if being a parent isn't hard enough to begin with!).

Keeping in regular contact with a diabetes education centre is crucial if you have a child, especially an infant, with diabetes. A diabetes educator and dietitian can provide invaluable assistance. Also, these centres may allow you to access additional services such as that of a social worker. Not all diabetes education centres specialize in children with type 1 diabetes, so ask them if this is their particular area of expertise; if it isn't, they'll gladly refer you to a centre that has this expertise. You should also have a pediatrician with particular expertise in young children with diabetes. If you don't, your family physician or your diabetes educator can refer you to one.

Preschoolers are beginning the process of separating from their parents and typically want to do things by themselves. (Most parents are very familiar indeed with their child's "I can do it! I can do it!" refrain.) This separation process makes giving injections and testing blood glucose more challenging for you, the parent. You need to encourage your little one to participate as much as they can, but you must be in control. (Indeed, you *are* the boss.) Your child can help, for example, by getting the blood glucose testing supplies and pressing the button on the lancing device (refer to Chapter 9). The diabetes educator can guide you toward other age-appropriate ways your child can be involved in managing her diabetes.

If you have other children, they may feel jealous of the extra attention that you pay to their sibling with diabetes, or they may fear that they, too, will develop diabetes. These feelings could cause your other children to misbehave or act out. Remember to include them in the education, and, if possible, let them help when they can.

Your Primary School-Aged Child Has Type 1 Diabetes

When children go to school, they interact with other children and want to fit in. A child with diabetes may feel embarrassed and may be reluctant to tell other children that he has diabetes. Or your child may have told his friends, but they didn't know how to handle the information. This is where your newfound expertise with diabetes can be invaluable. You can educate your child's friends about diabetes, and maybe speak to their parents as well.

As time goes on, your child is going to separate from you further. He may insist on giving the insulin injections and doing the blood tests. Although you should encourage your child to be involved, do not let your child be fully responsible. You must always supervise your child to ensure that he is doing things properly.

Because your child may feel uncomfortable letting peers know about the diabetes, he may avoid testing glucose and giving insulin when friends are around. At this stage, too, fast food may replace some proper, healthy nutrition. Meet with the diabetes nurse educator and dietitian regularly so you and your child learn how to deal with these and other challenges.

Blood glucose targets for a primary school-aged child

For children ages 6 to 12, the CDA target before-meal blood glucose readings are 4.0 to 10.0 mmol/L and the target A1C is up to 7.5 percent. (A target A1C of up to 8.0 percent is acceptable if this higher target is required in order for your child to avoid hypoglycemia.) The higher end of this target range is suitable for a 6-year-old, but you should aim for the lower end the older your child gets.

Because your child requires insulin therapy, he or she will be at risk of hypoglycemia. There are a number of ways to reduce this risk, the strategy depending, in part, on what time the low blood glucose occurs.

These are ways you can reduce your child's risk of *overnight* hypoglycemia:

- ✔ Give your child a bedtime snack containing carbohydrate and protein. A snack made with cornstarch is particularly helpful. Because cornstarch breaks down slowly, it provides glucose over a longer period of time. Your child's dietitian can provide you with cornstarch-containing recipes. You can also find some tasty ones in the book *Food and Diabetes,* by Doreen Yasui and Doreen Hatton of the British Columbia Children's Hospital.

- ✔ Measure your child's blood glucose at bedtime and increase the amount of the bedtime snack if the glucose level is under target.

- ✔ Occasionally check your child's blood glucose at 3 a.m.

- ✔ Ask your child if she has symptoms such as nightmares, headaches, and unexplained sweating, which might be clues to nighttime low blood glucose.

These are ways you can reduce the risk of *daytime* hypoglycemia:

✔ Be sure your child doesn't skip meals or scheduled snacks.

✔ Have your child check his or her blood glucose before exercising and, if below target, take extra carbohydrate according to the planned duration and intensity of exercise.

✔ If your child tends not to finish meals, speak to your diabetes educator about occasionally using rapid-acting insulin *after* rather than *before* meals. (We discuss insulin therapy in Chapter 13.)

Mature siblings and, of course, parents should be aware of symptoms of hypoglycemia and know how to treat it, including knowing how and when to use glucagon. In Chapter 5 we discuss using glucagon to treat *severe* hypoglycemia. As we mention in the preceding section, glucagon can also be given in smaller amounts ("mini-dose glucagon") to treat *mild* or *impending* hypoglycemia in those who can't or won't ingest carbohydrates. The mini-dose to be given will depend on your child's body weight. Speak to your pediatrician or diabetes educator to find out the appropriate mini-dose for your child.

Meeting with primary school teachers and administrators

Seeing as your child spends so much time in school, this environment must be set up suitably. Schoolmates will likely not have much, if any, knowledge of diabetes (especially type 1 diabetes), and your child's teacher may have no or limited experience as well. We encourage you to meet with your child's teacher and the appropriate school administrators to review issues such as these:

✔ **When to monitor blood glucose and who can help your child with this task:** This discussion should also include where testing will take place and where (and how) to dispose of lancets.

✔ **Who will supervise the child with the task of giving insulin:** This applies whether the insulin is given by injection or via an insulin pump.

✔ **Who will supervise a younger child during meals and snacks:** No, not simply supervising to make sure that food fights don't break out! Rather, someone needs to make sure the youngster is actually ingesting the wonderful nutrients she has on her plate and in her cup.

✔ **How to recognize and treat hypoglycemia:** And, importantly, knowing when to call 9-1-1.

> ✔ **How to recognize hyperglycemia and what school staff should do if they suspect it is present:** Calling you — the parent — is an appropriate first step if your child is feeling perfectly well. But, if your child is at all unwell — especially if he is vomiting — the safest and best thing for the school to do is call an ambulance immediately.

> ✔ **Why your child must be allowed to have a water bottle and snacks at her desk:** Your child needs ready access both to water (to maintain hydration) and to snacks (to treat low blood glucose).

Your child can — and should — participate in any and all school activities, including academics, sports, and field trips. This will require additional expertise, however, on the part of school officials and chaperones. Again, you, the parent, can help out by teaching them what you have already learned.

The Canadian Diabetes Association, in order to "acknowledge and clarify the essential partnership among parents or caregivers, students and school personnel in the care of students with type 1 diabetes in the school system," has created the helpful and detailed *Standards of Care for Students with Type 1 Diabetes in Schools.* This document can be found online at `www.diabetes.ca/files/StandardsofCare.pdf`.

Your diabetes educator is an invaluable resource to help you familiarize your child's teacher and, most important, schoolmates about diabetes and how it affects your child. For example, Ian is blessed to work with wonderful diabetes educators at the Charles H. Best Diabetes Centre (`www.charleshbest.com`) who, in addition to their already myriad duties, have developed a school program in which they visit a child's school and give class presentations. It has been an overwhelming success. Ask your child's diabetes educator if they would consider doing the same. If they would like, have them call the Best Centre (905-620-0360) to learn more about the program.

Your Adolescent Has Type 1 Diabetes

Your adolescent with diabetes may provide some of your biggest challenges. (As if adolescence isn't tough enough — even with perfect health.)

An adolescent can have excellent blood glucose control, but it certainly isn't easy. To have excellent control means the teen must follow proper lifestyle therapy (nutrition and exercise) and pay regular attention to blood glucose monitoring and insulin adjustment. As you can imagine, most adolescents, eagerly seeking independence and freedom, are not thrilled with this. (And who could blame them?) Yet, for all of that, adolescence and the teenage years don't have to mean that diabetes gets neglected.

For children 13 years of age or over, the Canadian Diabetes Association recommends target blood glucose levels before-meals of 4.0 to 7.0 mmol/L, two-hour after-meal of 5.0 to 10.0, and an A1C 7 percent or less. (For adolescents who can achieve lower targets without undue hypoglycemia, the CDA recommends aiming for even lower blood glucose targets: before-meal blood glucose of 4.0 to 6.0, two-hour after-meal blood glucose of 5.0 to 8.0, and an A1C of 6 percent or less.)

The hormonal changes that occur in puberty can result in loss of blood glucose control; however, appropriate adjustments of insulin therapy can help to compensate. And speaking of hormonal changes, adolescent girls must be made aware of issues surrounding contraception. Unintended pregnancy in an adolescent is always a problem; unintended pregnancy in an adolescent with diabetes is even more of a problem. Appropriate members of the health care team should address these concerns. (We discuss diabetes and pregnancy in Chapter 7.)

You can help your adolescent with diabetes in many ways:

- ✔ Make sure that he knows you have certain expectations — expectations born of love and concern — in terms of his management of the diabetes.

- ✔ Be supportive and understanding — even when she goes through periods when she is less attentive to her diabetes than she should be. But make sure your teen knows that you're far from indifferent to that inattention. Encouragement often works better than nagging or lecturing (though, of course, these measures also have their occasional role, as any parent knows).

- ✔ Remind him that he need never be ashamed of diabetes. In its very essence, it is a simple hormone shortage. What shame is there in that?

- ✔ Keep an eye out to make sure your teen isn't missing insulin doses. Teenage girls sometimes skip insulin doses (with consequent hyperglycemia) because they have learned that it results in weight loss. Skipping insulin doses is dangerous and must be avoided.

- ✔ Review, in a non-judgmental way, your adolescent's blood glucose levels and assist with insulin adjustment. (And discuss with your child the option of you sharing responsibility for recording blood glucose results.)

- ✔ As your child grows, gradually transfer to him the responsibility for looking after the diabetes — based on your child's ability and interest. This may be the most important way you can help your child in the long term. (This is often the toughest task on this list.)

Up to 10 percent of teenage girls (and some teenage boys) with diabetes have an eating disorder, such as anorexia nervosa or bulimia. These disorders can result in malnutrition and, usually, poor blood glucose control. The teen may deny that the problem exists. If your adolescent has erratic glucose control, a high A1C, and/or seems to be focusing undue attention on weight, you should consider the possibility of an eating disorder and discuss it with your teen and your teen's doctor.

Sometimes, adolescents will share things with their diabetes educator that they may not readily share with you, even though they know you love them dearly and care about their health. Indeed, diabetes educators often say that children of this age spend their whole first visit talking about everything in their lives *except* the specifics of their diabetes. But that's okay. To help children with their diabetes, knowing them as people *first* and people with diabetes *second* is essential. Diabetes is, after all, but one component of their existence. A pediatric diabetes educator who knows "how the adolescent ticks" will be in a far better position to know how best to help with the diabetes.

Your Young Adult Child Has Type 1 Diabetes

By the time children reach their late teens, they are young adults and should be the ones in charge of their diabetes. But even then, your son or daughter still needs a support system.

Regrettably, what often happens is that teenagers "graduate" from a pediatric diabetes program (where they have started to feel very out of place as they sit amongst the younger — and smaller — children in the waiting room) and fail to hook up with an adult program or with an adult diabetes specialist. The single most important thing you can do to assist your young adult child with diabetes is to help ensure the appropriate transition of care. We discuss transition of care in the next section.

If your young adult child is heading off to post-secondary school and will have a roommate, your child should teach the roommate

- ✔ How to recognize if your child has hypoglycemia.

- ✔ How to help your child if he or she has hypoglycemia. This should include knowing where appropriate snacks are kept and how to give glucagon. If the roommate isn't comfortable giving glucagon, at the very least he or she should be reminded what situations require a call to 9-1-1.

- ✔ To be aware that, if your child has been drinking alcohol and is acting drunk, he or she may, in fact, be hypoglycemic, not inebriated. (Or, indeed, may be both inebriated *and* hypoglycemic.)

Transitioning Care: Moving from Pediatric to Adult Diabetes Specialist Care

As we discuss in the preceding section, a big problem for young adults with type 1 diabetes is that when they outgrow pediatric care, they fail to have their diabetes care transferred to adult diabetes specialists and educators. Sometimes this is because the young adult has moved away and doesn't seek out new health care providers. Sometimes it's because they are so busy with other things (school, work, relationships, and so forth) that finding a new physician, diabetes educator, and dietitian is simply not on the radar. And sometimes (fortunately less and less often) the pediatric diabetes team hasn't discussed (or arranged) transition of care with the person and it "simply didn't happen."

The problem with failed transition of care is that the young adult can take years to be re-engaged with diabetes health care providers. During this period of time, blood glucose control is often poor and, given sufficient time, diabetes complications may develop. Also, the young adult with diabetes will be missing out on being screened for (and treated for) diabetes complications.

Robert last saw his pediatrician, diabetes educator, and dietitian ten years ago, when, turning 18, he had "graduated" from pediatric care and moved out-of-town to attend university. For the next ten years he didn't see any health care provider. Now, at the age of 28 and newly engaged, his fiancée prompted him to see a family doctor who immediately referred him to Ian. Robert's fiancée attended the appointment with him. "I'm getting married in a couple of months," Robert announced with a broad smile, "and my fiancée wants me to look after myself better. She's worried about me. She twisted my arm to come." Ian remembers replying, "That's wonderful. It's great to have such a supportive person working with you. That is always a huge help." Unfortunately, Robert was found to have not only very poor blood glucose control (his A1C was a whopping 12 percent), but he also had evidence of early eye damage (retinopathy) and early kidney damage (microalbuminuria). Ian shared the disappointing news with Robert and his fiancée. They were devastated. But, Robert was highly motivated. By working with Ian and new diabetes educators, and with the support of his fiancée, Robert's blood glucose control quickly improved and his diabetes complications did not worsen.

Robert's scenario is all too common. With successful transition of care, he would have remained in contact with a diabetes health care team, would likely have had far better blood glucose control, and as a result may not have developed diabetes complications.

Here are ways you and your young adult child can help to ensure a smooth transition of care from the pediatrician and pediatric care diabetes educator and dietitian to their adult diabetes counterparts:

✔ A year or so before your child turns 18 (and therefore likely would have to leave the pediatric team's care), start discussing with the pediatric team what arrangements will be made for transitioning to adult care.

✔ If the pediatric team, as your child turns 18, hasn't yet made arrangements for transition of care, ask your child to ask them to make these arrangements. (Or, if your young adult child consents, ask on his behalf.) If the pediatric team is unable to arrange referral to an adult diabetes education team, your teen's family physician can make the arrangements.

✔ If your young adult child is moving to another city, her current pediatric team may be able to arrange for adult diabetes care in that other city. If your child has already moved away before any transition arrangements have been made, encourage your child to contact the local hospital to find out the names of adult diabetes specialists located in the region. Your child will likely require a referral to the specialist from another physician. If your child does not have a family physician, she can get a referral from a walk-in-clinic, emergency department physician, or any other physician.

It is not enough for young adults with type 1 diabetes to be referred to an adult diabetes program. Whenever possible, they should be referred to *a type 1 program*. The needs of adults living with type 1 diabetes are very different from the needs of adults with type 2 diabetes, and they need the help of a team that has expertise with type 1 diabetes. (Some communities — particularly small towns — may not have dedicated type 1 programs; in these situations the local diabetes health care providers, by virtue of necessity, likely have good knowledge about type 1 diabetes.)

If your child is away at college or university, but comes home often for Christmas, spring break, summer holidays, and the like, transitioning to adult diabetes health care in your home town may be a good option. Appointments with these providers can be scheduled for whenever your child is in town. In-between visits home, non-urgent needs can often be addressed by phone, e-mail, video conferencing, and so forth. (Ian has patients in colleges and universities in all sorts of places in Canada and the United States, and even overseas.)

One often overlooked, but very important aspect of successful transition of care is preparing the teenage child (and you, the parent, too!) for the differences between pediatric and adult diabetes care. These are important differences for your child and you to know:

✔ You may think of your child as your little one, but now that he's 18 years of age, he's legally an adult. He is not only free to make his own decisions, but the physician (and any other health care provider) is legally bound to honour his decisions.

✔ As your child is now an adult, the diabetes specialist will see her in private (unless your child specifically requests that a parent or some significant other remain in the room). This is often the first time your child has met in private with a doctor, and it may be stressful — especially for the parent.

When your adult child has her first appointment with the new diabetes specialist, she can ask the doctor if you can join them . . . preferably *after* the doctor has interviewed and examined your child. Difficult as this may be, joining them after the consultation is far better than being there during the consultation if your adult child is going to get the full assessment she needs and deserves. (Not many 18-year-olds are going to be fully open about smoking, alcohol, drug use, or sexual activity if their parent is in the room.)

✔ Your adult child will be expected to be the one in charge of booking appointments (and remembering to attend them!), going for lab tests, filling prescriptions, and so on.

✔ The doctor can no longer speak to you about your adult child's medical information without your child's expressed permission. That means no phone conversations or e-mail exchanges with you *unless* your child has specifically given the doctor permission to share information with you.

Sick Day Solutions for Your Child with Type 1 Diabetes

Children with type 1 diabetes are susceptible to all the usual childhood illnesses, but diabetes complicates their care.

An illness can affect glucose levels in opposite ways:

✔ *Blood glucose levels go up* when an infection is present. In this situation, higher doses (and extra injections) of insulin are required.

✔ *Blood glucose levels go down* if nausea and vomiting are present and foods and liquids aren't staying down. In this situation, lower doses of insulin are required.

Because a sick child's insulin requirements can go up *or* go down, when your child is ill you need to measure his blood glucose as often as every two to four hours. If his blood glucose level is elevated you also need to check his blood ketone level (refer to Chapter 9). If his blood glucose levels are significantly elevated (above 12.0 mmol/L or so), he may require additional rapid-acting insulin. If his blood glucose levels are in the lower range of normal, he will need smaller doses of insulin. Clearly no single "sick day solution" is available. The best solution depends on the specific situation you're facing.

If your sick child's blood glucose levels are elevated and ketones are present in the blood (0.6 mmol/L or higher) get your child to the nearest hospital emergency department immediately.

The fact your child isn't eating well doesn't necessarily mean that she requires less insulin; depending on the child's blood glucose levels, she may need *more* insulin than usual. Some of the sickest patients we've ever seen are those that became sick, had high blood glucose levels, and needed more insulin. But because they weren't eating well, the patient (or, in the case of children, their caregivers) mistakenly assumed that — despite the elevated blood glucose — because they were not eating well, they needed less insulin.

A key element of diabetes education is teaching you, the parent, what to do if your child becomes unwell. The diabetes educators will spend considerable time making sure you know how to keep your sick child safe. *Never* feel that you are left to your own devices to manage your sick child's diabetes. Indeed, trying to manage things on your own is unsafe! When your child is ill, the pediatrician, diabetes educator, and, if necessary, the nearest emergency department are there to help you.

Screening Tests for Organ Injury in Children and Adolescents with Type 1 Diabetes

The Canadian Diabetes Association recommends the following testing schedule for children with type 1 diabetes (refer to Chapter 6 for a detailed discussion on organ injury, how to prevent it, and how to test for it):

- **Blood pressure:** Your child's blood pressure should be checked at least twice per year.

- **Eye testing:** At the age of 15 (then at least annually), your child should have an eye examination by an expert eye professional if your child has had diabetes for at least five years. (Sometimes the frequency of screening can be changed to every two years, depending on your child's particular circumstances, such as blood glucose control and eye health.)

✔ **Kidney testing:** At the age of 12 (then annually), a urine sample should be tested for albumin/creatinine ratio (ACR) if your child has had diabetes for more than five years.

✔ **Lipid testing:** If your child is less than 12 years of age, lipid testing (including cholesterol and triglycerides) is required only if some additional risk factor (such as obesity) for cardiovascular disease is present. At 12 years of age, her lipids should be tested, then retested five years later (earlier than that if necessary).

✔ **Nerve testing:** At the onset of puberty (then annually), your child should have his feet tested (by using, for example, a thin nylon rod as we describe in Chapter 6) if he has had diabetes for more than five years. These painless tests can be done in the doctor's office and take but a moment to perform.

✔ **Thyroid testing:** Because the risk of thyroid disease is higher with type 1 diabetes, your child's thyroid function should be tested (by measuring, on a blood sample taken at a laboratory, the child's TSH level and thyroid peroxidase antibody) at the time of diabetes diagnosis, then at least every two years thereafter.

Because the risk of celiac disease is higher with type 1 diabetes, your child should be tested (with a blood test at a laboratory) if he or she *has symptoms* of celiac disease. Whether to test a child with type 1 diabetes who does *not* have symptoms of celiac disease is controversial. We discuss celiac disease in Chapter 6.

Summer Camps for Children with Type 1 Diabetes

One resource that can be tremendously valuable for you and your child with type 1 diabetes is a diabetes summer camp. Run by the Canadian Diabetes Association (CDA), these "D-Camps" ("D" for diabetes, naturally) are located in a number of regions across Canada and provide a safe, well-managed — and fun! — place where your child with diabetes can go and be in the majority. (This is likely the only time your child with diabetes will be in a place where having diabetes puts them in the majority.) He or she can learn a great deal about diabetes while enjoying all the pleasures of a summer camp environment. (Certainly not a minor benefit is the opportunity for you to have time off — for perhaps the first time in years.) You can find more info about the CDA D-Camps at www.dcamps.ca.

CDA camps offer assistance with camp fees. Contact the camp nearest you for more information.

Of course, you may instead be looking at sending your child to a regular day camp program. This is perfectly reasonable, but some advance planning is important. In particular, consider doing the following:

✔ Speak to the camp director to make sure the camp can safely accommodate your child.

✔ Find out if the camp has a nurse on site.

✔ Arrange for your child to have a mature counsellor.

✔ Meet with the counsellor before the start of camp to make sure he or she has the necessary knowledge to look after your child. In particular, talk about how to deal with blood glucose testing, how to prepare for extra activity, how to tell if your child may be experiencing hypoglycemia and, especially, how to treat hypoglycemia including how and when to use a glucagon kit.

✔ Make sure that your child will receive the necessary snacks (and, of course, meals) at the appropriate times.

✔ Send a kit of important supplies with your child to camp. The kit should include blood glucose monitoring equipment, snacks, a glucagon kit, and, if your child will need to give insulin during the day, necessary insulin supplies.

✔ Make sure other staff — such as swim instructors and lifeguards — know that your child has diabetes.

✔ Find out if the camp has had other children in the past — or currently — with diabetes. If so, consider speaking to their parents to find out if things went well or, if not, why not.

✔ Ensure that your child wears a medical alert bracelet.

Your diabetes educator may have experience with regular day camps that have looked after children with diabetes. Give your educator a call and ask.

Your Child Has Type 2 Diabetes

The epidemic of obesity has led to a higher prevalence of type 2 diabetes in children than has ever been seen before. Indeed, depending on the community, up to 25 percent (or, in some communities, even more) of children with diabetes have type 2 diabetes. This was virtually unheard of until recently.

The Canadian Diabetes Association recommends screening children for type 2 diabetes with a fasting blood glucose level drawn at a lab if they are at increased risk of type 2 diabetes. (In some circumstances a glucose tolerance test is ordered instead of a fasting blood glucose.) Specifically, the CDA recommends screening for type 2 diabetes every two years in children with *any* of the following:

- Three or more of the following risk factors in children who have *not* yet reached puberty (two or more of the following risk factors in children who *have* reached puberty):

  - They are obese. (Obesity for a child is defined as having a body mass index — BMI — at or above the 95th percentile for the child's age and gender. You can find a pediatric BMI calculator by searching online.)

  - They are a member of a high-risk population group (that is; being of Aboriginal, African, Asian, Hispanic, or South Asian ancestry).

  - They have a family history of type 2 diabetes and/or were exposed to diabetes while they were inside the mother's uterus (that is, the mom had diabetes while pregnant with the child).

  - They have evidence of insulin resistance (refer to Chapter 3), such as having acanthosis nigricans, high blood pressure, abnormal lipids, polycystic ovary syndrome, or excess fat in the liver (NAFLD or non-alcoholic fatty liver disease). (We discuss these conditions in Chapter 6.)

- They have prediabetes (refer to Chapter 4).

- They take certain types of medicines ("atypical antipsychotics") used to treat psychiatric disease.

Like children with type 1 diabetes, those with type 2 diabetes may be afraid of being stigmatized and may neglect healthy living practices to "be like everyone else" when it comes to eating (junk food), watching (too much) television, and so forth.

The CDA target A1C (refer to Chapter 9) for most children with type 2 diabetes is 7.0 percent or less. The first therapy for a child with type 2 diabetes is intensive lifestyle measures (diet, weight control, exercise), but pills (typically metformin, but glimepiride may be used instead; refer to Chapter 12) and insulin (Chapter 13) may be necessary. The metformin or insulin may be withdrawn after the benefits of lifestyle measures have taken effect.

You must help your obese child to lose weight or, at the very least, to not gain further inappropriate weight. Contact a dietitian to figure out the food that your child can eat to grow and develop without inappropriate weight gain. One of the most helpful techniques is to take the child into the super-market and point out the difference between unhealthy foods (such as those rich in fat) and those that are nourishing. Another is never to use foods such as cake and candy as rewards. Finally, if you keep problem foods out of the house, your child is much less likely to eat them.

If your child with type 2 diabetes becomes unwell, you need to be sure that he or she is drinking enough liquids. Clear liquids (like caffeine-free teas and soft drinks) are usually best. As long as your child can hold down clear liquids, you can generally continue to take care of your child at home. However, if your child's blood glucose level is particularly high or your child is very unwell, seek medical attention. If your child can't keep down even clear fluids, dehydration becomes a real concern and you should take your child to the hospital.

Your Child Has MODY

An unusual type of childhood diabetes goes by the name *MODY,* which stands for *maturity onset diabetes of the young.* This is a genetic condition leading to diabetes that has some features of type 1 diabetes and some features of type 2 diabetes. For example, affected children aren't obese on the one hand (as they would be if they had type 2 diabetes), yet aren't prone to ketoacidosis on the other (as they would be if they had type 1 diabetes). MODY exists in several forms, and the treatment depends on which type is present.

Although the term *MODY* remains in common use, it is being phased out and replaced by the names of the specific genetic defects in the various types (for example, *Chromosome 20, HNF-4alpha* is the new name for *MODY1*). *MODY* may be not be as scientifically precise, but it sure is a heck of a lot easier to say (and remember)!

Chapter 15

Diabetes in Special Groups: The Elderly and Aboriginal Populations

Although everyone living with diabetes faces some of the same challenges such as keeping one's blood glucose in control, certain populations face their own unique hurdles. In Chapter 7 we look at diabetes in pregnancy and in Chapter 14 we discuss diabetes in children. In this chapter we address diabetes in two other special populations: the elderly and Aboriginal populations.

Diabetes and the Elderly

Everyone wants to live a long time, but no one wants to get old. Nevertheless, as someone once said, getting old is better than the alternative! Woody Allen says the one advantage of dying is that you don't have to do jury duty. We think we'd rather do jury duty.

Defining *elderly* is the first problem. Although some medical studies have defined elderly as being as young as 60 (egads!), and although every year the definition seems to change, it's probably fair to say that about the age of 70 is the beginning of elderly. Using that definition, more than 20 percent of the Canadian population will be elderly by the year 2020. And one-fifth or more of that group will have developed diabetes.

Elderly people with diabetes are hospitalized 70 percent more often than the general elderly population. Even without hospitalization, elderly people with diabetes have special problems. In this chapter, we look at those problems and the best ways to handle them.

Recognizing that every person — including every elderly person — is unique, the Canadian Diabetes Association recommends that "otherwise healthy elderly people with diabetes should be treated to achieve the same (blood glucose), blood pressure and lipid targets as younger people with diabetes." On the other hand, if you are elderly *and* have poor health or limited life expectancy, such stringent targets would be inappropriate.

Bring a second set of ears with you when you see the doctor, pharmacist, diabetes educator, or, for that matter, any other member of your health care team. Diabetes and its management are complex, and having someone else listen in on the conversation will provide you with an additional resource later on.

Diagnosing diabetes in the elderly

Like so much else in the world of medicine, debate and uncertainty abound over why developing diabetes becomes increasingly likely as we get older. Some experts have suggested that aging itself leads to diabetes, but the main factor that causes diabetes may not be the number of years people have under their belts but rather the number of inches under their belts. That, of course, is a very encouraging piece of news because it means that if you can keep your weight under control as you get older, you can help to protect yourself from developing diabetes.

Depending on their mental functioning, elderly people who have developed high blood glucose may or may not recognize the onset of typical symptoms such as increased urination and greater thirst. Instead, their main symptoms may be loss of appetite, weight loss, confusion, urinary incontinence, or weakness and lethargy. Because symptoms like weakness and lethargy are so non-specific, the cause can initially go unrecognized. And a doctor or patient may easily (and understandably) attribute urinary incontinence to prostate problems in elderly men or bladder problems in older women.

If you have an elderly relative who is, for no apparent reason, fatigued, suffering from malaise, losing weight, or just has "the dwindles," neither your relative nor yourself should just chalk this up "to old age." Specific causes — including diabetes — need to be sought out. Ask your relative to go to the doctor for a diabetes test. Or, if necessary, go to the doctor's appointment with your relative and ask the doctor on their behalf. (Of course, all this also applies to *you* if it is you so-affected.)

Evaluating intellectual functioning

Knowing the intellectual functioning of an elderly individual with diabetes is extremely important because managing the disease requires a number of different skills. The person has to follow a special diet, administer medications properly, and test the blood glucose, for example. Studies have shown that elderly people with diabetes, for uncertain reasons, have a higher incidence of *dementia* (loss of mental functioning) than people without diabetes. If a person with diabetes also has dementia, performing these tasks is much more difficult for them.

If necessary, a physician can formally assess an elderly person's mental functioning by administering certain types of tests. When required, psychologists can conduct even more sophisticated testing. Testing helps with knowing whether the patient can be self-sufficient or will need help. Some people now living alone with no assistance are a danger to themselves and would benefit from an assisted-living situation. Elderly people are often fiercely independent and — as millions of members of the "sandwich" generation know — changing their living situation can be very difficult.

Dealing with eye problems

Elderly people with diabetes are more prone to eye problems that people without diabetes can also get, including cataracts, macular degeneration, and glaucoma. And they also are at risk of eye disease unique to diabetes: diabetic retinopathy. (See Chapter 6 for more information on these eye problems.)

Many elderly people don't receive the eye care they require. Everyone with diabetes — especially the elderly, who can have a whole variety of different eye problems — must see an eye specialist routinely. Removal of a cataract — a simple outpatient procedure nowadays — may make all the difference in the world.

Coping with urinary and sexual problems

Urinary and sexual problems are very common in elderly people with diabetes and greatly affect quality of life. An older person with diabetes may have weakness of the bladder muscle leading to retention of urine, followed by overflow incontinence when the bladder fills up. An older person may be unable to get to the bathroom fast enough. A chronically distended bladder can also lead to frequent urinary tract infections.

Almost 60 percent of men over the age of 70 have erectile dysfunction, and 50 percent have no *libido* (desire to have sex). The elderly take an average of seven medications daily, some of which may affect sexual function. Many elderly women with diabetes also experience sexual dysfunction. We discuss the causes for sexual dysfunction in men and women in Chapter 6.

To have sex at any age, you need sexual desire and the physical ability to perform, you need a willing partner, and you need a safe, private place. For the elderly, any or all of these may be missing.

Treating sexual dysfunction isn't always necessary if you and your partner are okay with the situation as it is. If not, however, a number of effective therapies are available (refer to Chapter 6).

Regrettably, elderly people are sometimes seen as asexual — even by members of the medical profession who should know better. For this reason you may have to take the initiative and bring up the issue of your sexual difficulties when you visit your physician.

Monitoring foot problems

If you have peripheral neuropathy and/or impaired blood supply to your feet due to hardening of the arteries (*peripheral arterial disease*) you are at high risk of diabetes foot complications including foot ulcers, gangrene, and even amputations. Therefore, you need to take extra precautions to protect your feet.

It is essential that you check your feet daily. Look for areas of skin breakdown, blackened discolouration (especially of the toes), or open sores. If you cannot see your feet well enough to check them, ask a close friend or relative to check for you. If that isn't feasible (or even if it is), speak to your family physician about having a foot care professional (podiatrist, chiropodist, or foot care nurse) keep regular tabs on your feet including cutting your toenails for you.

If ever you find even the slightest evidence to suggest you may have a foot infection seek immediate medical attention. Foot infections in a person with diabetes — especially an elderly person with diabetes and peripheral arterial disease — can progress very rapidly, so time is of the essence.

Refer to Chapter 6 for more information on preventing and treating foot problems.

Considering treatment for high blood glucose

Goals for a very elderly, debilitated person with diabetes and a short life expectancy are different from those for a person with diabetes who is elderly but physiologically strong and could live for 15 or 20 more years. A 65-year-old person has a life expectancy of at least 18 more years — plenty of time to develop complications of diabetes.

In a broad sense, blood glucose control in an elderly person has two possible main objectives depending on your particular situation:

- **For a frail elderly person:** In this situation any undue restrictions are inappropriate and, indeed, perhaps even cruel, so the goal is to maintain blood glucose levels in a range that will prevent symptoms and minimize the risk of hypoglycemia. The goal for before-meal blood glucose levels is 5.0 to 12.0 mmol/L; the goal for A1C is up to 8.5 percent.

- **An elderly person who is generally healthy and has a good life expectancy:** In this situation the goal is to keep blood glucose levels in a range that will minimize the risk of developing complications. The goal for before-meal blood glucose levels is 4.0 to 7.0 mmol/L, and two hours after meals is it 5.0 to 10.0 mmol/L; the goal for A1C is 7.0 percent or less. (Refer to Chapter 9.)

Every elderly person with diabetes can treat his or her blood glucose control successfully (even if not easily).

Avoiding hypoglycemia is especially important in the elderly (particularly the frail elderly) and takes precedence over almost any other aspect of blood glucose control. If you (or your loved one with diabetes) are experiencing episodes of hypoglycemia, be sure to contact your physician to have your therapy adjusted.

Nutrition therapy

Healthy nutrition is a cornerstone of good diabetes care for the elderly, just as it is in the younger population.

In addition to the intellectual function required to understand and prepare proper meals, the elderly may have other problems eating healthfully:

- They may have poor vision and be unable to see to read or cook.

- Their ability to taste and smell may be decreased, so they may lose interest in food.

- ✔ They often have a loss of appetite, especially if they live alone after the loss of a spouse or if they're depressed.
- ✔ They may have arthritis that makes cooking more difficult.
- ✔ They may have poor teeth or a dry mouth, either of which make eating more difficult.
- ✔ They may have low income and be unable to afford the healthful foods they require.

Any one of these problems may be enough to prevent proper eating, and as a result, nutrition and, ultimately, the general health of an elderly person are at risk.

As we say throughout this book, even when obstacles to good diabetes management are present, they're never insurmountable. If you're facing some of the hurdles in the previous list and are unsure how to deal with them, we recommend you visit with the dietitian.

One of Ian's pet peeves is that far too many elderly, frail individuals with diabetes are maintained on highly restrictive diets. Especially when a person may not have many years of life ahead, this is simply unnecessary and unfair. If you (or your loved one) are in this situation, speak to your nutritionist (or, if you don't have one, your physician who can refer you to one) and have your diet liberalized. Your diabetes therapy can be adjusted in other ways to deal with any worsening of your blood glucose control that might then arise.

Because elderly individuals don't always get complete nutrition from food, unless you're sure you're eating very well (refer to Chapter 10), taking a daily multivitamin would be a good idea.

Exercise therapy

An elderly person who can exercise will derive many benefits from it, including improved blood glucose control, better blood pressure and lipids, and, importantly, a better sense of well-being. Because elderly people have more coronary artery disease, arthritis, eye disease, neuropathy, and peripheral arterial disease, exercise may need to be very limited or is sometimes not possible. Nonetheless, even if an elderly person can't walk at all, the person may still be able to do resistance exercises while sitting in a chair. (Refer to Chapter 11 for more on exercise.)

Because elderly people are more likely to have other health issues, and in particular, heart problems (which may not be diagnosed), speak to your physician before starting a new exercise program to determine that it's safe for you.

Medication therapy

If lifestyle therapy with diet and exercise isn't controlling blood glucose levels, then medications to lower blood glucose become necessary. (We discuss non-insulin antihyperglycemic medications in Chapter 12 and insulin therapy in Chapter 13.) Elderly people often have many specific considerations that make taking these medications more complicated:

- The person may not be able to read the prescription label or dose to be dialed up on an insulin pen device.

- The person may have difficulties thinking and be unable to take the medicine properly.

- The person may have physical limitations that prevent taking medication, especially insulin.

- Older people often have decreased kidney function, making some drugs last longer or build up to excessive levels.

- The person may have poor nutrition and be more prone to hypoglycemia.

For all these reasons, your physician must take great care in selecting the appropriate types and doses of your medicines. Also, your pharmacist will need to spend the extra time required to sit down with you and review your medications and how to take them.

When selecting the best medicine to reduce blood glucose levels for an elderly person, a variety of choices exist:

- **Metformin:** For most people with type 2 diabetes — including elderly individuals — metformin is a good choice unless you have poor kidney function (as determined by a blood test). Metformin does not cause hypoglycemia, which makes it particularly well suited to people at risk for this. We discuss metformin and the other medicines in this list in Chapter 12.

- **Sulfonylureas:** These medications need to be used cautiously as they can cause hypoglycemia. If a physician prescribes a sulfonylurea, you should start with a low dose and slowly increase it. The preferred sulfonylureas are gliclazide and glimepiride — rather than glyburide — because they are less likely to cause low blood glucose.

- **Actos (pioglitazone):** A member of the TZD drug family, this medication can be helpful, but, because it can cause heart failure in susceptible individuals, it needs to be used cautiously and only if you have normal heart function. Also, TZD medication increases the risk of certain types of bone fractures in women.

✔ **GlucoNorm (repaglinide):** If you have irregular eating habits, this is a good medication choice because you only take it when you're eating a meal and, compared to some other diabetes medications, it is less likely to cause hypoglycemia.

✔ **DPP-4 inhibitors:** These medications can be a good choice because they're safe, very well tolerated (side effects are rare), and do not cause hypoglycemia. A GLP-1 analogue can also be used.

✔ **Insulin:** If insulin is used, although the same basic principles apply to the elderly as they do to younger individuals, Levemir or Lantus insulin are generally preferred over NPH because they're less likely to cause hypoglycemia.

A seven-day pill dispenser (organizer) is an invaluable tool for people who are taking a number of different medicines. We recommend you ask your pharmacist to prepare your medicines for you in these containers. Ian and Dr. Heather McDonald-Blumer discuss this and other related topics regarding safe and effective use of medications in *Understanding Prescription Drugs For Canadians For Dummies* (Wiley).

Before you leave the doctor's office or pharmacy, discuss your medicines with your doctor (and your pharmacist) and, in particular, determine what side effects might occur.

Diabetes and Aboriginal Peoples

Aboriginal peoples in Canada include First Nations, Inuit, and Métis populations. Although type 2 diabetes has become increasingly prevalent in all communities across Canada, the problem has reached truly epidemic proportions among Aboriginal peoples. The reasons for this high rate aren't known for certain, but lifestyle changes (including increased calorie consumption, reduced exercise, and increased levels of overweight and obesity — including among Aboriginal children) are likely at least partly responsible, as are genetic factors.

Considering the extent of the problem

An estimated 12 percent of First Nations peoples living on reserves have diabetes, and 25 percent of those over the age of 45 are affected. These rates are far above those of the Canadian population as a whole (which has an average rate of 7.5 percent or so), and it is thought that the prevalence is going to increase further.

Aboriginal children and adolescents are affected by type 2 diabetes at much higher rates than their non-Aboriginal counterparts. Also, Aboriginal women are more than twice as likely as non-Aboriginal women to develop gestational diabetes (refer to Chapter 7).

Inuit people actually have prevalence rates that are below average for the Canadian population, though even in this group, the number of people with diabetes is increasing.

Not only are diabetes prevalence rates high, but evidence suggests that Aboriginal people with diabetes have an increased risk (compared to non-Aboriginal people with diabetes) of certain diabetes complications such as coronary artery disease, high blood pressure, retinopathy, and kidney damage. (We discuss these complications in Chapter 6.) Also, compared with non-Aboriginal communities, in Aboriginal communities the diagnosis of diabetes is more likely to be delayed, diabetes education services may be less readily available, and important health care services such as dialysis may be less accessible. (In some cases people may need to travel long distances to receive appropriate treatment, or even move their entire family.)

Screening for diabetes for Aboriginal peoples

Because of the high prevalence and early onset of diabetes in Aboriginal peoples, the Canadian Diabetes Association (CDA) recommends early and frequent diabetes screening if one or more additional risk factors (refer to Chapter 4 for a discussion of diabetes risk factors) are present. In this circumstance, the CDA recommends the following screening schedule:

- **For adults:** Every one to two years.
- **For children:** Every two years beginning at the age of 10 or puberty.

Looking at how Aboriginal peoples are combatting the problem

Having recognized the extent and severity of the problem, Aboriginal communities are now tackling the problem on a number of fronts. Here are some initiatives taking place in some regions:

- Teaching diabetes prevention strategies in elementary schools
- Organizing field trips to the local grocery store to teach about food selection

✔ Introducing programs to increase physical fitness

✔ Establishing health services programs geared specifically toward Aboriginal health issues and concerns

✔ Banning junk food from schools

✔ Getting local stores to promote healthy foods over snack foods

Clearly, non-Aboriginal communities would be well served by following the lead set by these Aboriginal communities and adopting similar healthy-living strategies.

Aboriginal people living in larger urban areas can contact the National Association of Friendship Centres (www.nafc.ca), which can provide helpful advice regarding available treatment resources.

Chapter 16

Special Circumstances: Employment, Insurance, Safe Driving, and Preparing for Disaster

....

In This Chapter

▶ Dealing with the workplace

▶ Discovering insurance options

▶ Driving safely

▶ Being ready in case disaster strikes

....

*I*f you have diabetes you can do almost anything, including almost any type of work. Airline pilot? Check. Justice of the Supreme Court? Check. Race-car driver? Check. Mechanic, teacher, bus driver, lawyer? Check, check, check, and check! You name it, and you can almost certainly do it (assuming you have the requisite skills of course). Ensuring your employer knows it too, however, can sometimes be a challenge. In this chapter we look at these and other issues surrounding employment for people living with diabetes. We also look at important issues concerning diabetes and driving, insurance, and how you can prepare yourself for when a disaster — natural or otherwise — strikes.

Employing Both You and Your Rights

Although it happens less and less, as a person with diabetes you may run into discrimination when you try to get a job. It can happen for a number of reasons, all with little-to-no justification. Part of it relates to prospective employers having worries about safety when a person with diabetes works for them. They may also have concerns that you will have needs that interfere with your ability to perform your job or that you will require the workplace to be modified in cumbersome or inconvenient ways. Like virtually all aspects of discrimination, discrimination against people with diabetes is based on ignorance.

Fighting for your rights

Canadians with diabetes have protections that citizens of other countries often do not. Section 15.1 of the Canadian Charter of Rights and Freedoms states:

> *Every individual is equal before and under the law and has the right to the equal protection and equal benefit of the law without discrimination and, in particular, without discrimination based on race, national or ethnic origin, colour, religion, sex, age or mental or physical disability.*

Although considering diabetes as a disability isn't appealing, this designation does give you certain legal protections under the Charter.

Ian recalls chatting with the mother of a 10-year-old boy with type 1 diabetes. An active, outgoing, athletic, and bright child, he had just read in a newspaper story that diabetes was a disability. He brought the article over to his mother and asked, "Mom, what's a disability?" His mother was speechless. Looking at her "I can do anything" child, she could only smile in wonder. (Which reminds Ian of the story a colleague shared: One of his young patients e-mailed his mother after getting hired for his first-ever job: "Dear Mom, I'm working, even though my pancreas isn't.")

Other groups and organizations actively campaign for your rights, including the Canadian Medical Association, which has an official policy position that "previous blanket discrimination in the workplace . . . should now be replaced with a case-by-case review."

The Canadian Diabetes Association's position statement advises that

- ✔ A person with diabetes should be eligible for employment in any occupation for which he or she is individually qualified.

- ✔ A person with diabetes has the right to be assessed for specific job duties on his or her own merits based on reasonable standards applied consistently.

- ✔ Employers have the duty to accommodate employees with diabetes unless the employer can show it to cause undue hardship to the organization.

Employers cannot say that *any* cost they incur is an "undue hardship." This provision is not meant to be used as an excuse to avoid hiring people with diabetes. As you know, most people with diabetes — likely including yourself — don't need particularly special treatment from their employers. Usually all that's necessary is a few extra minutes per day to test blood glucose and take medication, as well as appropriate breaks for snacks and meals.

When you're going for a job interview, you don't have to inform your prospective employer that you have diabetes, or, for that matter, tell the employer anything else about your health unless the health issues are directly related to a specific job requirement or you are applying for a "safety-sensitive" position, such as working as a police officer or firefighter (see the next section). As well, after you're hired, you don't need to provide medical information unless your employer needs it to accommodate your specific needs appropriately.

The Canadian Human Rights Commission document, *A Place for All: A Guide to Creating an Inclusive Workplace* (www.chrc-ccdp.ca/pdf/chrc_place_for_all.pdf), is designed to assist both employers and employees in understanding their legal rights and responsibilities in setting up an accommodating workplace.

Affecting your ability to work

In part because of the now-established rights that people with diabetes have achieved, virtually no organizations will issue an outright ban on hiring you just because you have diabetes. People with diabetes work just about anywhere and everywhere. And they function as effectively and efficiently as anybody else. Of course!

As we mention in the previous section, however, some (not many, mind you, but some) exceptions apply to your usual employment rights. If you're applying for a safety-sensitive position (such as firefighting or police work), the inherent unpredictability of these jobs may work against your being hired. Nonetheless, no blanket or uniform policy across Canada exists, and each fire department and police force determines its own hiring practices.

Ian has many police officers and paramedics among his patients. Having diabetes has not interfered with their ability to get hired or do their jobs. He also has a number of firefighters in his practice, however, they were generally diagnosed after they had been hired. Would they have been hired anyway? Impossible to know. Will diabetes potentially jeopardize these firefighters' jobs? That, too, is impossible to answer, although our personal observation is that a shift in job description is not unusual (for example, being moved to a supervisory role).

The following factors, among others, may influence your ability to get and keep a safety-sensitive job:

- ✔ The policies of a given force

- ✔ Any earlier precedents of the force

- ✔ The knowledge and comfort levels of the health staff and administrators regarding diabetes

- ✔ Your overall blood glucose control and tendency toward hypoglycemia (especially, severe hypoglycemia) and your general state of health

- ✔ Your ability to perform the required tasks

The last two items on this list seem far and away the most important to us. Each person is different. And that includes each person with diabetes.

If having hypoglycemia is, potentially, especially hazardous for your particular line of work, we strongly recommend you look at getting a continuous glucose monitoring system. We discuss continuous glucose monitoring in detail in Chapter 9.

The Canadian Forces have the wise policy of making decisions on a case-by-case basis, which is as it should be. Their general policy, however, is that

- ✔ If you already have diabetes when you apply for a position with the Canadian Forces, they're unlikely to hire you.

- ✔ If you develop type 2 diabetes after you're already enrolled, you'll likely be "retained without career restrictions."

- ✔ If you develop type 1 diabetes after you're already enrolled, you'll "normally be released" or you "may be accommodated for a three-year period, then released."

The most important point is that, with a few exceptions such as those we describe, you can do pretty much anything if you have diabetes. You can climb mountains — literally and figuratively. And as for employment, almost no jobs exist in Canada that you cannot both obtain and perform.

Exploring your avenues of recourse

If you feel you've been discriminated against because of your diabetes, regarding employment or prospective employment, you have several avenues of recourse:

- If discrimination occurs in federal jurisdiction, you can file a human rights complaint with the Canadian Human Rights Commission. Information on this is available on their website (www.chrc-ccdp.ca).

- If discrimination occurs outside of federal jurisdiction, you can file a complaint with the human rights commission in the appropriate province or territory.

- The Canadian Diabetes Association (CDA) has a National Advocacy Council, composed of both volunteers and staff, mandated primarily to "act on broad policy matters which can have a positive impact for many people affected by diabetes." The Council "offers advice and guidance," but in general is looking at the "big picture." So unless your concern has national implications, given their limited resources, they may not be able to take on your particular case. If you have a concern you want addressed, start by contacting your local CDA branch and go from there.

Sometimes the best way to change discrimination is by lifting the veil of ignorance and educating your employer. If you aren't successful at teaching your employer about diabetes, you may wish to share the CDA resource *Diabetes in the Workplace: A Guide for Employers and Employees* (www.diabetes.ca/about-us/what/position-statements/discrimination/workplace).

Insuring Your Health

This book is all about steps you can take to ensure your good health. As hard as that can seem at times, *in*suring your health can be even more difficult.

Thankfully, Canadians have a publicly funded, universal health care program, so fundamental health care is available to you regardless of your income. As for life, disability, and travel insurance, things get more difficult. The protections offered to you by human rights laws that we talk about earlier in this chapter don't apply in the same way for insurance policies. Indeed, when you're applying for insurance, you can expect to be asked if you have diabetes, and you must tell the truth; otherwise, any policy you are granted may be revoked and you will not be paid any insurance benefits.

The Canadian Diabetes Association has formed corporate partnerships to make getting insurance easier for you. You can find out more about diabetes-related insurance issues by visiting these two helpful pages on the CDA website:

- **Insurance guidelines:** www.diabetes.ca/diabetes-and-you/living/guidelines/insurance

- **Frequently asked questions:** www.diabetes.ca/get-involved/helping-you/advocacy/faq/insurance

Life insurance

Having diabetes does not automatically exclude you from obtaining life insurance, though it does make it more difficult. Of course, if you develop diabetes while you're already covered, you'll have an easier time than if you're applying for insurance (or an increase in your coverage) after you have been diagnosed (what insurance companies refer to as having a "pre-existing condition").

Insurance companies make their determination about your insurability on a case-by-case basis, meaning that they'll look at you as an individual and make their decision on more than the simple fact of your diabetes. They'll look at what kind of therapy you're receiving, what kind of glucose control you have, whether you have complications from your diabetes, and so forth.

If you are approved for a policy, you'll likely find that your premiums are higher, for the same level of benefits, than those of a person without diabetes.

If you look after your health well, you may live longer (and be healthier) than people without diabetes who don't look after themselves well. Hopefully, insurance companies will take this into account when they assess your insurability.

Bear in mind that different insurance companies have different policies (so to speak), so if one place turns you down, try somewhere else. Another thing you can do is to go through a licensed insurance broker who can act on your behalf, deal with multiple insurers, and try to help you obtain an appropriate policy.

Disability insurance

Unless you had disability insurance before you were diagnosed with diabetes, you will likely find it difficult (though not impossible) to find an insurance company that will offer you a policy. If you are otherwise in excellent health, your odds of successfully finding an insurer will be, as you might imagine, far greater.

Travel insurance

Travel insurance is much easier to obtain than disability insurance; however, you will need to carefully scrutinize any policy to see what is excluded from coverage. You may find that if you become ill with a diabetes-related condition, you won't be covered.

Driving When You Have Diabetes

Few adults in Canada get by without ever having to drive somewhere. (And of course, if you're a teenager, you have to drive *everywhere!*) We're so dependent on our cars to get us to work or the movies, grocery shopping or the hardware store, doctors' appointments or dentists' appointments, that for most people, losing their licence is not just inconvenient, it can be downright devastating. In this section we look at the measures you can take to help preserve your licence, and, if you have lost it, what steps you can take to regain it.

Determining if you're medically fit to drive

Most people who don't know better may assume that if you have diabetes you are at much higher risk of having a car accident. Of course, at one time, most people assumed the world was flat, too. The truth is that medical studies do not show convincing evidence that having diabetes increases your risk; in fact, one study even showed that people with type 1 diabetes had a lower risk than drivers without diabetes who were under the age of 30. How about that! Nonetheless, provincial and territorial bodies have the important and appropriate task of ensuring that drivers are safe to operate motor vehicles, so you may have to overcome a number of hurdles.

Your ability to obtain and retain a licence depends on a number of factors, including the way your diabetes is being treated. This section looks at those issues specific to your diabetes (of course, non-diabetes factors may also affect your fitness to drive). The recommendations in this section are based on those established by the Canadian Diabetes Association (www.diabetes. ca/diabetes-and-you/living/guidelines/commercial-driving). Note that these CDA recommendations are just that — recommendations — and not legally binding rules or regulations.

Taking necessary precautions

The CDA recommendations include the following for *all* drivers with diabetes:

- ✔ Have your fitness to drive assessed based on your personal situation (that is, the decision about your suitability to drive should be made on a case-by-case basis).
- ✔ Keep a log of your blood glucose results.
- ✔ Ensure that you are up-to-date on how to avoid hypoglycemia and how to treat it if it occurs.

- Measure your blood glucose level immediately before and at least every four hours during long drives. If you have hypoglycemia unawareness (refer to Chapter 5) you should test more often. (Ian recommends pulling into a rest stop and testing hourly during long drives, even though that may seem like quite a hassle. Trust us: Getting into an accident because of hypoglycemia is a much bigger hassle.)

- Always have your hypoglycemia treatment nearby. (The trunk of your car isn't nearby! We recommend you keep treatment *on your person* or, if that's not possible, *right beside you in easy reach*. Digging around in your purse while you're driving on the expressway isn't easy or safe. Nor is reaching over to the glove box.)

- Don't drive if your blood glucose level is less than 4.0 mmol/L. If your level is between 4.0 and 5.0 mmol/L, ingest some carbohydrate before you resume driving. (Admittedly erring on the side of caution, Ian recommends following the memorable dictum: "Don't drive if you're under five." Five in this case is 5.0 mmol/L.)

- Don't resume driving until at least 45 minutes have passed since you treated an episode of hypoglycemia.

Pull off the road and stop in a safe area if you think you may be hypoglycemic. Don't keep driving!

Applying for a commercial licence

As you might imagine, obtaining and maintaining a professional driver's licence is much trickier if you have diabetes, especially if you're taking insulin therapy. Nonetheless, your suitability to drive should be judged on a case-by-case basis, and indeed, licensing bodies increasingly recognize this, we're pleased to say.

When you first apply for a commercial licence, the appropriate governing body will review your request and base its decisions on many different factors. These factors include, importantly, your blood glucose control (especially whether or not you're having problems with hypoglycemia) and whether you have complications from your diabetes.

This section discusses commercial licence issues *in Canada*. As licensing requirements differ in the United States, if you will be driving a commercial vehicle into the United States, look into their specific requirements, rules, and regulations.

CDA recommendations for commercial licence requirements

To assist both individuals with diabetes and governments, the CDA has developed recommendations. Like the CDA recommendations in the preceding section, these aren't legally binding rules or regulations. If you want to apply for a commercial licence, you should contact the appropriate licensing body to see what their specific requirements are, but they'll likely want you to do — as a minimum — the following things as suggested by the CDA:

✔ Complete a questionnaire that pays particular attention to both your risk of having hypoglycemia and how often you may have been experiencing hypoglycemia. (You can get a sample questionnaire from the CDA.)

✔ Have your diabetes specialist perform a full assessment of your health status.

✔ Have a full eye exam performed by your eye specialist.

✔ Obtain documentation from your diabetes education centre proving that you have attended their program.

✔ Have a recent A1C result.

✔ Have a record of your blood glucose measurements (taken at least twice daily) dating back six months (or less, of course, if you were diagnosed less than six months ago). Preferably, your record will be a downloaded log from your meter.

CDA exclusion criteria for maintaining a commercial licence

The Canadian Diabetes Association's *exclusion criteria* (that is, those things that, if present, would prevent you from holding a commercial licence) include your having

✔ An episode of severe hypoglycemia within the past six months.

✔ Ongoing hypoglycemia unawareness (refer to Chapter 5).

✔ Poorly controlled blood glucose levels (hyperglycemia or hypoglycemia).

✔ The recent introduction of insulin or, if you're already on insulin, a change in your type of insulin or the frequency that you give it.

✔ Significant visual impairment.

✔ Peripheral neuropathy or cardiovascular disease (refer to Chapter 6) that's severe enough that it could affect your ability to drive.

✔ Inadequate frequency or reliability of blood glucose monitoring.

✔ Inadequate knowledge of the causes, symptoms, and treatment of hypoglycemia. (Don't worry, we have yet to see this determined by a quiz or essay! It's an impression that your health care providers would make based on your discussions. Besides, you and anyone with diabetes absolutely have to know all about hypoglycemia anyway. If you don't, read Chapter 5 and, in addition, ask your health care team to review this crucial subject with you.)

Your physician's duty to report

Physicians are trained always to look out for the best interests of their patients. And that is as it should be. Physicians are also bound — quite rightly — by rules of confidentiality. However, exceptions apply to the way that physicians normally practise. Indeed, in most areas of Canada it is the law that doctors have to report (to the appropriate licensing body) a patient that the physician feels is unsafe to operate a motor vehicle. This is a terribly difficult position for physicians to be in, as the person being reported is invariably and understandably very upset. Even worse, it's often emergency room physicians who have to make this report, and they don't have the benefit of a previous relationship with the patient. Reporting patients is one of the most difficult and unpleasant tasks that doctors face.

Keeping your driver's licence

If you have diabetes and lose your licence, the most likely reason would be that you had an episode of hypoglycemia while you were driving that led either to a collision or to your being pulled over by police because of erratic driving. (This, of course, is one of the most important reasons for you to wear a medical alert, so that those who come to your aid can quickly recognize that you have diabetes and that you are not intoxicated.) Hypoglycemia bad enough to lead to this situation usually only happens if you're treated with insulin (rather than non-insulin antihyperglycemic medications) and is much more likely to occur if you have type 1 diabetes.

Many things about having diabetes are unfair, but perhaps least fair of all is that the better your glucose control is, the more prone you are to hypoglycemia. Nonetheless, that's a fact of diabetes life and you have to work around it to protect you and your licence. Fortunately, most of the time you can avoid episodes of severe hypoglycemia while driving by taking a few relatively simple steps. (We list the measures recommended by the CDA earlier in this section.)

In Ian's experience, these are the most important measures you can undertake to avoid losing your licence:

- ✔ Never drive unless you have checked your blood glucose level immediately before you're about to drive, to ensure that it's not low. (As we mention earlier in this section, Ian recommends following the "don't drive if you're under 5" dictum.)

- ✔ Check your blood glucose levels hourly during long drives to ensure your blood glucose is at a safe level. Never assume your blood glucose levels are normal just because you do not feel low. You must test to be sure.

✔ Keep treatment for low blood glucose on your person or in very easy reach and ingest it if you have *any* suspicion whatsoever that you are low.

✔ If you suspect you're low get off the road *immediately*! Never say to yourself, "Oh, I think I might be getting low; if I start to feel worse I'll pull off the road." If you think your levels are low, get off the road immediately! Your licence may depend on it. More importantly, your life (and the lives of others) may depend on it.

Regaining your driver's licence

Though each province and territory has its own policies, if you lose your licence because of an incident that occurred when you were hypoglycemic, in Ian's experience the following are the two most important things the licensing body will look for in considering your request to reinstate your licence:

✔ Evidence of satisfactory blood glucose control as reflected by a carefully kept and accurate (preferably downloaded) log of your readings for the preceding few months. The record should show an absence of frequent or severe hypoglycemia. (*Note:* Hyperglycemia is not as dangerous as hypoglycemia when it comes to the safety of your driving.)

✔ A letter from your diabetes specialist or a copy of your diabetes specialist's records that reflect your ongoing co-involvement in managing and following your therapy.

Preparing for When Disaster Strikes

Of all the horrors (and there were so many) associated with Hurricane Katrina, one Ian found particularly gut-wrenching was the story of people with diabetes who risked death because they had run out of insulin and, isolated in their flood-ravaged homes, were unable to obtain more. Though hurricanes are not a common occurrence in Canada, many other forms of severe weather do occur and it is therefore essential that you, as a person with diabetes, take special precautions to protect yourself in the event of a calamity.

These are the things you should have on hand so that you're prepared if disaster strikes:

✔ An up-to-date list of all your health conditions and all the medicines — including the doses — you're taking. (During a disaster your health records — including your doctor's files and your pharmacist's data — may be unavailable.)

✔ At least a few days' supply of non-perishable, diabetes-friendly foods.

✔ At least a three-day supply of bottled water.

✔ A source of carbohydrate to treat hypoglycemia. (Refer to Chapter 5.)

✔ At least a two to four weeks' supply of your diabetes medications (including your insulin and other antihyperglycemic medications) and testing supplies (including lancets, test strips, a meter — or even two — and an extra battery). This means making sure you have these extra quantities of these essential items with you as, for example, you head up to the cottage for that winter getaway in snow country.

✔ An insulated container for storing your insulin to keep it from being exposed to temperature extremes.

✔ A glucagon emergency kit (if you're taking a medicine — such as glyburide or insulin — that can cause hypoglycemia). (For more about glucagon, refer to Chapter 5.)

✔ A first-aid kit that contains bandages, dressings, and topical medications (such as an antibiotic cream or ointment) to treat cuts, abrasions, and so on.

In a disaster, you should never walk barefoot (as is the case in all circumstances anyhow).

Part V
The Part of Tens

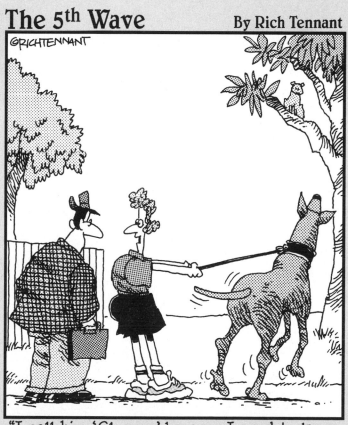

The 5th Wave   By Rich Tennant

@RICHTENNANT

"I call him 'Glucose,' because I need to keep him under control every day."

In this part . . .

*J*ust ahead, a Letterman-worthy top ten list of the most important ways you can ensure you remain healthy with your diabetes. We also look at frequently asked questions posed by people with diabetes.

Chapter 17

Ten Ways to Stay Healthy and Avoid Complications

In This Chapter

▶ Learning for life

▶ Living healthfully

▶ Monitoring your numbers

▶ Keeping an eye on your vision and your feet

▶ Mastering your medicines

*W*e're thrilled you're reading this chapter because here we discuss the top ten things you need to know to stay healthy with your diabetes. If we were given a podium high enough and a speaker loud enough, these are the key messages we would shout out for all to hear.

If you don't have diabetes yourself and are reading this book on behalf of someone you love who does (which many of our readers tell us is the case), even if your loved one chooses not to read the whole book, please insist he or she looks at this chapter. Blame us for your insistence.

Following the advice on these pages could be the difference between disability and early death or a long and healthy life. More than two-thirds of diabetes complications are avoidable when people follow the ten points we discuss in this chapter. We consider it a tragedy, one that frustrates us and saddens us, that people are getting sick and even dying because they don't know the information in this chapter. We wrote this book — and particularly this chapter — to change things.

These ten points are, indeed, the ten most important ways that you can stay healthy and lead a full and active life with your diabetes. And these measures are readily available to each and every person with diabetes. But — and this is a very big *but* — remember one other crucial point: Even if you follow just a portion of the recommendations in this chapter, you're still making headway. Even if you don't meet all your targets for weight control, blood glucose, blood pressure, and so forth, that doesn't mean you've failed and it doesn't mean it was all for naught. Any improvement in your weight or exercise or blood pressure or glucose levels or any of the other items we list here will help reduce your likelihood of developing complications. So be proud of your work and your successes and, for those things lagging behind, well, striving toward additional goals is always good to do.

Learn for Life

Every day, the two of us read professional journals or attend lectures or go to conferences, all with the express purpose of educating ourselves about how best to look after people with diabetes. And the family physicians we work with do the same. As do the diabetes educators and dietitians. As do the podiatrists and the pharmacists and all the other professionals whose mission is to help you stay healthy. Your whole diabetes team is always learning. You, too, are a part of your diabetes team. So that means you also have to do your share of leaning.

The more you know, the better your odds are of being healthy. Ian's motto — right on the homepage of his website (www.ourdiabetes.com) — guiding his professional life is "Rule your diabetes; don't let it rule you!" Your continued education is the single most important factor in allowing you to do this. Don't be in the dark. Know what you should eat. Know how you should exercise. Know what your blood pressure is and what it should be, what your lipids are and what you are aiming for. Know what the best medicines are and how to safely and effectively use them. Whoever said "ignorance is bliss" surely didn't have diabetes. Or, if they did, they likely came to rue the day they said it.

Don't be a passive partner in your diabetes care; be actively involved. You can learn from the other members of your health care team (especially from your diabetes educator and dietitian). You can learn by reading this book, reviewing (reputable) websites such as that of the Canadian Diabetes Association (CDA) at www.diabetes.ca, and attending meetings of your local CDA branch. Until diabetes has a cure, learning needs to be a part of your life. It's that simple.

The Internet has a lot of misinformation, so you must be careful to check out a recommendation before you start to follow it. Even information on reliable sites may not be right for your particular problem.

Eat Earnestly

The most important point about a "diabetic diet" is that it is a healthy diet for anyone, with diabetes or without. You shouldn't feel like a social outcast because you're eating the right foods. And you shouldn't feel guilty if occasionally you eat the wrong foods either, for that matter. *Remember:* There is no such thing as cheating. A healthy diabetes meal plan is not a crash diet, a high-protein diet, a grapefruit diet, or any other fad diet. A diabetes meal plan is a lifelong program of healthy, well-balanced eating.

You can follow a diabetes meal plan wherever you are, not just at home. Every menu has something that's appropriate for you. If you're invited to someone's home, let that person know you have diabetes and that you can eat only a limited amount of carbohydrate and fat. If that fails, then limit the amount you eat. And if that's somehow not possible, then accept the fact that your diet won't always be perfect (and whose is?) and go on from there.

Follow a healthy diet designed by both you and your dietitian and you'll have an excellent foundation in your plan for good health. Ignore proper nutrition and you'll be destined to have poor glucose control; indeed, any and all blood glucose-lowering medications (including insulin) are much less effective without a proper diet. Your destiny is in your hands — and in your mouth.

Refer to Chapter 10 for more on your diet.

Exercise Enthusiastically

If we were to tell you that we had a treatment for you that is free, would only have to be taken once per day, and could help keep your blood glucose levels under control, reduce your blood pressure, improve your lipids, reduce your stress level, help prevent heart attacks, and lower your risk of dying over the next ten years by one-half, you would not only want it, you would demand it! Okay then, it's yours. Exercise.

Preferably daily (or at least most days of the week). Preferably for at least 25 minutes per day. Make exercise as much a part of your life as breathing. The key to success with exercise? Finding the type you like and sticking with it. You don't need to run the Boston Marathon or swim across Lake Ontario (though you are welcome to if you want); something as simple (and inexpensive) as a daily walk is highly therapeutic.

Refer to Chapter 11 for more on exercise.

Give the Heave-Ho to Harmful Habits

You go to the grocery store . . . but forget your wallet at home. You buy a brand-new computer printer . . . and don't have the right cable. You have a breakaway . . . and mishandle the puck. We all have our missteps — opportunities and circumstances that we manage to mess up. But most of these are small miscues or, at worst, temporary setbacks. Having diabetes may be no piece of cake (well, actually, you can have a piece of cake, but that's another story), but with careful management you can lead a full, active, and long life. What a shame that smoking can wreck all that.

Smoking is bad enough for a person without diabetes, but if you have diabetes, smoking makes almost every complication more likely to occur. In essence, smoking rots your arteries. You place yourself at enormous risk of a heart attack, stroke, blindness, amputations . . . ; the list goes on and on. But you can change the odds. Quit smoking now and you can markedly improve your likelihood of avoiding these complications. Some things in life are beyond one's control. Smoking isn't one of them. Millions of Canadians have quit smoking. So can you.

Does it seem unfair that after you were diagnosed as having diabetes, all those well-meaning people (family, friends, doctors, nurses, dietitians . . .) asked you to change your diet, your exercise, your weight, and, if you smoke, your tobacco use, too? Well, if you think so, then you may also think it unfair that we will now ask you to moderate your drinking. No more than two (for women) or three (for men) a day. Tops. Your health is our raison d'être. No apologies for that.

Refer to Chapter 6 for tips on quitting smoking. Refer to Chapter 10 for more on alcohol and diabetes.

Controlling Your Numbers: Optimizing Your Blood Glucose, Blood Pressure, Cholesterol, and Kidney Function

You can rest assured that your doctor knows your average blood glucose (as reflected by your A1C level), your blood pressure, your cholesterol, and your kidney function. Yet despite this, most Canadians with diabetes don't have all these levels under control and as a result are developing often-avoidable complications. Clearly something's wrong with this picture.

We won't go into all the many factors here, but will point out one particularly important and easily correctable one: Most people with diabetes don't know their own numbers, and as a result don't know when they are above target (we discuss targets in the following sections), and thus, also don't know when they need to take corrective action.

"If it ain't broke, don't fix it," some people say. Okay, we'll go along with that. But what if you don't know that it's broke? What then? Your blood glucose, blood pressure, cholesterol, and kidney function tests all belong to *you*. Indeed, they're part of you. And you need to know them. Period.

Now that we've, hopefully, convinced you (perhaps you didn't need convincing), let's look at the numbers you should be targeting and what to do if you are exceeding them.

Blood glucose levels

High blood glucose is a toxin to your body. It can lead to blindness, kidney failure, and nerve damage. But you're clearly not just waiting around for bad things to happen; if you were, you wouldn't be reading this book. To prevent high blood glucose from damaging your body, be sure to test your blood glucose regularly. (Refer to Chapter 9.) Your blood glucose target is 4.0 to 7.0 mmol/L before meals, and 5.0 to 10.0 mmol/L two hours after meals. Your A1C target is no more than 7 percent. If your A1C is above 7 percent despite good before-meal readings, then your two-hour, after-meal target is 5.0 to 8.0 mmol/L. (These are the targets for the great majority of people with diabetes. As we discuss in other chapters, target values are different for children, pregnant women, and some elderly individuals.)

If your blood glucose levels are too high, speak to your health care team (particularly your diabetes educator, dietitian, family doctor, and, if you have one, your diabetes specialist) about what changes can be made to your treatment plan to help get your blood glucose control where it should be.

Cholesterol

Low LDL cholesterol is good. High LDL cholesterol is bad. Now, which do you want for your birthday? Got the wrong gift? So trade it in. Don't accept a poor LDL cholesterol level. An optimal LDL will reduce your risk of cardiovascular disease, so an optimal LDL is what we're after. The CDA target is for the LDL level to be less than or equal to 2 mmol/L. Be sure to know your own LDL cholesterol level, and, if it is above target, speak to your physician to discuss how to make it better. She may recommend a visit to the dietitian, a change to your exercise program, or medication. We discuss cholesterol further in Chapter 6.

Blood pressure

Among the nasty things that high blood pressure causes are strokes, eye damage, heart attacks, and kidney failure. Quick: What was your blood pressure the last time your doctor checked it? And was that within the CDA target? If you know these two answers, congratulations. If you don't, then we're again thrilled that you're reading this. Your blood pressure should be less than 130/80. If your value is higher than this, speak to your doctor about how you can bring it into target. We discuss blood pressure in detail in Chapter 6.

Kidney function

You can markedly reduce the likelihood of diabetes ever causing damage to your kidneys if you keep your blood glucose and blood pressure under control. Your doctor should be monitoring your kidney function by testing your blood to measure your eGFR (normal is equal to or greater than 60 mL/min) and your urine to measure your albumin/creatinine ratio (ACR; normal is less than 2 mg/mmol). If your values are exceeding this, effective treatment is available as we discuss in Chapter 6.

See Your Eye Doctor

You may have 20/20 vision; heck, you may be able to see a speck of dust at 100 paces — but what you can't see is the back of your eyes. Only a skilled eye professional can determine the true health of your eyes. Don't be misled into thinking that your visual acuity (as reflected by your need for — and the strength of — prescription lenses) has anything to do with the health of your eyes. It doesn't. See your eye doctor regularly so you can, well, continue to see your eye doctor.

Refer to Chapter 6 for more on eye care.

Fuss Over Your Feet

We walk, on average, about 184,000 kilometres (115,000 miles) in our lifetime. That's over four trips around the equator (well, okay, we realize that those darn oceans would keep getting in the way, but you know what we mean). So if you want to keep those lovely lower appendages of yours up to this task, you gotta look after 'em. Having diabetes means that your feet are at risk of damage including ulcerations, infections, and even gangrene and, potentially, amputation. But these devastating complications are largely avoidable. Show your feet you care by looking after them with all the helpful measures we discuss in Chapter 6. Go ahead; love your feet. It's okay, really. In fact, it's essential.

Master Your Medicines

You may have noticed that your success with diabetes is based on a combination of things, including knowledge, lifestyle treatment, and medicine use. Although no one wants to take medicines, you cannot underestimate their importance. Indeed, with each passing year, physicians are asking people with diabetes to take more and more medications. The reason is simple: These medicines can keep you healthy and even save your life. Most people with diabetes need to take medicines to accomplish one or more of the following:

- ✔ **Optimize blood glucose:** If you have type 2 diabetes, this usually requires metformin, often with one or two other blood glucose-lowering medicines, one of which may be insulin. (Insulin is always necessary if you have type 1 diabetes.) (Refer to Chapter 12.)

- ✔ **Optimize blood pressure:** This usually requires an ACE inhibitor or ARB along with one, two, or even three other types of blood-pressure-lowering medication. (Refer to Chapter 6.)

- ✔ **Optimize LDL cholesterol:** This usually requires a statin and sometimes another medicine as well. (Refer to Chapter 6.)

- ✔ **Prevent heart attacks and strokes:** If you have or are at high risk of cardiovascular disease, you should be taking a statin and either an ACE inhibitor or an ARB. (Refer to Chapter 6.)

- ✔ **Prevent kidney failure:** If you have evidence of diabetes-related kidney malfunction, you should be taking an ACE inhibitor or ARB. (Refer to Chapter 6.)

- ✔ **Prevent pneumonia:** (At least this isn't a pill you have to remember to take!) Many people with diabetes fall ill each year from pneumonia. But you can reduce your risk for developing pneumonia by getting vaccinated against influenza and pneumoccoal pneumonia. (Refer to Chapter 6.)

(More controversial is whether or not people with diabetes should routinely take ASA to prevent heart attacks. We discuss this in Chapter 6.)

"My goodness!" you might (and should) say. "That could be seven or more different types of medicine to take every day." No one should tell you that's not a big deal. It *is* a big deal. But lying in a hospital bed with a stroke or an amputation or a dialysis machine at your side is, by far, a bigger deal. We have the means to keep you healthy and to help you live a long, full life. And those means include medicines. Don't think of the pills you need to swallow or the insulin you need to inject each day as an anchor dragging you down. Think of them as a life preserver lifting you up!

Help Your Doctor Help You

Your family doctor went through four or more years of post-secondary undergraduate studies then four years of medical school then two or more years of further training for one simple reason: Your doctor is a glutton for punishment! (Please don't tell your doctor we said that. We really, *really* didn't mean it.)

Your doctor did all this training because he wanted to be suitably equipped to help you stay healthy. But without your help, all that training is largely wasted. Having diabetes is not like having appendicitis. If you have appendicitis, all you have to do is lie on an operating table while the anesthetist puts you to sleep and the surgeon takes out your diseased organ. If you have diabetes, on the other hand, you have to be an active and involved partner, working with your doctor by regularly attending appointments, sharing with your doctor how you are doing with your nutrition program and your exercise, what your blood glucose levels are, what your blood pressure is (when, for example, using a machine at a drug store), if you are missing doses of your medicines or believe you're having side effects from them, if you're experiencing symptoms such as chest pain or shortness of breath, erectile dysfunction or vaginal discharge, numbness or burning in your feet, and so on.

Your doctor relies on you to work with her for the common goal of keeping you healthy. Without your help, your doctor may just as well take those diplomas off the wall and burn them. And that we do truly mean.

Don't Try to Do It Alone

In the previous section we discuss how you and your doctor can successfully work together. And, as we discuss in Chapter 8, many other health care professionals, including diabetes educators, dietitians, podiatrists, eye specialists, pharmacists, and others, are not only available to help you, but are keen to help you. Also, never underestimate the importance of your *family's* involvement on your health care team. If someone else in the home does the cooking, take that person with you when you meet with the dietitian. Have family members learn how to help you if your blood glucose level is low. If you can't inspect your own feet, ask a loved one to look for you. And if, at times, you're feeling frustrated or even fed up with the hassles of living with diabetes from day to day (we'd never deny that having diabetes can be a hassle), seeking the comfort of a loved one is often the best medicine of all.

Chapter 18

Ten Frequently Asked Questions about Diabetes

Though every person with diabetes is unique — and needs to be treated as such — some questions do come up remarkably often. Sometimes it's because the answer isn't obvious (for instance, why in the world blood glucose levels would go up overnight even if you haven't been eating), and sometimes it's because the answer isn't easy to find (for example, how to get your doctor to be a more effective communicator). This chapter looks at the ten most commonly asked questions that we hear in our offices. (And we even supply the answers!)

Why Are My Blood Glucose Levels Higher When I Get Up in the Morning than When I Go to Bed?

Having higher blood glucose levels in the morning than when you went to sleep the night before can seem like quite a conundrum. Did you take an unremembered stroll to the fridge at 3 a.m.? Not likely, unless you're one very hungry sleepwalker. Was it an overly big snack at bedtime that made your readings go up? Improbable, unless your snack was so huge that it would make Dagwood Bumstead proud. No, the answer lies within your body, not within your fridge or pantry.

Beginning about 3 a.m., your body starts to increase production of hormones such as cortisol and growth hormone, which are important for normal metabolism but which can, in a person with diabetes, lead to the release of glucose from the liver. This is called the *dawn phenomenon*.

Although this is a common problem, it's not one we take, ahem, lying down. You can try non-insulin blood glucose-lowering medications. But if first thing in the morning is the only time that your blood glucose level is elevated, then the most successful strategy is to take a dose of long-acting (Lantus, Levemir) or intermediate-acting (NPH) insulin at bedtime. (Sometimes Lantus and Levemir are given at other times.)

If you're having this problem despite already taking bedtime insulin, then a simple solution may be to increase your insulin dose. Be sure to discuss this possibility with your physician or diabetes educator.

We discuss insulin issues in detail in Chapter 13.

Why Are My Blood Glucose Levels All Over the Place?

If you're like most people with diabetes (especially type 1 diabetes), you will have experienced times when, despite your best efforts, your glucose control seemed a mess. High one minute, low the next. High for a couple of days, low for the next two. Up and down, down and up, for no apparent rhyme or reason.

But of course there *is* a reason; there's *always* a reason. Figuring out the reason is just a matter of detective work. Sometimes doctors and patients naively think that the only concerns in terms of glucose control are what you eat, how you exercise, and what medicines you take. Although these are the most important factors, many other things can influence blood glucose control. These influences include your stress level, your stomach function, your menstrual cycle, and more.

We discuss these issues in detail in Chapter 9.

Why Are My Blood Glucose Levels Getting Worse as Time Goes By?

Few things are as frustrating to a person with type 2 diabetes as finding that, despite following a proper diet (with occasional indiscretion — which is perfectly fine, by the way), taking more and more pills, and exercising regularly (okay, maybe irregularly, but doing some anyhow), one's blood glucose levels are progressively worsening. If you have been in this situation, you probably asked yourself, "What am I doing wrong?"

The answer is, probably nothing.

The problem is that diabetes is a progressive disease. This means that despite your (and our) best efforts, your pancreas is going to have a hard time keeping up. In fact, the day your type 2 diabetes was diagnosed, your pancreas was already running at only half normal function, and with each passing year it's likely to lose more and more of its ability to produce insulin. The net result is that, with all likelihood, you're going to require more and more medicine to control your glucose levels as time goes by. Worsening pancreas function is also the reason that the majority of people with type 2 diabetes will eventually require insulin therapy. That's not a sign that *you* have failed; it's a sign that *your pancreas* has. And that, of course, is not your fault.

What's the Difference between an A1C Level and a Blood Glucose Level?

One of the most important tests in assessing overall glucose control is also one of the least understood.

Your A1C (hemoglobin A1C) indicates what your average blood glucose level has been over the preceding three months. A1C is measured in percentage (unlike blood glucose, which is measured in mmol/L), and the result represents the proportion of your *hemoglobin* (the substance in your red blood cells that carries oxygen) that's permanently attached to glucose. The higher your average glucose readings over the preceding few months, the more glucose your hemoglobin is exposed to and the higher your A1C will be. Because it's an entirely different test from the one for blood glucose level, an A1C of 7 percent, for example, does *not* mean that your average blood glucose level is 7.0 mmol/L. (In fact, an A1C level of 7 percent indicates your average blood glucose is 8.6 mmol/L).

We discuss the A1C in detail in Chapter 9.

I Used to Be on Pills, but Now I'm on Insulin. Does that Mean I've Developed Type 1 Diabetes?

No, you still have type 2 diabetes. We can say that you have *insulin-treated* diabetes, but that's not the same as having type 1 diabetes.

When You're on Insulin, You're on It Forever, Right?

With the exception of a brief "honeymoon" period that some people experience shortly after the onset of type 1 diabetes, if you have type 1 diabetes, then yes, you need to be on insulin. And yes, it will be forever (or until we have a cure).

If you have type 2 diabetes and, despite appropriate lifestyle and non-insulin antihyperglycemic medications, your blood glucose control is still not what it should be, then yes, you really need to be on insulin. And yes, it will likely be forever. But if you're starting out with much to improve in your lifestyle, then you have a good chance that with diet, exercise, and weight loss, your non-insulin blood glucose-lowering medications will start to work better. Sometimes they work effectively enough that you may end up being able to come off insulin.

I'm Watching My Diet, So Why Is My Cholesterol Level High?

Some people can eat a bacon double cheeseburger and have normal cholesterol levels. And other people could order a veggie burger and have abnormal cholesterol levels. The difference? Genetics. Some people are simply genetically programmed to have a liver that manufactures excess cholesterol. Indeed, all of us produce the bulk of our cholesterol *within* our bodies. If you have a body that tends to over-produce cholesterol, you can combat this by following a proper diet, exercising, and getting your blood glucose control in order — but often this is not sufficient. Our genes are very strong. Often that helps us. Sometimes it doesn't.

We discuss cholesterol levels in detail in Chapter 6.

Why Do I Need Blood Pressure Pills If My Blood Pressure Is Good?

Your doctor may ask you to take blood pressure medication even when your blood pressure is good for two reasons:

✔ "Good" blood pressure is seldom good enough.

✔ Certain types of blood pressure pills also have other important roles to play that are separate from and independent of their blood pressure-lowering function.

If you have diabetes, then your risk of cardiovascular, kidney, and eye disease is high enough that your blood pressure can't just be good or okay. It has to be terrific. Great. Spectacular. Marvellous. You get the idea. *Optimal* blood pressure will go a lot further in keeping you healthy than will *good* blood pressure. And to achieve optimal blood pressure (less than 130/80), blood pressure medicines are often required.

ACE inhibitors and ARBs are commonly called *blood pressure pills;* however, studies have shown that these medicines do more than just lower blood pressure. Indeed, even if your blood pressure is within target to begin with, these medicines can lower your risk of a heart attack (if you're at high risk). They can also help prevent deterioration in your kidney function (if you have evidence of kidney damage). We discuss these topics in detail in Chapter 6.

How Can I Get My Doctor to Be More Communicative?

Congratulations. That you have asked this question tells us that you want to be an active participant in your health care. You aren't content to assume that everything must be okay because your doctor hasn't told you otherwise. You want to know your blood pressure and your cholesterol levels. You want to know your last A1C and whether your eye doctor observed any retinopathy.

Even if your doctor does not necessarily always show it, you can be quite confident that your doctor is absolutely thrilled that you're interested enough in your health to be actively involved in managing your diabetes. Nonetheless, some doctors are not particularly good communicators.

If you're feeling in the dark, you can follow several steps to obtain more information. We suggest trying these in the order they are listed, proceeding to the next step if the earlier one didn't meet with success:

1. **Let your doctor know you're interested.** Perhaps your doctor simply doesn't realize that you want to know the specifics of your results. Your first step should always be to simply let your physician know that you are keenly interested in your health and would like to know as much as possible about it. Your doctor will likely be overjoyed.

2. **Ask specific questions.** "Doctor, what is my blood pressure?" is more likely to get you a specific number than is asking "Doctor, how's my pressure?" which would likely be met with "It's fine."

3. **Ask for copies of your lab results.** You are fully entitled to knowing what your lab results are (heck, it's your blood and urine after all!). You are similarly entitled to having a copy of them provided to you. Usually, simply discussing your results with your doctor is sufficient; however, if you feel that this isn't providing you with enough in the way of specifics, then ask your doctor for a photocopy of your results. When you ask for these, we recommend you word your request in a non-threatening way; otherwise, your doctor may feel that you are second-guessing her judgment (which you may be, but there's no benefit to you if your doctor feels defensive). Try something like "Doctor, I like to keep tabs on my lab results. Can I have a photocopy for my records?" (Ian has a stamp which he imprints on lab requisitions advising the lab to provide a copy of the results directly to the patient, if the patient requests a copy.)

4. **Ask other members of your health care team.** If none of the previous steps has succeeded, try asking other members of your health care team. It may well be that if one of your physicians (say, for example, your diabetes specialist) is not readily forthcoming, another one may be (for example, your family physician). Your diabetes educator is another person to try, because he or she may have received copies of lab results or consultation letters from your physician(s). (In some Canadian jurisdictions, patients can access their own lab results online; Ian wishes this was true of all regions of Canada!)

Will 1 Always Have Diabetes?

We're sure you can tell why we saved this question for last; it is far and away the most difficult question we are ever asked. The quick answer is a simple "we don't know" — and, of course, we don't. The more complicated answer is (and this is our personal and highly subjective guess) the following:

✔ It's only a matter of time before a cure for type 1 diabetes is found. We don't know what shape this will take (perhaps islet cell transplants will get perfected, perhaps gene therapy will be refined, perhaps stem cell research will find an answer . . .) and we don't know when this will happen, but happen it will.

✔ If you have type 2 diabetes, the situation is much trickier, and we don't foresee a cure on the horizon. The factors leading to type 2 diabetes are complex and far from completely understood. It's highly unlikely that we're dealing with a single cause for which we can find a single cure. On the other hand, more and better treatment options are rapidly emerging. Even if we can't undo your diabetes, it's likely that we'll be able to offer such effective therapy that your diabetes will become less and less difficult for you to deal with. (It is worth noting, however, that if a cure for type 1 diabetes is found which is based on the body recovering its ability to make sufficient insulin, then this cure may also be applicable to people living with type 2 diabetes.)

Although a cure for diabetes is not imminent, rapid improvements in insulin pump therapy and continuous glucose monitoring are being made. The development of an artificial pancreas (composed of an insulin pump, as we discuss in Chapter 13; a continuous glucose monitoring system, as we discuss in Chapter 9; and a miniature and portable computer interface) is indeed on the horizon. Imagine how developing an artificial pancreas will revolutionize diabetes management! Though not a cure, it will be the next best thing. To learn more about current work on developing an artificial pancreas visit www.artificialpancreasproject.com.

As diabetes specialists, we're always full of hope. Every day, research comes out revealing new insights into the condition. And the pace at which new and better therapies are emerging is simply astounding. The single greatest advantage to you in having a disease that's so common is that this stimulates research scientists to put tremendous resources into finding ways to help you.

When we look back at our careers and see what medical science knows now that it did not when we first began our practices, we can only marvel at the progress we've made in our quest to keep people with diabetes healthy. Thousands of scientists — people who have dedicated their entire careers to this cause — are looking for a cure. Not just finding a new drug to control diabetes, but an honest-to-goodness cure. How can we be so certain? Because we read their research papers, and hear them speak, and meet them all the time.

Part VI
Appendixes

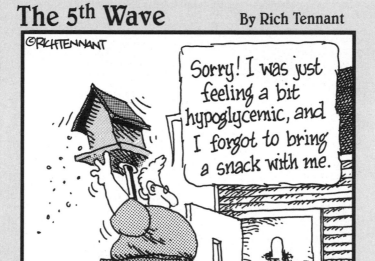

The 5th Wave   By Rich Tennant

Sorry! I was just feeling a bit hypoglycemic, and I forgot to bring a snack with me.

In this part . . .

Although your body may have but one appendix,
Diabetes For Canadians For Dummies has three! In
the first appendix we look at the food group system. After
you have digested that (or before, or indeed at any time),
you can take a gander at Appendix B, which lists a few
important websites. You can also head over to Appendix C,
which provides a quick-reference glossary of those
words — both obscure and not so obscure — that you
may be uncertain about.

Appendix A

The Food Group System

In This Appendix

▶ Looking at the Canadian Diabetes Association Food Group System

▶ Using food choices to create your diet

*I*n this appendix, you discover the method that dietitians in Canada are using to help their patients eat the right number of calories from the correct energy sources while still eating a variety of foods. Although many thousands of different foods are available, each one can be broken down on the basis of the energy source (carbohydrate, protein, or fat) that is most prevalent. This basic feature underlies nutrition planning, as you see here.

We look at the general principles of meal planning (and snacks, too!). Just remember that you need to see a dietitian to create a nutrition program that fits with your specific needs. (We discuss the role of dietitians as part of your health care team in Chapter 8.)

To assist people with diabetes in choosing healthy foods for their meals and snacks, the Canadian Diabetes Association (CDA) has developed *Beyond the Basics: Meal Planning for Healthy Eating, Diabetes Prevention and Management*. In this system, foods are divided into seven groups according to the amount of carbohydrate, protein, and fat they contain. Here are the groups:

✔ Grains and Starches

✔ Fruits

✔ Milk and Alternatives

✔ Other Choices (sweet foods and snacks)

✔ Vegetables

✔ Meat and Alternatives

✔ Fats

Each group includes many different food choices. The amount specified beside each food in the tables that follow represents one choice from that group and can be interchanged with any other choice in the same group. This system is highly effective, as long as you're keeping track of the amounts you're eating from the different groups.

Listing all food sources in this space isn't possible, but you can obtain a list of just about all the foods you might eat by ordering *Beyond the Basics* from the CDA (www.diabetes.ca or 800-226-8464). You can learn more about this publication at www.diabetes.ca/for-professionals/resources/nutrition/beyond-basics.

In the United States they use a similar concept, but they use the word *exchanges* rather than choices.

In the remainder of this appendix we look at each of the seven food groups. We then discuss a sample nutrition plan.

Grains and Starches

Table A-1 lists food choices for Grains and Starches. Each choice contains about 15 grams of carbohydrate, 2 grams of protein, and 68 calories. *Beyond the Basics* recommends high-fibre starch choices. On food labels, look for 4 grams or more of fibre per serving or greater than a 15-percent daily value.

Table A-1	Grains and Starches Food Choices
Food	*Serving*
Cereals, Grains, Pasta	
Bran cereals	125 mL (1/2 cup)
Cooked cereals	175 mL (¾ cup)
Shredded wheat biscuit	1
Wild rice (cooked)	75 mL (⅓ cup)
Pasta (cooked)	125 mL (½ cup)
Puffed wheat	375 mL (1½ cup)
Rice (cooked)	75 mL (⅓ cup)
Shredded wheat (bite size)	125 mL (½ cup)

Food	Serving
Bread	
Bagel small	½
Breadsticks	2
English muffin	½
Wiener	½, bun
Hamburger	½ bun
Pita	15 cm (6"), ½
Raisin bread	1 slice
Tortilla	15 cm (6"), 1 round
White or whole wheat bread	1 slice
Crackers/Snacks	
Soda crackers	7
Graham crackers	3
Matzoh	15 cm (6"), 1
Melba toast	4 slices
Triscuits	5
Rusks	2
Starchy Vegetables	
Corn (kernel)	125 mL (½ cup)
Corn on the cob	½ medium
Potato (baked or broiled)	½ medium
Plantain	75 mL (⅓ cup)
Starchy Foods with Fats	
Waffle	1
Tea biscuit	1
French fries	10
Pancake	10 cm (4"), 1
Croissant	1 small
Mashed potatoes	125 mL (½ cup)

Fruits

All fresh, frozen, and canned fruits as well as unsweetened juices are in this group. Choose whole fruit and eat the edible skins as much as possible for the benefit of fibre, vitamins, and minerals. Each Fruits choice (see Table A-2) contains about 15 grams of carbohydrate, 1 gram of protein, and 64 calories of energy.

Table A-2	Fruit Choices
Food	*Serving*
Fresh and Canned Fruit	
Apple	1 medium
Applesauce, unsweetened	125 mL (½ cup)
Apricots	4
Banana	1 small
Blackberries	500 mL (2 cups)
Blueberries	250 mL (1 cup)
Cantaloupe	250 mL (1 cup)
Cherries (fresh)	15
Cherries (canned)	125 mL (½ cup)
Figs, fresh	2 small
Fruit cocktail	125 mL (½ cup)
Grapefruit	1 small
Grapes	250 mL (1 cup) or 15
Honeydew	250mL (1 cup)
Kiwi	2 medium
Mango	125 mL (½ cup)
Nectarine	250mL (1 cup)
Orange	1 medium
Papaya	250 mL (1 cup)
Peach	1 large
Peaches (canned in light syrup)	125 mL (½ cup)
Pear	1 medium
Pear halves (canned, in light syrup)	125 mL (½ cup)
Persimmon	½
Pineapple (fresh)	175 mL (¾ cup)
Pineapple (canned in light syrup)	125 mL (½ cup) or 2 rings
Plum	2 medium
Raspberries	500 mL (2 cups)
Strawberries	500 mL (2 cups)
Tangerine	2 medium
Watermelon	250 mL (1 cup)

Food	Serving
Dried Fruit	
Apple	4 rings
Apricots	8 halves
Dates	2
Pear	½
Prunes	3
Raisins	25 mL (2 Tbsp.)
Fruit Juice	
Apple	125 mL (½ cup)
Grape	75 mL (⅓ cup)
Grapefruit	125 mL (½ cup)
Orange	125 mL (½ cup)
Pineapple	125 mL (½ cup)
Prune	75 mL (⅓ cup)

Milk and Alternatives

The different kinds of milk vary only in their fat content. The carbohydrate and protein content remain the same. One Milk and Alternatives choice (see Table A-3) contains about 12 grams of carbohydrate, 8 grams of protein, and from trace to 8 grams of fat (skim milk contains trace grams fat and 80 calories; 1-percent milk has 2 grams fat and 98 calories; 2-percent milk has 5 grams fat and 125 calories; and homogenized milk has 8 grams fat and 152 calories).

Table A-3	Milk and Alternatives Choices
Food	*Serving*
Milk (skim, 1%, 2%, or homo)	250 mL (1 cup)
Chocolate milk	125 mL (½ cup)
Evaporated milk	125 mL (½ cup)
Powdered milk, skim	50 mL (4 tbsp.)
Plain or artificially sweetened yogurt	175 mL (¾ cup)

Other Choices (sweet foods and snacks)

Sugar, and food with added sugar such as candy, Popsicles, and regular jam can be part of a healthy meal plan. This group consists of common snack foods and treats. Choose these foods in moderation as many lack fibre, vitamins, and minerals, and may contain a lot of fat. Current recommendations suggest no more than 10 percent of the total calories you consume be supplied by sugar. For example, if you are on a 2,000-calorie-per-day meal plan, your recommended amount of carbohydrate in the form of sugar would be 50 grams. Each choice in this group (see Table A-4) contains 15 grams of carbohydrate, generally very small amounts of protein (except for milk-based items), and from 0 to 12 grams of fat. Calorie values vary from approximately 77 to 164.

Table A-4	Other Choices
Food	*Serving*
Popcorn, air popped, low fat	750mL (3 cups)
Honey/molasses/corn syrup/maple syrup/ white or brown sugar	15 mL (1 Tbsp.)
Milk pudding, skim, no added sugar	125 mL (½ cup)
Regular jam, jelly, or marmalade	15 mL (1 Tbsp.)
Hard candy	5 small
Popsicles	1 bar
Ice cream	125mL (½ cup)
Oatmeal granola bar	1 bar (28 grams)
Muffin, small	1
Potato chips	10
Chocolate chip cookies	2

Vegetables

Vegetables are rich in nutrients, contain no fat, contain typically small, but variable amounts of protein (depending on the particular vegetable), and, with the exception of those that are richer in carbohydrates (parsnips, sweet peas, squash, and beets, which should be limited to half-cup portions at a meal), can be eaten in unlimited quantities in a healthy diet. Potatoes and corn are included in the Grains and Starches group due to their carbohydrate content.

These are examples of vegetables that can be eaten in unlimited quantities:

✔ Asparagus

✔ Beans, string, green, or yellow

✔ Bok choy

✔ Broccoli

✔ Brussels sprouts

✔ Cabbage

✔ Cauliflower

✔ Celery

✔ Cucumber

✔ Lettuce

✔ Mushrooms

✔ Okra

✔ Onion

✔ Peppers, green, red, and yellow

✔ Spinach

✔ Tomato (tomato is, technically, a fruit, but since it fits best here, we're sneaking it into this list)

✔ Zucchini

Meat and Alternatives

One choice of Meat and Alternatives (see Table A-5) contains no carbohydrate (except for legumes; that is, beans and lentils), about 7 grams of protein, 3 grams of fat, and 55 calories of energy. Legumes are low in fat and high in fibre and are excellent protein sources. Each half-cup portion will provide 15 grams of carbohydrate.

Only lean Meat and Alternatives choices are listed here. All foods listed are cooked.

Table A-5	Meat and Alternatives Choices
Food	**Serving**
Meat and Poultry	
Beef: round, sirloin, flank, tenderloin, ground	30 grams (1 oz.)
Pork: fresh, canned, cured, or boiled ham, ground	30 grams (1 oz.)
Veal: all cuts except for cutlets	30 grams (1 oz.)
Poultry: chicken, turkey	30 grams (1 oz.)
Fish and Shellfish	
All fish, fresh and frozen	30 grams (1 oz.)
Crab, lobster	50 mL (1/4 cup)
Oysters	3 medium
Canned in water (tuna or salmon)	50 mL (1/4 cup)
Canned sardines	3 small
Fresh shrimp	5 large
Cheese	
Low fat (about 7% milk fat)	1 slice, 30 grams (1 oz.)
Cottage cheese	50 mL (1/4 cup)
Ricotta cheese	50 mL (1/4 cup)
Alternatives	
Egg, large	1
Legumes: beans and lentils	125 mL (½ cup)
Hummus	75 mL (⅓ cup)
Vegetarian patty/wiener	1
Peanut butter	25 mL (2 Tbsp.)

The following Meat and Alternatives choices are high in saturated fat (choose them less often):

✔ Bologna: 1 slice

✔ Canned luncheon meat: 1 slice

✔ Sausage: 1 link

✔ Weiner, hot dog: 1

✔ Salami: 1 slice

✔ Regular cheese (greater than 20-percent milk fat): 1 slice, 30 grams (1 oz.)

Fats

These foods (see Table A-6) have 5 grams of fat and little or no protein or carbohydrate per portion. Therefore, each choice contains 45 calories. The important thing in this category is to notice the foods that are high in cholesterol and saturated fats — and avoid them.

Table A-6	Fat Choices
Food	*Serving*
Unsaturated Fats	
Avocado	⅛ medium
Salad dressing, regular	5 mL (1 tsp.)
Margarine, regular, non-hydrogenated	5 mL (1 tsp.)
Salad dressing, low fat	25 mL (2 Tbsp.)
Margarine, light, non-hydrogenated	15 mL (1 Tbsp.)
Mayonnaise, regular	5 mL (1 tsp.)
Almonds	8
Cashews	5
Pecans	5 halves
Peanuts	10
Walnuts	2 whole
Sunflower seeds	15 mL (1 Tbsp.)
Pumpkin seeds	20 mL (4 tsp.)
Oil (corn, olive, soybean, sunflower, peanut)	5 mL (1 tsp.)
Olives, small	10
Saturated Fats	
Butter	5 mL (1 tsp.)
Bacon	1 slice
Coconut milk, canned	25 mL (2 Tbsp.)
Cream, half and half	45 mL (3 Tbsp.)
Cream, sour, regular	25 mL (2 Tbsp.)
Cream, heavy	15 mL (1 Tbsp.)
Cream cheese	15 mL (1 Tbsp.)
Gravy	25 mL (2 Tbsp.)
Lard	5 mL (1 tsp.)
Pâté, liverwurst	15 mL (1 Tbsp.)
Shortening	5 mL (1 tsp.)

Free Foods

These foods do not contain a significant amount of calories, so you can eat as much of them as you want without worrying about serving size (though, of course, if you eat a pound of chili powder you may regret it for other reasons!).

- ✔ **Drinks:** Bouillon, sugar-free drinks, club soda, coffee, and tea
- ✔ **Condiments:** Horseradish, mustard, pickles (unsweetened), and vinegar
- ✔ **Seasonings:** Basil, lemon juice, celery seeds, lime, cinnamon, mint, chili powder, onion powder, chives, oregano, curry, paprika, dill, pepper, salt, flavouring extracts (vanilla, for example), pimiento, garlic, spices, garlic powder, ginger, soy sauce, herbs, wine (used in cooking), lemon, and Worcestershire sauce

As we discuss in Chapter 10, a number of types of sugar-free candy, sugar-free gum, sugar-free jam or jelly, and sugar substitutes can, depending on their contents, be consumed fairly liberally. However, bear in mind that sugar alcohols vary in the degree to which they are absorbed into the body. Also, in high doses they can cause unpleasant gastrointestinal symptoms such as abdominal cramping and diarrhea.

Using "Beyond the Basics" to Create a Nutrition Plan

Having different foods in each group that can be interchanged makes creating a varied nutrition plan easy. The following menus show the amounts for diets of 1,500 (Table A-7) and 1,800 (Table A-9) calories.

Table A-7		1,500 Calories	
Breakfast	*Lunch*	*Dinner*	*Snack*
2 Grains and Starches choices	2 Grains and Starches choices	2 Grains and Starches choices	1 Grains and Starches choice
1 Fruits choice	1 Fruits choice	1 Fruits choice	1 Milk (1%) and Alternatives choice
1 Milk (1%) and Alternatives choice	2 Meat and Alternatives choices	3 Meat and Alternatives choices	

Breakfast	Lunch	Dinner	Snack
1 Meat and Alternatives choice	1 Fats choice	2 Fats choices	
2 Fats choices	Vegetables as desired	Vegetables as desired	

This menu provides 180 grams of carbohydrate, 82 grams of protein, and 49 grams of fat, keeping it in line with 50 percent of energy from carbohydrate, 20 percent of energy from protein, and 30 percent of energy from fat.

Translating this into food, you can have the menu in Table A-8 on one day.

Table A-8	A Sample Menu		
Breakfast	**Lunch**	**Dinner**	**Bedtime Snack**
2 slices toast	2 slices bread	1 medium potato	1 shredded wheat biscuit
1 pear	1 large peach	15 grapes	250 mL (1 cup) 1% milk
250 mL (1 cup) 1% milk	1 slice cheese (low-fat) & 1 slice ham	90 g (3 oz.) lean beef	
1 egg	5 mL (1 tsp) margarine	10 mL (2 tsp.) regular salad dressing	
2 tsp., non-hydrogenated margarine	Vegetables (such as lettuce, cucumber for sandwich)	Salad, as desired, and 125 mL(½ cup) peas	

For a 1,800-calorie diet, you could have the menu in Table A-9.

Table A-9	1,800-Calorie Sample Menu		
Breakfast	*Lunch*	*Dinner*	*Bedtime Snack*
2 Grains and Starches choices	3 Grains and Starches choices	3 Grains and Starches choices	1 Grains and Starches choice
1 Fruits choice	1 Fruits choice	2 Fruits choices	1 Milk (2%) and Alternative choice
1 Milk (2%) and Alternatives choices	2 Meat and Alternatives choices	3 Meat and Alternatives choices	
2 Meat and Alternatives choices	2 Fats choices	2 Fats choices	
2 Fats choices	Vegetables as desired	Vegetables as desired	

This diet provides 225 grams of carbohydrate, 96 grams of protein, and 61 grams of fat, again maintaining the 50:20:30 division of calories. Using the example of the 1,500-calorie diet, go ahead and try to make up an 1,800-calorie diet for yourself.

Appendix B

Straight Goods on a Tangled Web: Diabetes Websites Worth Visiting

· ·

In This Appendix

▶ Starting at the authors' websites

▶ Checking general sites about diabetes

▶ Getting a taste of websites with recipes for people with diabetes

· ·

*T*he Internet can be a great resource for just about anything, but, of course, as everyone knows, with the good comes the bad. One minute you're looking at a high-quality, reputable, well-maintained site like that of the Canadian or American diabetes associations, and the next click you're looking at Uncle Bob's Instant Diabetes Cure. The problem is not that great information isn't out there; the problem is trying to figure out which sites have it and which just pretend to.

In this appendix and throughout this book, we discuss sites that we have found particularly useful. You should be able to get answers to just about any questions that you have. However, you must be cautious. A website is offering information to many people; it doesn't know you and your unique needs. Therefore, don't make any major changes in your diabetes care without first checking with your health care team. Remember also that the Internet is constantly changing and growing, so the web addresses we mention — and the information they contain — may change.

If you want to stay abreast of new, worthwhile sites, one helpful way to do this is to periodically check the "links" pages of sites that you have come to know and trust.

Ian's and Alan's Websites

Start your search at our web pages:

- ✔ www.ourdiabetes.com
- ✔ www.drrubin.com

You can find general information and advice about diabetes, tips, new developments, and answers to questions.

General Sites

All-encompassing sites such as the following will tell you about diabetes from A to Z. In keeping with that, we list them alphabetically:

- ✔ **The American Diabetes Association (ADA):** This helpful site, www. diabetes.org, offers loads of information. But as you can imagine, it uses American units (for glucose, cholesterol, and so on), which can be confusing for those of us north of the 49th parallel. Also, it uses American guidelines, which at times can be quite different from Canadian ones.

- ✔ **Ask NOAH about Diabetes:** This site, www.noah-health.org, provides a large amount of information in both English and Spanish. It comes from the New York Online Access to Health, a partnership of New York institutions.

- ✔ **The Behavioral Diabetes Institute:** If you have a psychological issue relating to your diabetes, you may find help at this site (www. behavioraldiabetesinstitute.org), which is "dedicated to helping people with diabetes live long, healthy, and happy lives."

- ✔ **The Canadian Diabetes Association (CDA):** The CDA site, www.diabetes. ca, is particularly helpful because it looks at diabetes issues from a Canadian perspective. Canadian guidelines are the backbone of the supplied information, and, of course, this site uses Canadian (international, actually) units. Particularly helpful is the listing of resources (including addresses and phone numbers) available in your province or territory and even within your community.

- ✔ **The Diabetes Monitor:** This site, www.diabetesmonitor.com discusses every aspect of diabetes, including the latest discoveries.

- ✔ **MedLinePlus Drug Information:** You'll find excellent information at this site, www.nlm.nih.gov/medlineplus/druginformation.html. It provides clear and well-presented information on virtually any drug you're likely to be prescribed. It also provides detailed information on complementary and alternative medicines.

> ✔ **Online Diabetes Resources by David Mendosa:** On his site, www.mendosa.com/diabetes.htm, David Mendosa, a medical writer who lives with diabetes, has catalogued a vast amount of online information concerning diabetes. Also available are some excellent articles that he's written on various topics in diabetes.

Recipe Websites for People with Diabetes

You can find a number of excellent recipes online. We note particularly good ones here:

✔ **The American Diabetes Association (ADA):** The ADA site, www.diabetes.org, has an extensive list of recipes — enough to keep you full for ages.

✔ **The Canadian Diabetes Association (CDA):** Not as extensive as the ADA's list, but still food for thought, is the CDA's list of recipes at www.diabetes.ca.

✔ **Children with Diabetes:** At www.childrenwithdiabetes.com you'll find a huge collection of recipes including many submitted by their readers (which is good because they come personally recommended; however, it also means the recipes may not have been evaluated by a registered dietitian).

✔ **Diabetic Gourmet Magazine:** In this online magazine, www.diabeticgourmet.com, you'll find many recipes and even a rating system — you can vote thumbs up or down on last night's dinner. Of course, your kids will already have voiced their opinion without the computer.

✔ **The Vegetarian Resource Group:** This large site (www.vrg.org) is filled with information for vegetarians who have developed diabetes.

Appendix C

Glossary

A1C: A measurement of overall blood glucose control for approximately the last three months (also referred to as the hemoglobin A1C or HbA1C).

Acarbose: A non-insulin antihyperglycemic medication that lowers blood glucose by slowing the rate of absorption of glucose from the small intestine into the blood.

ACE inhibitor: A class of drug that lowers blood pressure, protects the kidneys, and reduces the risk of heart attack in people with diabetes. The (generic names for the) available ACE inhibitors are benazepril, captopril, cilazapril, enalapril, fosinopril, lisinopril, perindopril, quinapril, ramipril, and trandolapril.

Actos: See *pioglitazone.*

Amaryl: See *glimepiride.*

Amino acids: Compounds that link together to form proteins.

Antibodies: A type of protein formed — as part of the immune system — when the body detects something foreign such as bacteria.

Antihyperglycemic medication: Medicine that lowers blood glucose. Typically refers to non-insulin antihyperglycemic medication. Also known as oral hypoglycemic agents or medications.

Apidra: See *glulisine.*

ARB: A class of drug that lowers blood pressure, protects the kidneys, and reduces the risk of heart attack in people with diabetes. The (generic names for the) available ARBs are candesartan, eprosartan, irbesartan, losartan, telmisartan, and valsartan.

Aspart: A type of rapid-acting insulin.

Atherosclerosis: Narrowing of arteries due to deposits of cholesterol and other substances.

Autoimmune disorder: Disease such as type 1 diabetes and Hashimoto's thyroiditis in which the body's immune system mistakenly attacks its own tissues.

Autonomic neuropathy: Diseases of nerves that affect organs not under conscious control, such as the heart, lungs, and intestines.

Avandia: See *rosiglitazone.*

Basal insulin: The insulin taken to provide blood glucose control in-between meals including overnight. Basal insulin typically refers to long-acting insulin (Lantus, Levemir) or the moment-to-moment small amounts of insulin administered by an insulin pump.

Basal-bolus insulin therapy: Therapy that combines use of both basal and bolus insulin.

Beta cell: The insulin-producing cells of the pancreas.

Blood glucose meter: A small, portable machine that allows for moment-to-moment measurement of your blood glucose level.

Body mass index (BMI): A measure of whether or not you're at a healthy weight for your height.

Bolus insulin: Rapid-acting (or regular) insulin given with meals to prevent blood glucose levels from climbing too high after meals, and also given to reduce an elevated blood glucose level.

Byetta: See *exenatide.*

Carbohydrate: One of the three major energy sources. It is usually found in grains, fruits, and vegetables, and is most responsible for raising the blood glucose.

Carbohydrate counting: Calculating the amount of carbohydrate in food one is about to eat and giving an amount of rapid-acting insulin proportionate to that in order to prevent the carbohydrate from unduly raising one's blood glucose.

Cataract: A clouding of the lens of the eye.

Cholesterol: A fat-like substance that is needed in the body (for example, for the production of certain hormones), but if present in excess levels can contribute to the development of atherosclerosis. See also *high-density lipoprotein (HDL)* and *low-density lipoprotein (LDL).*

Creatinine: A substance in blood that reflects the approximate level of kidney function. Used to calculate the estimated GFR (eGFR), which is a more precise measure of how efficiently your kidneys are able to purify your blood.

Continuous glucose monitoring system: The continual measurement of glucose using a small catheter placed under the skin in conjunction with a transmitter and a receiver (display unit).

Dawn phenomenon: The tendency for blood glucose to rise in the early morning due to secretion of hormones that counteract insulin.

Degludec: A new, very long-acting basal insulin.

Detemir: A type of long-acting basal insulin.

Diabeta: See *glyburide.*

Diabetes mellitus: A disease in which the blood contains too much glucose due to insufficient or ineffective insulin. Typically abbreviated as *diabetes.*

Diabetologist: A physician who specializes in diabetes.

Dialysis: Artificial cleaning of the blood when the kidneys aren't working.

Diamicron: See *gliclazide.*

DPP-4 inhibitors: A class of non-insulin antihyperglycemic medication that works by promoting insulin release and suppressing glucagon production from the pancreas.

Dyslipidemia: Abnormal cholesterol and triglyceride levels in the blood.

Endocrinologist: A physician who specializes in diseases of the glands, including the adrenal glands, the thyroid, the pituitary, the parathyroid glands, the ovaries, the testicles, and the pancreas.

Exenatide: A type of *GLP-1 analogue.*

Fats: The most concentrated source of calories of the three major energy sources. Some fats come from animals and some from plants.

Fibre: A substance in plants that can lower fat and blood glucose and can help prevent constipation.

Food group system: A system — designed to facilitate diabetes meal planning — that divides foods into seven groups according to the amount of carbohydrate, protein, and fat they contain.

Fructose: The sugar found in fruits, vegetables, and honey.

Gastroparesis: A form of autonomic neuropathy involving nerves to the stomach that results in a slowing of the rate that the stomach expels food into the small intestine.

Gestational diabetes: Diabetes that develops during pregnancy and goes away when pregnancy ends, but that indicates one is at increased risk of later developing type 2 diabetes.

Glargine: A type of long-acting basal insulin.

Gliclazide: A type of sulfonylurea medication.

Glimepiride: A type of sulfonylurea medication.

GLP-1 analogues: A class of injectable antihyperglycemic medication that works by multiple mechanisms including promoting insulin release and suppressing glucagon production from the pancreas, as well as reducing appetite and slowing down how quickly food is expelled from the stomach.

Glucagon: A hormone secreted by the pancreas that stimulates glucose release from the liver and causes blood glucose levels to rise. Also available in a glucagon kit for injection into a person who is unconscious from hypoglycemia.

Glucobay: See *acarbose.*

GlucoNorm: See *repaglinide.*

Glucose: A form of sugar that is the body's main source of energy.

Glucose tolerance test: A test where you consume a sugar-rich drink and your glucose levels are measured several times to establish if you have diabetes.

Glulisine: A type of rapid-acting insulin.

Glumetza: A once-a-day formulation of metformin.

Glyburide: A type of sulfonylurea medication.

Glycemic index: The extent to which a given food raises blood glucose.

Glycogen: The storage form of glucose in the liver and muscles.

Health care team: The group of people who work together to keep you healthy. You, the person with diabetes, are the most important member of the team. Other members include your family doctor, your diabetes specialist, your diabetes educator, your dietitian, your eye doctor, your pharmacist, and, when necessary, other specialists (such as a social worker, podiatrist, dentist, cardiologist, kidney specialist, neurologist, emergency room physician, and so forth).

Hemoglobin A1C: See *A1C.*

High-density lipoprotein (HDL): A good form of blood cholesterol that helps to protect you from atherosclerosis.

Honeymoon phase: A brief period of time, typically lasting no more than a few weeks to a few months, experienced by some individuals where, shortly after the onset of type 1 diabetes, some pancreatic function is recovered and less insulin is required.

Humalog insulin: See *Lispro insulin.*

Hyperglycemia: Higher than normal blood glucose levels.

Hyperosmolar hyperglycemic state: A dangerous condition in type 2 diabetes of very high blood glucose associated with severe dehydration.

Hypoglycemia: Lower than normal blood glucose levels.

Impaired fasting glucose (IFG): A condition in which fasting blood glucose levels are higher than normal, but not high enough to establish a diagnosis of diabetes. See *prediabetes.*

Impaired glucose tolerance (IGT): A condition in which the blood glucose level is higher than normal — but not high enough to establish a diagnosis of diabetes — during the post-drink phase of a glucose tolerance test. Also see *prediabetes.*

Incretins: Hormones, made by the intestine, that are important in regulating blood glucose control.

Incretin mimetic: Medication that acts similarly to the body's naturally occurring incretin hormones.

Insulin: The key hormone, made by the beta cells of the pancreas, that permits glucose to enter cells.

Insulin pump: A device that delivers insulin into the body through a small catheter under the skin.

Insulin reaction: Hypoglycemia as a consequence of injected insulin.

Insulin resistance: A condition in which the body does not properly respond to insulin. This is typically present in people with type 2 diabetes.

Intensive diabetes management: The term typically applied to people with diabetes who are on three or more insulin injections per day or are using an insulin pump. (This term is, however, more appropriately used to refer to all people with diabetes, regardless of the type of treatment they are on, as long as the treatment is aimed at achieving optimal blood glucose control.)

Islet cells: The cells in the pancreas that make insulin, glucagon, and other hormones.

Long-acting insulin: Insulin which lasts up to 24 hours after being injected. (Insulin degludec is a new insulin which lasts longer than 24 hours.)

Januvia: See *sitagliptin.*

Ketoacidosis: An acute loss of control of diabetes with high blood glucose levels and breakdown of fat leading to acid production. Much more common in type 1 than type 2 diabetes.

Ketone: A breakdown product of fat formed when fat, rather than glucose, is being used for energy.

Lancet: A sharp needle to prick the skin for a blood glucose test.

Lantus: See *glargine.*

Laser treatment: Therapy that burns small areas at the back of the eye to prevent worsening of retinopathy.

Levemir: See *detemir.*

Linagliptin: A type of *DPP-4 inhibitor.*

Lipohypertrophy: Area of fatty deposit under the skin from overuse of an insulin injection site.

Liraglutide: A type of *GLP-1 analogue.*

Lispro: A type of rapid-acting insulin.

Low-density lipoprotein (LDL): A bad form of blood cholesterol that contributes to the development of atherosclerosis.

Macrosomia: An overly big baby. This is generally considered to be a newborn weighing more than 4000 grams (8.8 pounds).

Macrovascular complications: Damage to the heart, brain, or legs due to blockage of large blood vessels.

Metabolic syndrome: A combination of several conditions, typically including an overweight state, abnormal lipids, elevated blood pressure, and increased blood glucose that puts you at increased risk of cardiovascular disease.

Metabolism: The body's use of energy and nutrients to maintain good health.

Metformin: A type of non-insulin antihyperglycemic medication that lowers blood glucose by blocking release of glucose from the liver.

Microalbuminuria: Abnormal loss of a specific type of protein, called albumin, from the body into the urine.

Microvascular complications: Damage to the retina, nerves, or kidneys due to blockage of small blood vessels.

Monounsaturated fat: A form of fat from certain vegetable sources that does not raise cholesterol.

Nateglinide: A type of non-insulin antihyperglycemic medication that lowers blood glucose by stimulating insulin release from the pancreas.

Neovascularization: Formation within the eyes of abnormal, fragile blood vessels that are prone to bleeding.

Nephropathy: Damage to the kidneys.

Neuropathy: Damage to parts of the nervous system.

Non-insulin antihyperglycemic medication: Medications, other than insulin, used to lower blood glucose.

NovoRapid: See *aspart.*

NPH insulin: A type of intermediate-acting insulin.

Omega-3 fatty acids: A type of fat, found in certain fish and certain other foods, that may protect against the development of atherosclerosis.

Onglyza: See saxagliptin.

Ophthalmologist: A physician who specializes in diseases of the eyes.

Oral hypoglycemic agent: An older name for non-insulin antihyperglycemic medication.

Pancreas: The organ that is actively involved in digestion and metabolism and contains the insulin-producing islet cells.

Peripheral neuropathy: Damaged nerve fibres, typically in the feet, that cause pain and numbness.

Pioglitazone: A type of TZD (thiazolidinedione) medication.

Podiatrist: A type of health care professional who specializes in treating diseases of the feet.

Polydipsia: Excessive intake of water.

Polyunsaturated fat: A form of fat from certain vegetable sources that may lower HDL.

Polyuria: Excessive urination.

Post-prandial: After eating.

Prediabetes: A term that includes *impaired fasting glucose* and *impaired glucose tolerance.* Having prediabetes puts you at much greater risk of later developing diabetes.

Pre-prandial: Before eating.

Protein: One of the three major energy sources, the one usually found in meat, fish, poultry, and beans. Protein is necessary for the body to maintain healthy tissues.

Rapid-acting insulin: Insulin which starts to work within minutes of being injected and lasts only a few hours.

Regular insulin: A short-acting insulin.

Repaglinide: A type of non-insulin antihyperglycemic medication that lowers glucose by stimulating insulin release from the pancreas.

Retina: The part of the eye that senses light.

Retinopathy: Disease of the retina.

Rosiglitazone: A type of TZD (thiazolidinedione) medication.

Saturated fat: A form of fat from animals that raises cholesterol.

Saxagliptin: A type of DPP-4 inhibitor

Sitagliptin: A type of DPP-4 inhibitor.

Somogyi phenomenon (effect): A rapid increase in blood glucose to a high level in response to hypoglycemia occurring during the night. Recent scientific evidence suggests that this rarely, if ever happens.

Starlix: See *nateglinide.*

Statin: A class of drug that lowers cholesterol. The (generic names for the) available statins are atorvastatin, fluvastatin, lovastatin, pravastatin, rosuvastatin, simvastatin.

Sulfonylureas: A class of non-insulin antihyperglycemic medication, which works by stimulating insulin secretion from the pancreas.

Thiazolidinedione: A class of non-insulin antihyperglycemic medication, which works by reducing insulin resistance, thereby helping glucose enter into fat and muscle cells. Abbreviated as TZD.

Tresiba: See *degludec.*

Trajenta: See *linagliptin.*

Trans fatty acids: A type of fat, formed during food processing, that when consumed may worsen cholesterol levels and contribute to the development of atherosclerosis.

Triglycerides: A form of fat in the body.

TZD: See *thiazolidinedione.*

Index

● *N* ●

Notes

Notes

Notes

Notes

Notes

Notes

BUSINESS & INVESTING

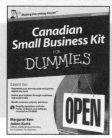

978-0-470-93652-8

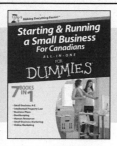

978-1-118-17282-7

Also available:
- Accounting For Canadians For Dummies 978-1-118-13346-0
- Bookkeeping For Canadians For Dummies 978-1-118-47808-0
- Building Wealth All-in-One For Canadians For Dummies 978-1-118-18106-5
- Business Plans For Canadians For Dummies 978-1-118-34912-0
- Flipping Houses For Canadians For Dummies 978-0-470-157336
- Investing For Canadians For Dummies 978-0-470-160299
- Personal Finance For Canadians For Dummies 978-0-470-679883
- Stock Investing For Canadians For Dummies 978-0-470-736845
- Trading For Canadians For Dummies 9780470677445

EDUCATION, HISTORY, & REFERENCE

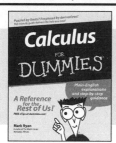

978-0-7645-2498-1

978-0-470-46244-7

Also available:
- Algebra For Dummies 978-0-7645-5325-7
- Art History For Dummies 978-0-470-09910-0
- Chemistry For Dummies 978-0-7645-5430-8
- English Grammar For Dummies 978-0-470-54664-2
- French All-in-One For Dummies 978-1-118-22815-9
- Statistics For Dummies 978-0-7645-5423-0
- World History For Dummies 978-0-470-44654-6

FOOD, HOME, & MUSIC

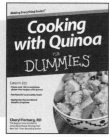

978-1-118-44780-2

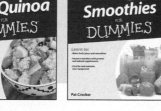

978-1-118-38749-8

Also available:
- 30-Minute Meals For Dummies 978-0-7645-2589-6
- Bartending For Dummies 978-0-470-63312-0
- Brain Games For Dummies 978-0-470-37378-1
- Butchery & Sausage Making For Dummies 978-1-118-37494-8
- Cheese For Dummies 978-1-118-09939-1
- Cooking Basics For Dummies 978-0-470-91388-8
- Gluten-Free Cooking For Dummies 978-1-118-39644-5
- Home Improvement All-in-One Desk Reference For Dummies 978-0-7645-5680-7
- Home Winemaking For Dummies 978-0-470-67895-4
- Ukulele For Dummies 978-0-470-97799-6
- Wine For Dummies 978-1-118-28872-6

Available wherever books are sold. For more information or to order direct: U.S. customers visit www.dummies.com or call 1-877-762-2974.
U.K. customers visit www.wileyeurope.com or call 0800 243407. Canadian customers visit www.wiley.ca or call 1-800-567-4797.

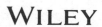

GARDENING

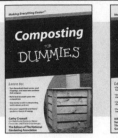

978-0-470-58161-2

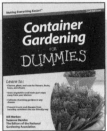

978-0-470-57705-9

Also available:

- ✔Gardening Basics For Dummies 978-0-470-03749-2
- ✔Organic Gardening For Dummies 978-0-470-43067-5
- ✔Sustainable Landscaping For Dummies 978-0-470-41149-0
- ✔Vegetable Gardening For Dummies 978-0-470-49870-5

GREEN/SUSTAINABLE

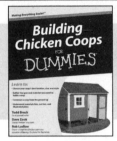

978-0-470-59896-2

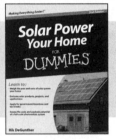

978-0-470-59678-4

Also available:

- ✔Alternative Energy For Dummies 978-0-470-43062-0
- ✔Energy Efficient Homes For Dummies 978-0-470-37602-7
- ✔Global Warming For Dummies 978-0-470-84098-6
- ✔Green Building & Remodelling For Dummies 978-0-470-17559-0
- ✔Green Cleaning For Dummies 978-0-470-39106-8
- ✔Green Your Home All-in-One For Dummies 978-0-470-59678-4
- ✔Wind Power Your Home For Dummies 978-0-470-49637-4

HEALTH & SELF-HELP

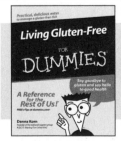

978-0-471-77383-2

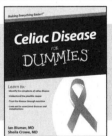

978-0-470-16036-7

Also available:

- ✔Acid Alkaline Diet For Dummies 9781118414187
- ✔Body Language For Dummies 978-0-470-51291-3
- ✔Borderline Personality Disorder For Dummies 978-0-470-46653-7
- ✔Breast Cancer For Dummies 978-0-7645-2482-0
- ✔Cognitive Behavioural Therapy For Dummies 978-0-470-66541-1
- ✔Diabetes Cookbook For Canadians For Dummies 9780470160282
- ✔Emotional Intelligence For Dummies 978-0-470-15732-9
- ✔Healthy Aging For Dummies 978-0-470-14975-1
- ✔Neuro-linguistic Programming For Dummies 978-0-470-66543-5
- ✔Understanding Autism For Dummies 978-0-7645-2547-6

HOBBIES & CRAFTS

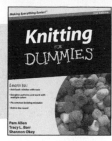

978-0-470-28747-7

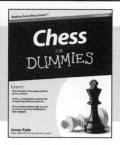

978-1-118-01695-4

Also available:
- Bridge For Dummies 978-1-118-20574-7
- Crochet Patterns For Dummies 97-0-470-04555-8
- Digital Photography For Dummies 978-1-118-09203-3
- Jewelry Making & Beading Designs For Dummies 978-0-470-29112-2
- Knitting Patterns For Dummies 978-0-470-04556-5
- Oil Painting For Dummies 978-0-470-18230-7
- Quilting For Dummies 978-0-7645-9799-2
- Sewing For Dummies 978-0-7645-6847-3
- Word Searches For Dummies 978-0-470-45366-7

HOME & BUSINESS COMPUTER BASICS

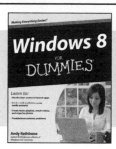

978-1-118-13461-0

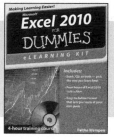

978-1-118-11079-9

Also available:
- Office 2010 All-in-One Desk Reference For Dummies 978-0-470-49748-7
- Pay Per Click Search Engine Marketing For Dummies 978-0-471-75494-7
- Search Engine Marketing For Dummies 978-0-471-97998-2
- Web Analytics For Dummies 978-0-470-09824-0
- Word 2010 For Dummies 978-0-470-48772-3

INTERNET & DIGITAL MEDIA

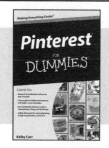

978-1-118-32800-2

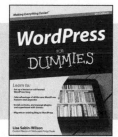

978-1-118-38318-6

Also available:
- Blogging For Dummies 978-1-118-15194-5
- Digital Photography For Seniors For Dummies 978-0-470-44417-7
- Facebook For Dummies 978-1-118-09562-1
- LinkedIn For Dummies 978-0-470-94854-5
- Mom Blogging For Dummies 978-1-118-03843-7
- The Internet For Dummies 978-0-470-12174-0
- Twitter For Dummies 978-0-470-76879-2
- YouTube For Dummies 978-0-470-14925-6

MACINTOSH

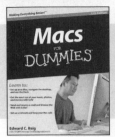

978-0-470-87868-2

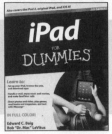

978-1118-49823-1

Also available:
- iMac For Dummies 978-0-470-20271-5
- iPod Touch For Dummies 978-1-118-12960-9
- iPod & iTunes For Dummies 978-1-118-50864-0
- MacBook For Dummies 978-1-11820920-2
- Macs For Seniors For Dummies 978-1-11819684-7
- Mac OS X Lion All-in-One For Dummies 978-1-118-02206-1

PETS

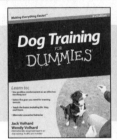

978-0-470-60029-0

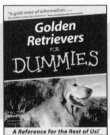

978-0-7645-5267-0

Also available:
- Cats For Dummies 978-0-7645-5275-5
- Ferrets For Dummies 978-0-470-13943-1
- Horses For Dummies 978-0-7645-9797-8
- Kittens For Dummies 978-0-7645-4150-6
- Puppies For Dummies 978-1-118-11755-2

SPORTS & FITNESS

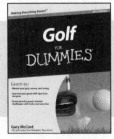

978-0-470-88279-5

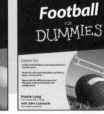

978-1-118-01261-1

Also available:
- Exercise Balls For Dummies 978-0-7645-5623-4
- Coaching Volleyball For Dummies 978-0-470-46469-4
- Curling For Dummies 978-0-470-83828-0
- Fitness For Dummies 978-0-7645-7851-9
- Lacrosse For Dummies 978-0-470-73855-9
- Mixed Martial Arts For Dummies 978-0-470-39071-9
- Sports Psychology For Dummies 978-0-470-67659-2
- Ten Minute Tone-Ups For Dummies 978-0-7645-7207-4
- Wilderness Survival For Dummies 978-0-470-45306-3
- Wrestling For Dummies 978-1-118-11797-2
- Yoga with Weights For Dummies 978-0-471-74937-0